Diabetes and Ocular Disease

Past, Present and Future Therapies

Lilly

This publication is made possible in part by a grant from Eli Lilly and Company.

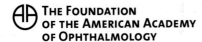

Diabetes and Ocular Disease

Past, Present, and Future Therapies

Edited by

Harry W. Flynn, Jr, MD

Department of Ophthalmology
Bascom Palmer Eye Institute
University of Miami School of Medicine

William E. Smiddy, MD

Department of Ophthalmology
Bascom Palmer Eye Institute
University of Miami School of Medicine

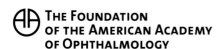

**THE FOUNDATION
OF THE AMERICAN ACADEMY
OF OPHTHALMOLOGY**

LEO

LIFELONG
EDUCATION FOR THE
OPHTHALMOLOGIST®

Library of Congress Cataloging-in-Publication Data

Diabetes and ocular disease : past, present, and future therapies / edited by Harry W. Flynn, Jr., William E. Smiddy.
    p. ; cm. — (Ophthalmology monographs ; 14)
    Includes bibliographical references and index.
    ISBN 1-56055-173-9
    1. Diabetic retinopathy. 2. Cataract. I. Flynn, Harry W. II. Smiddy, William E. III. American Academy of Ophthalmology. Foundation. IV. Series.
    [DNLM: 1. Diabetic Retinopathy—therapy. 2. Diabetic Retinopathy—diagnosis. WK 835 D5337 2000]
    RE661.D5 D46 2000
    617.7'1—dc21   99-044003

04 03 02 01 5 4 3 2 1

Printed in China

Contributors

Lloyd M. Aiello, MD
Beetham Eye Institute
Joslin Diabetes Center

Lloyd Paul Aiello, MD, PhD
Department of Ophthalmology
Joslin Diabetes Center
Harvard Medical School

William E. Benson, MD
Retina Service
Wills Eye Hospital

George W. Blankenship, MD
Penn State Geisinger
Health System

Gary C. Brown, MD
Retina Service
Wills Eye Hospital

Nauman A. Chaudhry, MD
Department of Ophthalmology
Bascom Palmer Eye Institute
University of Miami
School of Medicine

Emily Y. Chew, MD
National Eye Institute

Matthew D. Davis, MD
Department of Ophthalmology
and Visual Sciences
University of Wisconsin–Madison
Medical School

Frederick L. Ferris III, MD
National Eye Institute

Mitchell S. Fineman, MD
Retina Service
Wills Eye Hospital

Harry W. Flynn, Jr, MD
Department of Ophthalmology
Bascom Palmer Eye Institute
University of Miami
School of Medicine

James C. Folk, MD
Department of Ophthalmology
and Visual Sciences
University of Iowa
College of Medicine

Thomas W. Gardner, MD, MS
Departments of Ophthalmology
and Cellular and Molecular
Physiology
Penn State University
College of Medicine

Barbara E. K. Klein, MD, MPH
Department of Ophthalmology
and Visual Sciences
University of Wisconsin–Madison
Medical School

Ronald Klein, MD, MPH
Department of Ophthalmology
and Visual Sciences
University of Wisconsin–Madison
Medical School

Kean T. Oh, MD
Department of Ophthalmology
and Visual Sciences
University of Iowa
College of Medicine

Ingrid U. Scott, MD, MPH
Department of Ophthalmology
Bascom Palmer Eye Institute
University of Miami
School of Medicine

Gaurav K. Shah, MD
Retina Service
Wills Eye Hospital

Jay S. Skyler, MD
Departments of Medicine,
Pediatrics, and Psychology
University of Miami
School of Medicine

William E. Smiddy, MD
Department of Ophthalmology
Bascom Palmer Eye Institute
University of Miami
School of Medicine

Homayoun Tabandeh, MD
Department of Ophthalmology
Bascom Palmer Eye Institute
University of Miami
School of Medicine

Contents

Foreword by Arnall Patz, MD   *xvii*
Preface   *xix*
Acknowledgments   *xxi*

Chapter 1   PATHOGENESIS OF DIABETIC RETINOPATHY   **1**

Thomas W. Gardner, MD, MS
Lloyd Paul Aiello, MD, PhD

1-1   Retinal Anatomy and Physiology 1
    1-1-1   Neurons 1
    1-1-2   Glial Cells 1
    1-1-3   Blood Vessels 2
1-2   Preclinical Retinopathy 4
1-3   Nonproliferative Retinopathy 5
1-4   Macular Edema 9
1-5   Proliferative Retinopathy 10
1-6   Why Persons With Retinopathy Lose Vision 13
1-7   Conclusion 14
References 14

Chapter 2   EPIDEMIOLOGY OF EYE DISEASE IN DIABETES   **19**

Ronald Klein, MD, MPH
Barbara E. K. Klein, MD, MPH

2-1   Prevalence of Visual Impairment 19
2-2   Incidence of Visual Impairment 23
2-3   Risk Factors for Vision Loss and Legal Blindness 26
    2-3-1   Sex and Race 26
    2-3-2   Age and Duration of Diabetes 26
    2-3-3   Severity of Retinopathy and Macular Edema 29
    2-3-4   Other Risk Factors 29
2-4   Rehabilitation and Economic Costs of Blindness 29

2-5   Visual Acuity as Predictor of Death 30

2-6   Prevalence of Retinopathy in WESDR 32

2-7   Prevalence of Retinopathy in Other Studies 32

2-8   Incidence and Progression of Retinopathy 34

2-9   Risk Factors for Retinopathy 36

    2-9-1   Sex 36
    2-9-2   Race 36
    2-9-3   Genetics 37
    2-9-4   Age 38
    2-9-5   Duration of Diabetes 39
    2-9-6   Age at Diagnosis 40
    2-9-7   Puberty 40
    2-9-8   Hyperglycemia 42
    2-9-9   C-Peptide Status 44
    2-9-10 Exogenous Insulin 45
    2-9-11 Blood Pressure 45
    2-9-12 Proteinuria and Nephropathy 47
    2-9-13 Serum Lipids 47
    2-9-14 Cigarette Smoking 47
    2-9-15 Alcohol 48
    2-9-16 Body Mass Index 48
    2-9-17 Physical Activity 48
    2-9-18 Socioeconomic Status 48
    2-9-19 Pregnancy 49

2-10 Retinopathy, Comorbidity, and Mortality 49

2-11 Cataract 49

2-12 Glaucoma 53

2-13 Health Care Delivery 55

2-14 Conclusion 58

References 60

Chapter 3   **HISTORY OF EVOLVING TREATMENTS FOR DIABETIC RETINOPATHY**   **69**

George W. Blankenship, MD

3-1   Blood Glucose and Retinopathy 69
3-2   Light Energy for Treatment 70
3-3   Laser Photocoagulation 71
3-4   Mechanism of Action of Photocoagulation 72
3-5   Vitreous Surgery for Complications of Retinopathy 72
3-6   Clinical Trials 74
3-7   Conclusion 76
References 77

Chapter 4   **CLINICAL STUDIES ON TREATMENT FOR DIABETIC RETINOPATHY**   **81**

Frederick L. Ferris III, MD
Matthew D. Davis, MD
Lloyd M. Aiello, MD
Emily Y. Chew, MD

4-1   Photocoagulation 81
          4-1-1   Diabetic Retinopathy Study, 1971–1978 81
          4-1-2   Early Treatment Diabetic Retinopathy Study, 1980–1989 84
4-2   Vitrectomy 88
          4-2-1   Diabetic Retinopathy Vitrectomy Study, 1976–1983 88
4-3   Medical Approaches 89
          4-3-1   Blood Glucose Control 90
                    4-3-1-1 Diabetes Control and Complications Trial, 1983–1989 90
          4-3-2   Serum Lipid Lowering 92
          4-3-3   Blood Pressure Lowering 92
                    4-3-3-1 United Kingdom Prospective Diabetes Study, 1981–1998 92
          4-3-4   Aldose-Reductase Inhibition 92
                    4-3-4-1 Sorbinil Retinopathy Trial, 1983–1985 92
          4-3-5   Other Medical Investigations 92
4-4   Conclusion 93
References 94

Chapter 5 **PHOTOGRAPHY, ANGIOGRAPHY, AND ULTRASONOGRAPHY IN DIABETIC RETINOPATHY** **101**

Gaurav K. Shah, MD
Gary C. Brown, MD

5-1 Color Fundus Photography 101
5-2 Fluorescein Angiography 102
  5-2-1 Mild Nonproliferative Retinopathy 104
  5-2-2 Moderate Nonproliferative Retinopathy Without Macular Edema 105
  5-2-3 Moderate Nonproliferative Retinopathy With Macular Edema Not Clinically Significant 105
  5-2-4 Nonproliferative Retinopathy With Clinically Significant Macular Edema 105
  5-2-5 Severe Nonproliferative Retinopathy 108
5-3 Fluorescein Angioscopy 108
5-4 Ultrasonography 108
5-5 Conclusion 111
References 111

Chapter 6 **PHOTOCOAGULATION FOR DIABETIC MACULAR EDEMA AND DIABETIC RETINOPATHY** **115**

James C. Folk, MD
Kean T. Oh, MD

6-1 Symptoms and Medical History 115
  6-1-1 Macular Edema 116
  6-1-2 Proliferative Retinopathy 116
6-2 Clinical Evaluation 116
  6-2-1 Macular Edema 116
  6-2-2 Proliferative Retinopathy 116
6-3 Theoretical Considerations and Results in Photocoagulation 117
  6-3-1 Macular Edema 117
  6-3-2 Proliferative Retinopathy 121
6-4 Pretreatment Discussion 122
6-5 Lenses and Focusing 124
6-6 Laser Wavelengths 127
6-7 Laser Treatment Technique 128
  6-7-1 Macular Edema 128
    6-7-1-1 Complications of Treatment 136

6-7-2 Proliferative Retinopathy 137
6-7-2-1 Use of Anesthetic 137
6-7-2-2 Treatment Parameters 138
6-7-2-3 Single Versus Multiple Sessions 139
6-7-2-4 Intensity of Treatment 140

6-8 Postoperative Followup 143
6-8-1 Macular Edema 143
6-8-2 Proliferative Retinopathy 143

6-9 Special Cases 146
6-9-1 Macular Edema and Severe Retinopathy 146
6-9-2 Macular Edema and Cataract Surgery 148
6-9-3 Macular Edema and Traction 148
6-9-4 Proliferative Retinopathy and Traction 148
6-9-5 Proliferative Retinopathy and Hemorrhage 149

6-10 Patient Support 150
6-11 Conclusion 150
References 151

Chapter 7 VITRECTOMY FOR DIABETIC RETINOPATHY 155

William E. Smiddy, MD
Harry W. Flynn, Jr, MD

7-1 Surgical Indications 155
7-1-1 Media Opacities 155
7-1-2 Vitreoretinal Traction 159
7-1-3 Complications of Previous Vitrectomy 164

7-2 Surgical Objectives and Techniques 164
7-2-1 Media Opacities 165
7-2-2 Vitreoretinal Traction 165
7-2-3 Control of Hemorrhage and Reproliferation 168
7-2-4 Management of Severe Conditions 168
7-2-5 Instrumentation 168

7-3 Outcomes 169
7-3-1 Media Opacities 169
7-3-2 Vitreoretinal Traction 170
7-3-3 Complications of Previous Vitrectomy 171

7-4 Complications 171
7-5 Public Health Considerations 172
7-6 Conclusion 172
References 173

Chapter 8   MEDICAL MANAGEMENT OF DIABETIC RETINOPATHY   **181**

Jay S. Skyler, MD

8-1   Glycemic Control   181
        8-1-1   Epidemiologic Study   181
                8-1-1-1 Wisconsin Epidemiologic Study of Diabetic Retinopathy   181
        8-1-2   Intervention Studies   182
                8-1-2-1 Diabetes Control and Complications Trial   182
                8-1-2-2 Stockholm Diabetes Intervention Study and Meta-Analysis   184
                8-1-2-3 Kumamoto University Study   185
                8-1-2-4 United Kingdom Prospective Diabetes Study   185
        8-1-3   Current Recommendations   187
8-2   Blood Pressure Control   189
        8-2-1   Epidemiologic Studies   189
                8-2-1-1 Wisconsin Epidemiologic Study of Diabetic Retinopathy   189
                8-2-1-2 Hypertension in Diabetes Study   189
        8-2-2   Current Recommendations   192
8-3   Angiotensin-Converting Enzyme Inhibitors   192
        8-3-1   Intervention Study   193
                8-3-1-1 EURODIAB Controlled Trial of Lisinopril
                        in Insulin-Dependent Diabetes Mellitus   193
8-4   Dyslipidemic Control   194
8-5   Platelet Inhibitors   194
        8-5-1   Aspirin   194
        8-5-2   Aspirin Plus Dipyridamole   195
        8-5-3   Ticlopidine   195
8-6   Experimental Medical Therapies   196
        8-6-1   Aldose-Reductase Inhibitors   196
        8-6-2   Rheologic Agents   196
        8-6-3   Agents to Improve Capillary Fragility   197
        8-6-4   Histamine-Receptor Antagonists   197
        8-6-5   Inhibitors of Endothelial Cell Proliferation   197
8-7   Conclusion   197
References   198

Chapter 9   **CATARACT MANAGEMENT IN DIABETES**   **203**

Mitchell S. Fineman, MD
William E. Benson, MD

9-1   Preoperative Severity of Retinopathy 204
     9-1-1   No or Mild Retinopathy 204
     9-1-2   Nonproliferative Retinopathy Without Macular Edema 205
     9-1-3   Nonproliferative Retinopathy With Macular Edema 206
     9-1-4   Proliferative Retinopathy 206
9-2   Method of Cataract Extraction and Visual Acuity Outcome 208
     9-2-1   Extracapsular Cataract Extraction Versus Phacoemulsification 208
     9-2-2   Combined Cataract Extraction and Vitrectomy 209
9-3   Factors Affecting Visual Outcome 210
     9-3-1   Age 210
     9-3-2   Sex 210
     9-3-3   Previous Vitrectomy 210
9-4   Role of Posterior Capsulotomy 211
9-5   Treatment of Postoperative Macular Edema 211
9-6   Choice of Intraocular Lens 213
9-7   Conclusion 213
References 215

Chapter 10   **NONRETINAL ABNORMALITIES IN DIABETES**   **221**

Ingrid U. Scott, MD, MPH
Harry W. Flynn, Jr, MD

10-1   Corneal Diseases 221
10-2   Glaucoma 222
     10-2-1 Primary Open-Angle Glaucoma 222
     10-2-2 Angle-Closure Glaucoma 223
     10-2-3 Neovascular Glaucoma 224
     10-2-4 Blood-Associated Glaucoma 225
10-3   Lens Abnormalities 226
     10-3-1 Refractive Error 226
     10-3-2 Cataract 226

10-4   Optic Nerve Abnormalities 227

      10-4-1 Acute Optic Disc Edema 227
      10-4-2 Wolfram Syndrome 228
      10-4-3 Optic Nerve Hypoplasia 228
      10-4-4 Optic Atrophy 228

10-5   Cranial Nerve Abnormalities 229

10-6   Infectious Diseases 230

      10-6-1 Endophthalmitis 230
      10-6-2 Mucormycosis 231

10-7   Conclusion 232

References 233

Chapter 11   FUTURE THERAPIES FOR DIABETIC RETINOPATHY   239

Lloyd Paul Aiello, MD, PhD
Thomas W. Gardner, MD, MS

11-1   Historical Perspective 239

11-2   Growth-Factor Hypothesis of Neovascularization 242

11-3   Candidate Mediators of Neovascularization 244

11-4   Clinical Associations of VEGF in Proliferative Retinopathy 246

11-5   VEGF Induction of Diabetes-like Retinal Pathology 248

      11-5-1 VEGF in Proliferative Retinopathy 248
      11-5-2 VEGF in Nonproliferative Retinopathy 253
      11-5-3 VEGF in Ischemia-Induced Neovascularization 255

11-6   Basic Mechanisms and Targets 256

11-7   Role of Protein Kinase C 260

11-8   Protein Kinase C Inhibitors 261

11-9   Current Status of Novel Therapeutic Agents 263

11-10 Future Hurdles for Antiangiogenic Therapy 264

11-11 Conclusion 265

References 266

Appendix   **ABSTRACTS OF MAJOR COLLABORATIVE MULTICENTER TRIALS
FOR DIABETIC RETINOPATHY**   **275**

Compiled by
Nauman A. Chaudhry, MD
Homayoun Tabandeh, MD
Harry W. Flynn, Jr, MD

A-1   Diabetic Retinopathy Study (DRS) 275
A-2   Early Treatment Diabetic Retinopathy Study (ETDRS) 279
A-3   Diabetic Retinopathy Vitrectomy Study (DRVS) 290
A-4   Diabetes Control and Complications Trial (DCCT) 292
A-5   Sorbinil Retinopathy Trial (SRT) 296
A-6   United Kingdom Prospective Diabetes Study (UKPDS) 296

CME Credit   **299**

Answer Sheet   **300**

Self-Study Examination   **301**

Index   **317**

Foreword

Diabetes and Ocular Disease: Past, Present, and Future Therapies is an outstanding addition to the Academy's Ophthalmology Monographs series. The topics included in the monograph comprise a comprehensive and timely overview of the dramatic progress during the past three decades in treating diabetic retinopathy and other ocular complications of diabetes. The contributors are internationally recognized authorities on the subject matter of their chapters. The authors of the various chapters either served as chairs or played other leadership roles in the Diabetic Retinopathy Study (DRS), Early Treatment Diabetic Retinopathy Study (ETDRS), Diabetic Retinopathy Vitrectomy Study (DRVS), Diabetes Control and Complications Trial (DCCT), and other studies.

The monograph benefits from the high quality of the carefully selected photographs, well-executed drawings, and numerous tables. The uniform format of the visual program throughout the text is of great assistance to the reader. The book's thorough documentation provides the reader with plentiful references for further research. The appendix, which reprints the published abstracts of reports of the major clinical trials, is a valuable resource.

Because the monograph represents the culmination of the Academy's Diabetes 2000® project, it is appropriate to review briefly the history of the program. In 1988, Hunter R. Stokes, Sr, MD, then Academy Secretary for Governmental Relations, recognized the contribution the Academy could make by bringing patients into the system for more timely treatment of their diabetic retinopathy. The Committee of Academy Secretaries and the Academy Board of Trustees approved Dr Stokes' recommendation to launch the project, and I was invited to explore potential opportunities for the Academy membership. I appointed a task force consisting of John A. Colwell, MD, a diabetologist of national repute, and the chairs of the collaborative clinical trials. The task force drafted a mission statement and considered several avenues of endeavor, including educationally oriented programs.

The Academy Board of Trustees voted to focus Diabetes 2000 on education, and the project was assigned to Ronald E. Smith, MD, then Secretary for Continuing Education, as National Project Director. I served as National Chair and chair of the National

Scientific Advisory Board, which was constituted of the original task force. Dr Smith was succeeded by George W. Blankenship, MD, then José S. Pulido, MD, both of whom continued the tradition of excellent leadership as National Project Director.

The Symposium on the Treatment of Diabetic Retinopathy, held at the Airlie House in Virginia in 1968, led to the classification of diabetic retinopathy and the Diabetic Retinopathy Study (DRS). The National Eye Institute invited Matthew D. Davis, MD, to chair this multicenter clinical trial of photocoagulation treatment. The DRS proved that photocoagulation decreased the rate of visual loss from severe diabetic proliferative retinopathy. After 2 years, the rate of severe visual loss in patients with high-risk characteristics in the untreated group was 26% and only 11% in the treated group. As an early developer of the argon laser, I was one of those who believed that direct treatment of neovascularization of the disc should be tested. Early in the trial, focal treatment of disc neovascularization involved an increased risk of hemorrhage and so was discontinued. Panretinal photocoagulation as used in the DRS for high-risk proliferative diabetic retinopathy was proven to be highly successful and is the standard treatment employed today.

The DRS also provided a dividend in educating the ophthalmologic community about the importance of controlled clinical trials. The DRS stimulated interest in further multicenter trials on diabetic eye disease and subsequently on other ocular disorders. Leaders of the parent National Institutes of Health recognized that the success of the DRS fostered enthusiasm for clinical trials in other institutes.

There are more than 16,000,000 people with diabetes mellitus in the United States alone. This excellent monograph will serve as a resource for ophthalmologists, including residents and fellows, and for primary care physicians who care for diabetic patients. The book will prompt molecular biologists to consider areas where their basic research skills can contribute to the understanding of diabetic eye disease. Medical students will find the monograph useful in their course of study as well. Drs Flynn and Smiddy are to be congratulated on the superb organization of the volume and for selecting as chapter authors many of the pioneering leaders who have contributed so significantly to the current state of knowledge in treating this all-too-common disorder.

Arnall Patz, MD

Preface

Diabetes mellitus is a complex, multifactorial disease often associated with progressive retinopathy and visual loss. This monograph compiles current information from leading authorities regarding treatment strategies for diabetic eye disease. The emphasis of the chapter authors has been to provide practitioners of ophthalmology with an up-to-date, practical reference for the diagnosis and management of ocular disease in diabetic patients. The contributors have assimilated pertinent basic science and clinical information comprehensively, yet concisely, to include not only the guidelines established by the collaborative studies but also the concepts of disease mechanisms and clinical management that have subsequently evolved.

In 1989, the American Academy of Ophthalmology initiated the Diabetes 2000® project with the mission of eliminating preventable blindness from diabetic retinopathy. Over the decade of the 1990s, Diabetes 2000 encouraged collaboration among primary care physicians, allied health professionals, and ophthalmologists to ensure early detection and appropriate management of diabetic retinopathy. Diabetes 2000 initiatives included instructional courses and symposia at the Annual Meeting of the American Academy of Ophthalmology, state and local seminars on diabetic management, and literature through pharmacists and package inserts for raising awareness of diabetic eye disease among patients. Federally funded economic studies show that detection and treatment of diabetic eye disease saves, even at suboptimal care, $250,000,000 annually. The Diabetes 2000 project has achieved its goal of informing medical care providers and patients that diabetic retinopathy screening and appropriate treatment are an essential part of medical care for persons with diabetes. In January 2000, the Foundation of the Academy assumed responsibility under a new name: EyeCare America^{SM} Diabetes Project. The program is building on the success of the Diabetes 2000 project by focusing on the patient, as well as educating primary care physicians.

The educational objectives of this monograph are to

- Describe the pathogenesis of diabetic retinopathy
- Review the epidemiology of eye disease in diabetes
- Summarize the history of evolving treatments for diabetic retinopathy
- Outline the clinical studies on treatment for diabetic retinopathy
- Assess the use of photography, angiography, and ultrasonography in diabetic retinopathy
- Explain photocoagulation techniques for diabetic macular edema and diabetic retinopathy
- Analyze the use of vitrectomy for diabetic retinopathy
- Provide information on the medical management of diabetic retinopathy
- Demonstrate how cataract is managed in diabetes
- Identify nonretinal abnormalities in diabetes
- Explore future therapies for diabetic retinopathy
- Familiarize the reader with the major clinical trials for diabetic retinopathy

Harry W. Flynn, Jr, MD
William E. Smiddy, MD

Acknowledgments

A special thanks is extended to the many people who contributed to the completion of this monograph. Arnall Patz, MD, director emeritus of the Wilmer Eye Institute at Johns Hopkins Hospital, was selected to chair the Diabetes 2000® project. His guidance of the project was invaluable, and his foreword to this monograph is deeply appreciated. Pearl C. Vapnek provided outstanding expertise as our editorial adviser and major organizer for the book. Our secretaries, Iva Dhanpath and Lucy Rumpf, contributed greatly to organizing the written material, as well as contacting the contributors through countless faxes and emails. Finally, we extend our gratitude to the chapter authors for generously contributing their knowledge of both basic science mechanisms and clinical issues in diabetic retinopathy.

Harry W. Flynn, Jr, MD
William E. Smiddy, MD

CHAPTER 1

Pathogenesis of Diabetic Retinopathy

Thomas W. Gardner, MD, MS
Lloyd Paul Aiello, MD, PhD

This chapter reviews the clinical and cellular changes in the development and progression of diabetic retinopathy. Both the ocular and the systemic factors that influence retinopathy and, in particular, its vision-threatening aspects are emphasized. The roles of these factors in the treatment of diabetic retinopathy are discussed in this chapter and in Chapter 11, "Future Therapies for Diabetic Retinopathy."

1-1

RETINAL ANATOMY AND PHYSIOLOGY

The retina consists of three fundamental types of cellular elements: neurons, glial cells, and blood vessels (Figure 1-1).

1-1-1 Neurons

Together, the neurons and glial cells of the retina comprise more than 95% of the retinal mass. However, because they are transparent to visible light, their structure and function are not readily apparent on clinical examination. As demonstrated in Figure 1-1, the retina is primarily a neural tissue. Retinal neurons include photoreceptors, amacrine, bipolar, horizontal, and ganglion cells. The input from the first four types converge on the ganglia, and the ganglion cells' electrical output is conducted via axons of the nerve fiber layer and optic nerve. Disruption of any of the neurons interferes with vision, but built-in redundancy of these cells allows for many cells to be dysfunctional or lost before clinically detectable visual loss occurs. At least 50% of ganglion cells in an area must be lost before a clinically detectable visual defect is apparent, as in eyes with glaucoma.

1-1-2 Glial Cells

The glial cells of the retina—Müller cells and astrocytes—serve as support cells for the neurons and blood vessels.[1] They regulate extracellular ion concentrations, metabolize neurotransmitters, and provide balance of the nutrients to the neurons. For example, diminished levels of the neurotransmitter glutamate would impair synaptic transmission of electrical impulses. Excess glutamate, accumulated in response to retinal ischemia or diabetes, is toxic to neurons and may cause neuronal cell death.

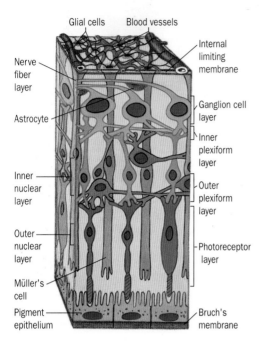

Glial cells   Blood vessels

Nerve fiber layer

Astrocyte

Inner nuclear layer

Outer nuclear layer

Müller's cell

Pigment epithelium

Internal limiting membrane

Ganglion cell layer

Inner plexiform layer

Outer plexiform layer

Photoreceptor layer

Bruch's membrane

Figure 1-1 *Anatomy of normal retina.*

In addition to their effects on neurons, astrocytes also play an important role in blood vessel function and in guiding development. Astrocytes play an important role in fetal vascular development and may influence new vessel growth.[2] Vascular endothelial growth factor (VEGF) appears to be the major cytokine involved in this process and is produced by astrocytes. Astrocytes also signal blood vessels to acquire barrier properties to form the blood–retina barrier[3] and influence the development of tight junctions in retinal endothelial cells.[4]

1-1-3 Blood Vessels

Impaired retinal vascular autoregulation is a feature of progressive diabetic retinopathy. The retinal circulation[5] consists of a progressive circuit of vessels that includes conduits into and out of the retina and microvessels (Figure 1-2A). The microcirculation includes precapillary arterioles, capillaries, and postcapillary venules. Arterioles possess smooth muscle, which allows the cells to change their radius and dynamically regulate local delivery of blood to the retina. The precapillary arterioles are the primary resistance vessels, whereas venules have a high density of receptors for vasoactive agents, such as histamine. The venules are primarily passive conducting tubes, which drain blood out of the retina.

Autoregulation is a general feature of blood vessels of the central nervous system that maintains appropriate blood delivery despite changes in systemic arterial pressure.[6] The retinal arterial vessels have smooth muscle, while capillaries, arterioles, and venules possess pericytes, which function as modified smooth muscle cells. These

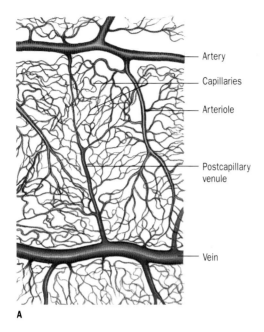

A

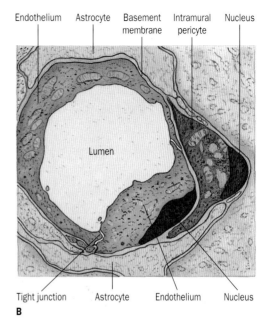

Endothelium Astrocyte Basement Intramural Nucleus
membrane pericyte

Tight junction Astrocyte Endothelium Nucleus

B

features allow the retinal circulation to autoregulate in response to systemic and local metabolic demands (Figure 1-2B). Blood vessels normally autoregulate in response to the partial pressure of carbon dioxide (Pco_2) and oxygen (Po_2). Arteriolar narrowing in patients with hypertension is a reflection of autoregulation to maintain normal intravascular (oncotic) pressure. The autoregulatory mechanisms and blood–retina barrier are overwhelmed in grade IV hypertension. As a result, blood, serous fluid, and lipid transudates (imprecisely called "exudates") may accumulate in the macula, and the optic disc may swell.

Under normal conditions, retinal blood flow balances nutrient delivery and waste removal with retinal metabolism. Diabetes, a systemic malfunction of carbohydrate, lipid, and protein metabolism, leads to vas-

Figure 1-2 *Retinal microcirculation. (A) Broad capillary-free zone is present around artery (red), and much narrower zone is seen about vein (blue). (B) Human retinal capillary shows endothelium with tight junctional complexes between adjacent cells, intramural pericyte, and basement membrane material with cavities.*

TABLE 1-1

Preclinical Retinopathy

Symptoms	Clinical Signs	Abnormal Test Results	Histopathology	Cellular Events
Usually none	Normal-appearing retina	Color perception: decreased blue-yellow sensation (deuter-anomaly)	Neural cell apoptosis	Decreased vascular tight-junction proteins
		ERG: decreased oscillatory potential amplitudes		Vascular basement membrane thickening
		Vitreous fluorometry: increased blood–retina barrier permeability		Glial cell reactivity: increased glutamate

cular damage and subsequent ischemia in tissues such as the retina. Thus, diabetic retinopathy is fundamentally the result of an imbalance between retinal metabolism and vascular supply.

1-2

PRECLINICAL RETINOPATHY

In patients with younger-onset (type 1) diabetes in whom the duration of diabetes is well known, the interval between diagnosis and development of any retinopathy (microaneurysms) in half the patients is 7 years.[7] In patients with older-onset (type 2) diabetes, it is more difficult to determine this interval between the development of diabetes and the development of retinopathy because approximately 7 years elapse between the onset of non–insulin-dependent diabetes and its diagnosis.[8] There is ample evidence that functional and anatomic changes occur before the onset of vascular lesions in both types of diabetes, as discussed below and shown in Table 1-1.

Diabetic patients with normal-appearing retinas generally lack specific visual symptoms. Nevertheless, sensitive testing methods have demonstrated subtle defects in neurosensory retinal function, including decreased blue-yellow color perception and contrast sensitivity.[9–12] In addition, the oscillatory amplitudes on the b-wave of the electroretinogram (ERG) may be reduced.[13] Multifocal ERG testing has demonstrated regional depression of the ERG in diabetic patients before the onset of vascular lesions.[14] These tests indicate dysfunction of the inner retina. Although the specific defect(s) that causes these functional changes is not known, such changes probably reflect dysfunction of inner retinal neurons. Nerve fiber layer defects may also be detected by red-free photography in diabetic patients with minimal or no vascular lesions.[15] More than 35 years ago, Bloodworth[16] and Wolter[17] showed that diabetes damages retinal ganglion cells in regions removed from vascular pathology. Together, these findings provide strong evidence that retinal function may be altered prior to the onset of vascular lesions and that diabetic retinopathy is not strictly a vascular disease.

Experimental studies of diabetic rats have demonstrated increased neural cell injury within 1 month of diabetes,[18] long before the onset of typical vascular lesions. This accelerated cell death results in loss of the ganglion cell and inner plexiform layers, with retinal thinning after 8 months. Reduced oscillatory potentials[19] and optic nerve axon size[20] in diabetic rats may be due to altered glutamate metabolism.[21,22] Because Müller cells and astrocytes are responsible for glutamate metabolism, glutamate accumulation implies that glial cells are defective. Glutamate is a well-recognized cause of neuronal cell death in cerebral ischemia, so-called glutamate excitotoxicity.[23,24]

Vascular changes, which may begin within 5 years of type 1 diabetes, include delayed leukocyte migration in the perifoveal capillaries,[25] increased blood–retina barrier permeability as detected by vitreous fluorometry,[26] and increased retinal blood flow compared to nondiabetic control subjects.[27] Studies in diabetic rats have shown increased blood–retina barrier permeability and alterations in retinal blood flow within 1 to 3 months.[28,29] These findings suggest that vascular autoregulation is impaired before vascular lesions appear.

Further evidence for early pathophysiologic abnormalities in the preclinical phase arises from studies in experimentally diabetic dogs. Engerman and Kern[30] showed that the intensive control of diabetes in dogs for the first 2.5 years determined the subsequent development of vascular lesions, whether or not the animals were subsequently treated with high or low doses of insulin to achieve tight or poor metabolic control, respectively. Thus, while this phase of diabetic retinopathy appears to be innocuous from a clinical standpoint, numerous cellular and metabolic processes are active that lead to the development of clinically evident nonproliferative diabetic retinopathy. The nature of these cellular processes is not well understood at this time.

1-3

NONPROLIFERATIVE RETINOPATHY

Nonproliferative diabetic retinopathy (NPDR) is defined and staged by ophthalmoscopic features such as vascular lesions, including microaneurysms, intraretinal hemorrhages, and vasodilation. Table 1-2 summarizes the manifestations of NPDR.

Implicit in these definitions is the theory of a primary vascular disorder. The definitions are useful clinically because they permit evaluation of ophthalmoscopically visible ocular risk factors for moderate and severe visual loss.

TABLE 1-2

Nonproliferative Diabetic Retinopathy

Symptoms	Clinical Signs	Abnormal Test Results	Histopathology	Cellular Events
None, blurred vision, or glare	Retinal vasodilation	Intravenous fluorescein angiography: vascular leakage and occlusion	Microaneurysms, intraretinal hemorrhages in nerve fiber layer and outer plexiform layer	Increased VEGF expression by neurons and glial cells
	Microaneurysms	ERG: depressed oscillatory amplitudes	Cytoid bodies, nerve fiber layer swelling	Vascular cell apoptosis
	Nerve fiber layer infarcts	Increased retinal blood flow	Neuronal loss and degeneration, lipid exudates and extracellular edema in outer plexiform layer	
	Intraretinal hemorrhages			
	IRMAs		Glial cell occlusion of capillaries	
	Venous beading			
	Retinal depression sign			

Some younger patients (<45 years) also exhibit focal depressions in the macular reflex, the "retinal depression sign" (Figure 1-3).[31] This sign results from small retinal depressions that reflect light away from the observer so that the macula appears slightly darker than the surrounding retina. The sign is best observed by slit-lamp biomicroscopy and is also noted on fundus photographs, particularly with red-free filters. The thinning may result from macular ischemia and/or nonischemic neuroretinal degeneration (apoptosis). This finding may explain paracentral scotomas and may be confused with epiretinal membranes or macular edema.

Fluorescein angiographic–evident vascular leakage and capillary closure in the mid-peripheral retina may represent shunting of retinal blood flow into the posterior pole, where it increases the propensity for developing diabetic macular edema (DME).[32] Capillary closure is a characteristic element of progressive NPDR, but it is unclear if formed vascular elements—erythrocytes, leukocytes, or platelets—initiate vascular occlusion. Histopathologic studies have shown that glial cells migrate through the vessel wall and occlude vascular lumens in patients with diabetic retinopathy.[33] Whether this is a primary event related to glial cell proliferation or secondary to intraluminal capillary plugging is not known. Basement membrane thickening is a characteristic histopathologic feature and may be a primary step in capillary closure, but its cause is also unknown.

It has long been held that pericytes are particularly susceptible to the insults of diabetes and are lost more rapidly than endothelial cells. Although pericytes (and endothelial cells) clearly undergo cell death by apoptosis,[34] it is uncertain if pericytes are uniquely susceptible to diabetes. The original light microscopic study[35] of trypsin digest preparations did not indicate the anatomic regions from which the images were taken, gave no statistical analysis of pericyte dropout or other morphologic lesions, and did not determine whether pericyte loss occurred in areas without microaneurysms. Another study[36] questioned whether pericytes are lost first or preferentially in diabetic retinopathy.

Cotton-wool spots have long been considered to represent focal microinfarcts of the nerve fiber layer.[37] However, cotton-wool spots have also been described in patients without clinical or fluorescein angiographic evidence of vascular occlusion[38] and may resolve without nerve fiber layer loss. Hence, they possibly result from impaired axonal transport, particularly in patients with poorly controlled diabetes.

The biochemical and cellular events that initiate vascular lesions in diabetic retinopathy are complex and are also uncertain in humans. Most of the information is derived from studies in animals with experimental diabetes induced by streptozotocin or alloxan, or in vascular cell culture experiments. While it is clear that intensive treatment of diabetes in humans or animals significantly delays the onset and progression of retinopathy,[39] it is not known whether the development of retinopathy represents a direct effect of insulin, a consequence of

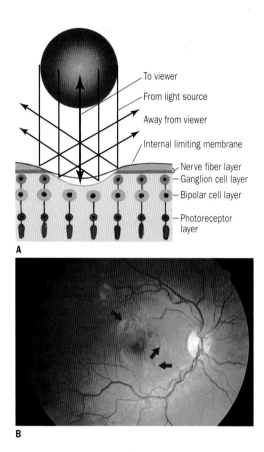

Figure 1-3 *(A) Focal retinal depressions reflect light away from observer, so area appears relatively darker than normal regions. (B) Fundus photograph of retinal depression.*

hyperglycemia, or another metabolic derangement associated with diabetes. The metabolic pathways that have been associated with diabetic retinopathy include activation of the polyol pathway, nonenzymatic glycosylation, and activation of the β_2 isoform of protein kinase C (PKC-β_2).[40,41]

Increased glucose metabolism via the polyol pathway,[42] first suggested as a cause of cataracts in diabetes, has also been considered to account for diabetic retinopathy and peripheral neuropathy. The hypothesis is that increased glucose metabolism via this pathway results in the accumulation of sorbitol, reduction of *myo*-inositol, and/or reduction in activity of sodium-potassium-ATPase, which may account for vascular dysfunction. Aldose reductase is a key enzyme in the polyol pathway. However, specific vascular functional abnormalities, such as barrier breakdown or capillary closure, have not been fully explained by this hypothesis. Studies of aldose-reductase inhibitors in diabetic dogs[43] and rats[44] have shown conflicting results. A clinical trial of an aldose-reductase inhibitor did not show a benefit on slowing retinopathy progression,[45] but the duration of the study was short (3 years).

Another theory for the development of diabetic retinopathy involves vascular damage by advanced glycosylation end products. According to the concept of nonenzymatic glycosylation,[46] sugar molecules bond covalently to reactive molecules and cause alterations in the functions of proteins, nucleic acids, and cells, such as macrophages.

This reaction gives rise to the glycohemoglobin (hemoglobin A_{1c}) test, which measures diabetes control over a 2- to 3-month period. This mechanism has been proposed to account for cross-linking of long-lived proteins, such as collagens, which are found in vascular basement membranes and vitreous. Collagen cross-linking may reduce the turnover of collagen and allow for basement membrane thickening or may contribute to vitreous collagen contraction. An inhibitor of nonenzymatic glycosylation is being tested in humans with diabetic nephropathy.

Another metabolic mechanism involves a specific molecule in signal transduction cascades. Protein kinase C adds phosphate molecules to serine or threonine residues of cytoplasmic proteins (Figure 1-4). Activation of PKC-β_2 has been observed in retinas of diabetic rats[40] in response to vascular endothelial growth factor/vascular permeability factor (VEGF/VPF).[41] This enzyme also phosphorylates other proteins in the signal transduction cascade of VEGF/VPF and histamine, and is associated with alterations in retinal blood flow and blood–retina barrier breakdown.[47] Inhibition of PKC-β_2 with an oral agent reduces retinal and renal vascular dysfunction in experimental diabetes,[48] and is now in phase III clinical trials.

VEGF/VPF is produced primarily by nonvascular retinal cells, including ganglion cells, Müller cells, and astrocytes.[49] This finding suggests that the increased vascular permeability may be the consequence of vasoactive compounds from the neural retina acting secondarily on the microvasculature and supports the theory that diabetic retinopathy may not be a primary vascular disease.

1-4

MACULAR EDEMA

The physiologic factors that govern the development of DME are similar to those involved in tissue edema elsewhere in the body. Increased intravascular hydrostatic pressure tends to drive fluid across the vascular wall—Starling's law (Figure 1-5).[50] Autoregulatory vasodilation of arterioles causes intravascular pressure in the arterioles to decrease and venules to increase—Poiseuille's law. Increased hydrostatic pressure induces arterial and venular diameters to increase—Laplace's law—and blood vessel length and tortuosity to increase. These physiologic relationships are consistent with the clinical signs of vascular dilation and tortuosity in diabetic retinopathy. Serial observations in patients with diabetes have shown that retinal vascular diameter and length increase prior to the onset of DME. These parameters improve following macular photocoagulation for DME[51] and after panretinal photocoagulation for proliferative diabetic retinopathy.[32]

In addition to altered autoregulation of vascular flow, the intrinsic integrity of the blood–retina barrier is impaired. Studies with differential vitreous fluorometry in humans show that breakdown of the inner blood–retina barrier (formed by tight junctions between endothelial cells) predominates over changes in the outer barrier (tight junctions between retinal pigment epithelial cells) in early DME.[52] The outer barrier breaks down in patients with chronic DME. The proteins that comprise the tight junctions between vascular endothelial cells are reduced in early experimental diabetes,

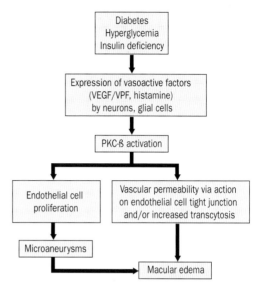

Figure 1-4 *Possible mechanism for development of NPDR.*

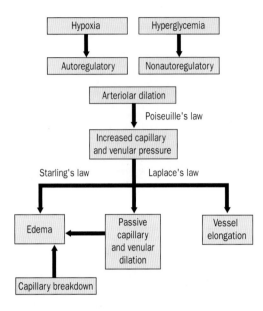

Figure 1-5 *Relationship of altered vascular physiology to development of macular edema. Capillary occlusion with resulting nonperfusion has been confirmed as capillary dropout. Resulting retinal hypoxia produces autoregulatory arteriolar vasodilation with reduced pressure fall in arterioles and increase of capillary and venular hydrostatic pressure. Vessels dilate and increased capillary hydrostatic pressure leads to edema development, according to Starling's law.*
Redrawn from Kristinsson JK, Gottfredsdottir MS, Stefansson E: Retinal vessel dilatation and elongation precedes diabetic macular oedema. Br J Ophthalmol 1997;81:274–278, with permission from the BMJ Publishing Group.

and this may account for increased vascular permeability.[53] As such, the hemodynamic abnormalities in the retina are analogous to those that occur in the kidney in earlier diabetes, that is, increased renal blood flow and increased glomerular permeability, with resultant albuminuria.[54]

Microaneurysms are the most characteristic ophthalmoscopic features of diabetic retinopathy. They occur throughout the posterior pole and are often first noted temporal to the macula. Their importance lies in their association with the retinopathy severity and as sources for leakage of fluid and lipid transudates. Histologically, they are outpouchings of the capillaries, with focal endothelial cell proliferation and pericyte loss, often adjacent to areas of nonperfusion. The factors that contribute to microaneurysm formation likely include structural features (loss of supporting pericytes and astrocytes), hemodynamic alterations (increased capillary intramural pressure), and local production of vasoproliferative factors, such as VEGF. Like cotton-wool spots, retinal thickening, and hemorrhages, microaneurysms can wax and wane through the course of retinopathy.[55]

Systemic factors, such as poor diabetes control, systemic arterial hypertension, hyperlipidemia,[56] and hypoalbuminemia, may all contribute to the development of DME.

1-5

PROLIFERATIVE RETINOPATHY

Proliferative diabetic retinopathy (PDR), defined by neovascularization of the optic disc, retina, and/or iris, may be an aberrant attempt to compensate for the capillary clo-

TABLE 1-3

Proliferative Diabetic Retinopathy

Symptoms	Clinical Signs	Abnormal Test Results	Histopathology	Cellular Events
None, reduced vision, nyctalopia, or floaters	Retinal signs: neovascularization of optic disc, retina, and/or iris, retinal vasodilation, beading, and IRMAs	Intravenous fluorescein angiography: severe capillary closure and hyperfluorescence of neovascularization with leakage	Glial cell proliferation and epiretinal membranes	Vitreous collagen cross-linking
	Vitreous signs: vitreous cells, contraction, and opacification of posterior hyaloid face, partial posterior vitreous detachment with epiretinal membranes, and tractional retinal detachment	Dark adaptation: impaired	Endothelial cell proliferation	Endothelial cell mitosis
		Ultrasonography: partial posterior vitreous detachment with vitreoretinal adhesions; retinal detachment	Intraretinal hemorrhage	Glial cell proliferation
			Cystoid macular edema	Occluded capillaries
			Neuronal loss	
			Retinal detachment	

sure and retinal hypoxia in eyes with severe NPDR. Table 1-3 outlines the features of PDR. The new vessels grow perpendicular to the plane of the retina into the scaffolding provided by the vitreous cortex, typically at the junction of perfused and nonperfused retina (Figure 1-6) from the venules. In contrast to normal retinal vessels, which are ensheathed by glial cells, neovascularization is associated with reactive glial cells,[57] which may allow endothelial cell tight junctions to become leaky, with resultant hyperfluorescence noted on fluorescein angiography.

PDR, like wound healing in other tissues, first involves angiogenesis (neovascularization), followed by remodeling of the wound, with subsequent fibrosis, and even-

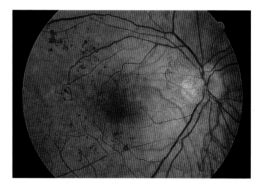

Figure 1-6 *Growth of neovascularization at margin of perfused and nonperfused retina.*

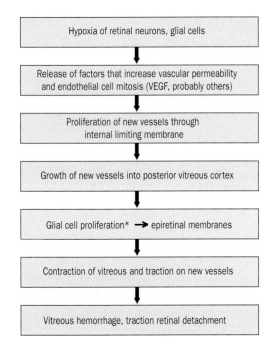

Figure 1-7 *Mechanisms of PDR. *Point at which glial cell proliferation begins is not known, and may occur at same point as endothelial cell proliferation.*

tual replacement of the vascular tissues by collagen. The natural history of untreated PDR includes fibrosis, which induces traction on the neovascularization. Subsequent contraction may induce preretinal hemorrhage, vitreous hemorrhage, and traction retinal detachment. Panretinal photocoagulation modifies the healing response by reducing the neovascular proliferation, avoiding the development of fibrotic elements.

The cellular events that lead to neovascularization include retinal hypoxia, elaboration of factors that stimulate endothelial cell proliferation, and vitreous contraction (Figure 1-7).[58] A number of factors have been implicated in the pathogenesis of retinal neovascularization, including growth hormone, insulin-like growth factor 1 (IGF-1), basic fibroblast growth factor (bFGF), and VEGF/VPF. As noted above, VEGF/VPF is produced by cells in the neurosensory retina and acts by specific endothelial cell surface receptors to induce retinal neovascularization. VEGF/VPF levels are increased in the vitreous of eyes with neovascularization and diminish after panretinal photocoagulation.[59] Inhibition of VEGF/VPF action by antisense oligonucleotides that inhibit VEGF/VPF messenger RNA or by antibodies that bind the protein before it can activate its receptors reduces neovascularization in experimental models.[60]

VEGF/VPF production is not unique to diabetic retinopathy; it is also increased in retinopathy of prematurity and other ocular neovascular processes, as well as in physiologic conditions (menstruation and wound healing) and in pathologic vascularization (tumors) throughout the body. The control of retinal angiogenesis is complex, and the molecular puzzle is still in the process of being unraveled.[61] Vitreous collagen cross-linking via nonenzymatic glycosylation may be the mechanism of vitreous contraction.

1-6

WHY PERSONS WITH RETINOPATHY LOSE VISION

Most ophthalmologists would concur that persons with diabetic retinopathy lose vision because of the visible vascular changes. Certainly, diabetes may lead to visual loss for a variety of reasons. These may be categorized into abnormalities of the media and neurosensory system, as shown in Table 1-4. The most common retinal features associated with visual impairment—macular edema and traction retinal detachment—are associated with prominent vascular abnormalities. Nevertheless, it is not certain that the vascular changes per se are causally related to the visual loss. As pointed out by Bloodworth,[16] "There is, as yet, no concrete evidence that capillary changes initiate the condition." In other words, because retinal neurons (not vessels) transduce vision, it follows that loss of neuronal function must accompany visual impairment.

Neuronal dysfunction occurs in primary retinal ischemic events (central retinal artery occlusion), but also results from retinal detachment, accumulation of retinal extracellular fluid (macular edema), or diabetic papillopathy. Thus, vision loss must ultimately involve retinal neurons.[62] Because diabetes likely has a direct effect on retinal neurons,[18] visual impairment may not require primary vascular abnormalities, as in glaucoma, photoreceptor dystrophies, or sphingolipidoses.

TABLE 1-4

Mechanisms of Visual Loss in Diabetes

Abnormalities of Ocular Media

Cornea: epithelial erosions

Lens: transient swelling associated with poor metabolic control; cataract

Vitreous: vitreous hemorrhage

Abnormalities of Neurosensory System

Retina: macular edema or ischemia; macular heterotopia; traction or rhegmatogenous retinal detachment; neuronal degeneration as direct effect of diabetes or secondary to vascular occlusion

Optic nerve: diabetic papillopathy; nonarteritic anterior ischemic optic neuropathy; axonal degeneration secondary to diabetes or to vascular lesions

1-7

CONCLUSION

Many steps in the pathogenesis of diabetic retinopathy are under intensive investigation. Diabetic retinopathy involves both vascular and neural elements of the retina from the early stages of diabetes through the development of PDR. Improved means of preventing visual loss in diabetes depend on a better understanding of the relationships between the neural retina and blood vessels and of how the normal relationships are disturbed in this disease.

REFERENCES

1. Stone J, Dreher Z: Relationship between astrocytes, ganglion cells and vasculature of the retina. *J Comp Neurol* 1987;255:35–49.

2. Zhang Y, Stone J: Role of astrocytes in the control of developing retinal vessels. *Invest Ophthalmol Vis Sci* 1997;38:1653–1666.

3. Janzer RC, Raff MC: Astrocytes induce blood–brain barrier properties in endothelial cells. *Nature* 1987;325:253–257.

4. Gardner TW, Lieth E, Khin SA, et al: Astrocytes increase barrier properties and ZO-1 expression in retinal vascular endothelial cells. *Invest Ophthalmol Vis Sci* 1997;38:2423–2427.

5. Wise GN, Dollery CT, Henkind P: *The Retinal Circulation*. New York: Harper & Row; 1971: 34–54.

6. Wise GN, Dollery CT, Henkind P: *The Retinal Circulation*. New York: Harper & Row; 1971: 108–111.

7. Klein R, Klein BEK: Vision disorders in diabetes. In: *Diabetes in America*. 2nd ed. NIH Publication 95-1468. Bethesda MD: National Institute of Health; 1995:311–338.

8. Harris MI, Klein R, Welborn TA, Knuiman MW: Onset of NIDDM occurs at least 4–7 yr before clinical diagnosis. *Diabetes Care* 1992;15: 815–819.

9. Sokol S, Moskowitz A, Skarf B, et al: Contrast sensitivity in diabetics with and without background retinopathy. *Arch Ophthalmol* 1985;103: 51–54.

10. Della Sala S, Bertoni G, Somazzi L, et al: Impaired contrast sensitivity in diabetic patients with and without retinopathy: a new technique for rapid assessment. *Br J Ophthalmol* 1985;69: 136–142.

11. Daley ML, Watzke RC, Riddle MC: Early loss of blue-sensitive color vision in patients with type I diabetes. *Diabetes Care* 1987;10: 777–781.

12. Hirsh J, Puklin JE: Reduced contrast sensitivity may precede clinically observable retinopathy in Type I diabetes. In: Henkind P, ed: *Acta: XXIV International Congress of Ophthalmology, San Francisco, 1982*. Philadelphia: JB Lippincott Co; 1983:719–724.

13. Coupland SG: A comparison of oscillatory potential and pattern electroretinogram measures in diabetic retinopathy. *Doc Ophthalmol* 1987;66:207–218.

14. Palmowski AM, Sutter EE, Bearse MA Jr, Fung W: Mapping of retinal function in diabetic retinopathy using the multifocal electroretinogram. *Invest Ophthalmol Vis Sci* 1997;38:2586–2596.

15. Chihara E, Matsuoka T, Oguar Y, Matsumara M: Retinal nerve fiber layer defect as an early manifestation of diabetic retinopathy. *Ophthalmology* 1993;100:1147–1151.

16. Bloodworth JMB: Diabetic retinopathy. *Diabetes* 1962;2:1–22.

17. Wolter JR: Diabetic retinopathy. *Am J Ophthalmol* 1961;51:1123–1139.

18. Barber AJ, Lieth E, Antonetti DA, et al, Penn State Retina Research Group: Neural apoptosis in the retina during experimental and human diabetes: early onset and effect of insulin. *J Clin Invest* 1998;102:783–791.

19. Sakai H, Tani Y, Shirasawa E, et al: Development of electroretinographic alterations in streptozotocin-induced diabetes in rats. *Ophthalmic Res* 1995;27:57–63.

20. Scott TM, Foote J, Peat B, Galway G: Vascular and neural changes in the rat optic nerve following induction of diabetes with streptozotocin. *J Anat* 1986;144:145–152.

21. Lieth E, Barber AJ, Xu B, et al, Penn State Retina Research Group: Glial reactivity and impaired glutamate metabolism in short-term experimental diabetic retinopathy. *Diabetes* 1998; 47:815–820.

22. Mizutani N, Gerhardinger C, Lorenzi M: Müller cell changes in human diabetic retinopathy. *Diabetes* 1998;47:445–449.

23. Lipton SA, Rosenberg PA: Excitatory amino acids as a final common pathway for neurologic disorders. *N Engl J Med* 1994;330:613–622.

24. Vorwek CK, Lipton SA, Zurakowski D, et al: Chronic low-dose glutamate is toxic to retinal ganglion cells: toxicity blocked by memantine. *Invest Ophthalmol Vis Sci* 1996;37:1618–1624.

25. Sander B, Larsen M, Engler C, et al: Early changes in diabetic retinopathy: capillary loss and blood–retina barrier permeability in relation to metabolic control. *Acta Ophthalmol* 1994;72: 553–559.

26. Krogsaa B, Lund-Andersen H, Mehlsen J, Sestoft L: Blood–retinal barrier permeability versus diabetes duration and retinal morphology in insulin dependent diabetic patients. *Acta Ophthalmol* 1987;65:686–692.

27. Grunwald JE, DuPont J, Riva CE: Retinal haemodynamics in patients with early diabetes mellitus. *Br J Ophthalmol* 1996;80:327–331.

28. Enea NA, Hollis TM, Kern JA, Gardner TW: Histamine H1 receptors mediate increased blood–retinal barrier permeability in experimental diabetes. *Arch Ophthalmol* 1989;107:270–274.

29. Bursell SE, Clermont AC, Oren B, King GL: The in vivo effect of endothelins on retinal circulation in nondiabetic and diabetic rats. *Invest Ophthalmol Vis Sci* 1995;36:596–607.

30. Engerman RL, Kern TS: Progression of incipient diabetic retinopathy during good glycemic control. *Diabetes* 1987;36;808–812.

31. Gardner TW, Miller ML, Cunningham D, Blankenship GW: The retinal depression sign in diabetic retinopathy. *Graefes Arch Klin Exp Ophthalmol* 1995;233:617–620.

32. Grunwald JE, Brucker AJ, Petrig BL, Riva CE: Retinal blood flow regulation and the clinical response to panretinal photocoagulation in proliferative diabetic retinopathy. *Ophthalmology* 1989;96:1518–1522.

33. Bek T: Glial cell involvement in vascular occlusion of diabetic retinopathy. *Acta Ophthalmol* Scand 1997;75:239–243.

34. Mizutani M, Kern TS, Lorenzi M: Accelerated death of retinal microvascular cells in human and experimental diabetic retinopathy. *J Clin Invest* 1996;97:2883–2890.

35. Cogan DG, Toussaint D, Kuwabara T: Retinal vascular patterns, IV: diabetic retinopathy. *Arch Ophthalmol* 1961;66:366–378.

36. de Oliveira F: Pericytes in diabetic retinopathy. *Br J Ophthalmol* 1966;50:134–143.

37. Yanoff M, Fine BS: *Ocular Pathology: A Text and Atlas.* Hagerstown: Harper & Row; 1975:397.

38. Roy MS, Rick ME, Higgins KE, McCulloch JC: Retinal cotton-wool spots: an early finding in diabetic retinopathy? *Br J Ophthalmol* 1986;70: 772–778.

39. Diabetes Control and Complications Trial Research Group: The effect of intensive treatment of diabetes on the development and progression of long-term complications in insulin-dependent diabetes mellitus. *N Engl J Med* 1993;329:977–986.

40. Koya D, King GL: Protein kinase C activation and the development of diabetic complications. *Diabetes* 1998;47:859–866.

41. Aiello LP, Bursell SE, Clermont A, et al: Vascular endothelial growth factor–induced retinal permeability is mediated by protein kinase C in vivo and suppressed by an orally effective β-isoform-selective inhibitor. *Diabetes* 1997;46: 1473–1480.

42. Greene DA, Lattimer SA, Sima AA: Sorbitol, phosphoinositides, and sodium-potassium-ATPase in the pathogenesis of diabetic complications. *N Engl J Med* 1987;316:599–606.

43. Engerman RL, Kern TS: Aldose reductase inhibition fails to prevent progression of retinopathy in diabetic and galactosemic dogs. *Diabetes* 1993;42:820–825.

44. McCaleb ML, McKean ML, Hohman TC, et al: Intervention with the aldose reductase inhibitor, tolrestat, in renal and retinal lesions of streptozotocin-diabetic rats. *Diabetologia* 1991;34: 695–701.

45. Sorbinil Retinopathy Trial Research Group: A randomized trial of sorbinil, an aldose reductase inhibitor, in diabetic retinopathy. *Arch Ophthalmol* 1990;108:1234–1244.

46. Brownlee M: Glycation and diabetic complications. [Lilly Lecture 1993] *Diabetes* 1994;43: 836–841.

47. Clermont AC, Aiello LP, Mori F, et al: Vascular endothelial growth factor and severity of NPDR mediate retinal hemodynamics in vivo: a potential role for vascular endothelial growth factor in the progression of nonproliferative diabetic retinopathy. *Am J Ophthalmol* 1997;124: 433–446.

48. Ishii H, Jirousek MR, Koya D, et al: Amelioration of vascular dysfunctions in diabetic rats by an oral PKC β inhibitor. *Science* 1996;272: 728–731.

49. Lutty GA, McLeod DS, Merges C, et al: Localization of vascular endothelial growth factor in human retina and choroid. *Arch Ophthalmol* 1996;114:971–977.

50. Kristinsson JK, Gottfredsdottir MS, Stefansson E: Retinal vessel dilatation and elongation precedes diabetic macular oedema. *Br J Ophthalmol* 1997;81:274–278.

51. Gottfredsdottir MS, Stefansson E, Jonasson F, Gislason I: Retinal vasoconstriction after laser treatment for diabetic macular edema. *Am J Ophthalmol* 1993;115:64–67.

52. Larsen M, Dalgaard P, Lund-Andersen H: Differential spectrofluorometry in the human vitreous: blood–retina barrier permeability to fluorescein and fluorescein glucuronide. *Graefes Arch Klin Exp Ophthalmol* 1991;229:350–357.

53. Antonetti DA, Barber AJ, Lieth E, et al: Vascular permeability in experimental diabetes is associated with reduced endothelial occludin content: occludin expression is decreased in experimental diabetic retinopathy. *Diabetes* 1998; 47:1953–1959.

54. Gardner TW, Lieth E, Antonetti DA, et al: A new hypothesis on mechanisms of retinal vascular permeability in diabetes. In: Friedman EA, L'Esperance FA, eds: *The Diabetic Renal-Retinal Syndrome.* 6th ed. Dordrecht, Netherlands: Kluwer Publishers; 1998:169–179.

55. Bresnick GH, Segal P, Mattson D: Fluorescein angiographic and clinicopathologic findings. In: Little HL, Jack RL, Patz A, Forsham PH, eds: *Diabetic Retinopathy.* New York: Thieme-Stratton; 1983:37–71.

56. Chew EY, Klein ML, Ferris FL III, et al: Association of elevated serum lipid levels with retinal hard exudate in diabetic retinopathy. ETDRS Report Number 22. *Arch Ophthalmol* 1996;114: 1079–1084.

57. Ohira A, de Juan E Jr: Characterization of glial involvement in proliferative diabetic retinopathy. *Ophthalmologica* 1990;201:187–195.

58. Casey R, Li WW: Factors controlling ocular angiogenesis. *Am J Ophthalmol* 1997;124: 521–529.

59. Aiello LP, Avery RL, Arrigg PG, et al: Vascular endothelial growth factor in ocular fluid of patients with diabetic retinopathy and other retinal disorders. *N Engl J Med* 1994;331:1480–1487.

60. Aiello LP: Vascular endothelial growth factor: 20th-century mechanisms, 21st-century therapies. *Invest Ophthalmol Vis Sci* 1997;38: 1647–1652.

61. Neely KA, Gardner TW: Ocular neovascularization: clarifying complex interactions. *Am J Pathol* 1998;153:665–670.

62. Lieth E, Gardner TW, Barber AJ, et al: Retinal neurodegeneration: early pathology in diabetes. *Clin Exp Ophthalmol,* in press.

CHAPTER 2

Epidemiology of Eye Disease in Diabetes

Ronald Klein, MD, MPH

Barbara E. K. Klein, MD, MPH

Diabetes, particularly diabetic retinopathy, is the leading cause of new cases of blindness in persons age 20 to 74 years in the United States.[1-6] Approximately 8% of those who are legally blind are reported to have diabetes as the cause, and it is estimated that more than 12% of new cases of blindness are attributable to diabetes. Of insulin-dependent patients with diabetes for 30 or more years, 12% are blind. Patients who have diabetic retinopathy are 29 times more likely to be blind than nondiabetic persons. Blindness due to diabetes is estimated to involve lost income and public welfare expense of $500 million annually.

2-1

PREVALENCE OF VISUAL IMPAIRMENT

Estimates of rates of legal blindness in the US have been reported by the National Society to Prevent Blindness from data of the Model Reporting Area (MRA) registry.[1-3] It was estimated that 7.9% of persons who were legally blind reported diabetes as the cause of their blindness.

Prevalence rates for diabetes-related legal blindness increased with increasing age to a maximum in patients age 65 to 74 years; thereafter, the rates declined, possibly due to higher death rates in the elderly diabetic population with other end-organ disease (Table 2-1). White females and nonwhite males and females had higher rates of legal blindness, compared with white males. Because the MRA registry data were based on self-reports and required registration at specific agencies in 16 states, the rates are thought to underestimate the actual prevalence of legal blindness by as much as 50%.[4]

The 1989 National Health Interview Survey (NHIS)[5] found that those with type 1 diabetes had higher self-reported frequencies of "blindness" and "trouble seeing" than those with type 2 diabetes in patients age <45 years. These data probably underestimate visual impairment, because the sensitivity of responses to questions about vision is low (about 32% to 45%).[6]

TABLE 2-1

Prevalence of Legal Blindness due to Diabetes and Retinopathy, by Age and Sex, US 1978

Age and Sex	No. of Cases of Legal Blindness due to Diabetes	% of Total Cases of Legal Blindness due to Diabetes	No. of Cases of Legal Blindness due to Diabetic Retinopathy	% of All Cases of Legal Blindness Attributable to Diabetic Retinopathy
Age (Years)				
<5	0	0	0	0
5–19	<50	<0.1	<50	<0.1
20–44	4,000	4.8	3,500	4.2
45–64	12,250	11.3	10,600	9.8
65–74	13,700	14.4	11,150	11.7
75–84	7,850	7.5	6,200	6.0
≥85	1,700	2.6	1,200	1.8
Sex				
Males	14,750	6.1	12,800	5.3
Females	24,750	9.7	19,850	7.7
Total	39,500	7.9	32,650	6.6

Note: *Data are estimated from MRA data 1970.*

Source: Vision Problems in the U.S.: A Statistical Analysis. *New York: National Society to Prevent Blindness; 1980.*

Population-based estimates of frequencies of impaired vision in diabetic patients were reported in the Wisconsin Epidemiologic Study of Diabetic Retinopathy (WESDR),[7] in which a standardized protocol for determination of visual acuity was used.[8] The objectives of the study were to describe the prevalence and severity of diabetic retinopathy, decreased vision, and other ocular and systemic conditions. The associations of these conditions with other personal and demographic characteristics in a geographically defined population in an 11-county area in southern Wisconsin were examined.[9–11] The participants and their diabetic management were typical of medical practice in Wisconsin: 452 physicians participated (98.9% of all physicians who offered primary care to diabetic patients in the 11-county area).

Of the 10,135 diabetic patients identified in this survey, all insulin-taking patients diagnosed at age <30 years (1210 patients, the younger-onset group with type 1 diabetes) and a probability sample of patients diagnosed as having diabetes at age

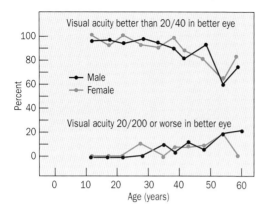

Figure 2-1 *Prevalence of no visual impairment and of legal blindness in insulin-taking persons diagnosed with diabetes at age <30 years, by age.*
Klein R: WESDR 1980–1982, unpublished data.

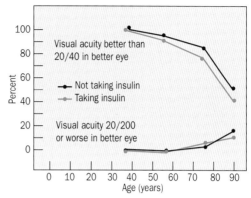

Figure 2-2 *Prevalence of no visual impairment and of legal blindness in persons diagnosed with diabetes at age ≥30 years, by age.*
Klein R: WESDR 1980–1982, unpublished data.

≥30 years (1780 patients, the older-onset group with type 1 and type 2 diabetes) were invited to participate in the examination phase of the study, conducted from September 1980 to July 1982. Of the younger-onset group, 92% had no impairment (best-corrected visual acuity in the better eye of better than 20/40).[7] The frequency of visual impairment increased with increasing age (Figure 2-1).

No cases of legal blindness were found in persons age <25 years. The rate of legal blindness increased with age in both males and females, reaching peaks of 14% and 20%, respectively, in persons age 65 to 74 years. In the older-onset group, rates of blindness increased with increasing age and accounted for 2.2% in patients not taking insulin and 1.6% in those taking insulin (Figure 2-2). The age-specific rates of legal blindness in both younger- and older-onset diabetic patients in the WESDR were higher

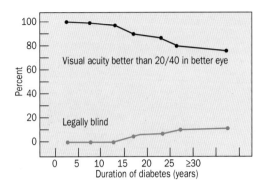

Figure 2-3 *Percent with visual acuity better than 20/40 and with legal blindness among insulin-taking patients diagnosed with diabetes at age <30 years, by duration of diabetes. Data are from WESDR 1980–1982.*

Klein R, Klein BEK, Moss SE: Visual impairment in diabetes. Ophthalmology *1984;91:1–9.*

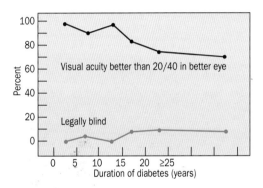

Figure 2-4 *Percent with visual acuity better than 20/40 and with legal blindness among patients diagnosed with diabetes at age ≥30 years, by duration of diabetes. Data are from WESDR 1980–1982.*

Klein R, Klein BEK, Moss SE: Visual impairment in diabetes. Ophthalmology *1984;91:1–9.*

than those estimated for the general US population in the First National Health and Nutrition Examination Survey (NHANES I)[12] or for all participants in the Framingham Eye Study (FES).[13]

Legal blindness was related to duration of diabetes in both younger- and older-onset participants in the WESDR (Figures 2-3 and 2-4).[7] In the younger-onset group, legal blindness first occurred in patients having diabetes for about 15 years or more and increased from 3% in those with 15 to 19 years' duration to 12% in patients with diabetes for ≥30 years. In the older-onset group, rates of legal blindness were lower, reaching only 7% in patients having diabetes for 20 to 24 years.

Diabetic retinopathy was partly or totally responsible for legal blindness (acuity of 20/200 or worse) in 86% of eyes of younger-onset patients with such severe impairment (Figure 2-5).[7] Diabetic retinopathy was less often a cause of legal blindness in the older-onset patients; other causes of visual impairment, such as macular degeneration or cataract, were more frequently responsible in this group.

In a study in Poole, England, 2% of 449 non–insulin-taking patients and 1% of 212 insulin-taking diabetic patients were legally blind.[14] In another population-based study in Oxford, England, in 1982, 28% of 188 patients age ≥60 years with known type 2 diabetes were visually impaired.[15]

In a Danish study, 3.4% of males and 2.6% of females in a cohort of 727 patients with type 1 diabetes diagnosed at age <30 years were legally blind.[16] Legal blindness was estimated to be 50 to 80 times higher in patients with diabetes. Proliferative diabetic retinopathy (PDR) was the primary cause of legal blindness in this study.

2-2

INCIDENCE OF VISUAL IMPAIRMENT

In data from the MRA registries, the incidence of legal blindness due to diabetes paralleled prevalence studies; it peaked at 45 to 64 years of age, decreased with age, and was higher for females.[1] Of new cases of legal blindness, 12.4% were attributed to diabetes, the majority due to diabetic retinopathy. Diabetic retinopathy was the third most common diagnosis responsible for legal blindness in patients of all ages and was the leading cause of new cases of blindness in patients age 20 to 74 years. No recent national population-based registry data are available in the US.

Data from the Radcliffe Infirmary Diabetes Clinic in England indicate that, for insulin-taking diabetic patients diagnosed at age ≤20 years, the incidence of blindness was 0.1% after 10 years, 1.6% after 20 years, and 3.5% after 30 years of diabetes.[17] For patients diagnosed at age ≥60 years, the incidence of blindness was 1.8% after 10 years and 5.5% after 20 years of diabetes. An 8-year incidence of 7.6 per 1000 patient-years in males and 10.2 per 1000 patient-years in females with type 1 diabetes was reported from Denmark.[16] In a later study in Oxford, England, 4.8% of those with type 2 diabetes and age ≥60 years at baseline became legally blind over a median period of 6 years.[15]

The frequency of change in rates of impaired vision in the WESDR is presented in Table 2-2.[18] Among those patients not impaired at baseline, the older-onset group taking insulin had the highest incidence of impaired vision (16.1%) or legal blindness (1.2%). The estimated annual incidence of

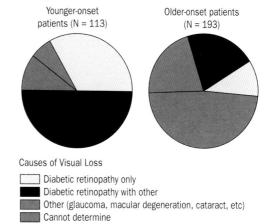

Causes of Visual Loss

☐ Diabetic retinopathy only
■ Diabetic retinopathy with other
▨ Other (glaucoma, macular degeneration, cataract, etc)
▨ Cannot determine

Figure 2-5 *Causes of visual loss (visual acuity 20/200 or worse) in diabetic patients. Data are from WESDR 1980–1982.*

Klein R, Klein BEK, Moss SE: Visual impairment in diabetes. Ophthalmology *1984;91:1–9.*

TABLE 2-2

Four-Year Incidence of Visual Impairment in Diabetic Patients, by Impairment Degree at Baseline Exam, WESDR 1980–1986

Impairment Degree	No. of Participants	Visual Impairment at Followup			
		None (%)	Mild (%)	Moderate (%)	Blind (%)
Younger-Onset					
None	832	95.3	2.8	1.4	0.5
Mild	26	26.9	42.3	15.4	15.4
Moderate	10	10.0	10.0	30.0	50.0
Blind	20	0	0	0	100.0
Older-Onset Taking Insulin					
None	423	83.9	10.6	4.3	1.2
Mild	27	29.6	22.2	40.7	7.4
Moderate	15	6.7	13.3	26.7	53.3
Blind	8	0	0	0	100.0
Older-Onset Not Taking Insulin					
None	454	91.0	5.5	2.9	0.7
Mild	29	20.7	31.0	31.0	17.2
Moderate	7	0	0	28.6	71.4
Blind	4	0	0	0	100.0

Source: *Moss SE, Klein R, Klein BEK: The incidence of vision loss in a diabetic population.* Ophthalmology *1988;95: 1340–1348.*

blindness reported in the WESDR was 3.3 per 100,000 population. This is higher than the estimated annual incidence rates of legal blindness due, in part, to diabetes of 1.6 to 2.1 per 100,000 persons in the general population derived from the MRA data.[1] Rates in the WESDR are comparable to those reported in the Rochester, Minnesota, study.[19] Interpolating back from 20 years in the Rochester population produces an estimated 4-year rate of legal blindness of 1.6% in all diabetic patients, compared with 2.2% in the WESDR study.

Few population-based data are available to determine trends in the frequency of decreased vision. Two studies in England, one in the county of Avon and the other in the county of Leicestershire, compared rates of registration for blindness benefits attrib-

TABLE 2-3

Ten-Year Incidences of Legal Blindness, Visual Impairment, and Doubling of Visual Angle, by Diabetes Group, WESDR 1980–1992

Group	Blindness No.	Blindness %	Visual Impairment No.	Visual Impairment %	Doubling of Visual Angle No.	Doubling of Visual Angle %
Younger-onset	868	1.8	832	9.4	880	9.2
Older-onset taking insulin	465	4.0	423	37.2	472	32.8
Older-onset not taking insulin	490	4.8	454	23.9	494	21.4

Source: *Moss SE, Klein R, Klein BEK: Ten-year incidence of visual loss in a diabetic population.* Ophthalmology *1994; 101:1061–1070.*

uted to diabetic retinopathy in 1985 with those recorded in England in 1965.[20-22] Registry data may be unreliable, however, due to underreporting, nonuniform disease classification, and inaccurate denominator determination. In Avon in 1985, blindness due to diabetes (1.8 registrations per 100,000) was similar to that in England in 1965 (1.6 registrations per 100,000).[20] This was attributed, in part, to the increase in the number of patients diagnosed as having diabetes since 1965. In Leicestershire, a significant decrease in the frequency of those registered as being blind between 1975 and 1985 was attributed to better local care and the increased use of laser photocoagulation.[21]

The WESDR cohort was re-examined 10 years after the baseline examination.[23] The 10-year incidences of legal blindness, impaired vision, and doubling of the visual angle by diabetes group are presented in Table 2-3.[24] There appeared to be a decrease in the estimated annual incidence of blindness in the three WESDR diabetic groups in the last 6 years compared with the first 4 years of the study (Table 2-4).[24]

TABLE 2-4

Annual Incidence of Blindness, by Diabetes Group, WESDR 1980–1992

Group	1980–1982 to 1984–1986 (%)	1984–1986 to 1990–1992 (%)	1990–1992 to 1995–1996 (%)
Younger-onset	0.38	0.05	0.18
Older-onset taking insulin	0.82	0.14	—
Older-onset not taking insulin	0.67	0.37	—

Sources: *Moss SE, Klein R, Klein BEK: Ten-year incidence of visual loss in a diabetic population.* Ophthalmology *1994;101:1061–1070.*

Moss SE, Klein R, Klein BEK: The 14-year incidence of visual loss in a diabetic population. Ophthalmology *1998;105:998–1003.*

Possible reasons for the decrease in the estimated annual incidence of blindness are not explained by changes in the incidence of PDR or an increased frequency of panretinal photocoagulation in the second 6-year period.[23] Higher frequencies of focal photocoagulation for macular edema and lens extraction for cataract in the second 6-year period of the study compared with the first 4 years may explain only part of the decrease in frequency of blindness over time. It is possible that early detection and treatment of PDR may have resulted in the decline in rates of legal blindness over the last 6 years of the study.

Because of the high death rate in older-onset diabetic persons in the WESDR, only the younger-onset group was re-examined at the 14-year followup.[25] The 14-year cumulative incidence of blindness was 2.4% (95% confidence interval [CI] 1.3% to 3.5%), the incidence of visual impairment was 12.7% (95% CI 10.3% to 15.2%), and the doubling of the visual angle was 14.2% (95% CI 11.7% to 16.7%). There appeared to be a small increase in the estimated annual rates of visual loss in the younger-onset group in the last 4-year period compared to the previous 6-year period.

RISK FACTORS FOR VISION LOSS AND LEGAL BLINDNESS

2-3-1 Sex and Race

In the WESDR, sex was not associated with the 10-year incidence of legal blindness, except for a slightly higher incidence in older-onset women not taking insulin than in older-onset men not taking insulin (5.8% versus 3.6%) and in older-onset women taking insulin than in older-onset men taking insulin (5.4% versus 2.3%).[24] Analyses of MRA registry data indicate that the highest rates of legal blindness due to diabetes occurred in nonwhite females; nonwhite males and white females were intermediate, and white males had the lowest rates.[4] In the Baltimore Eye Survey, legal blindness due to diabetic retinopathy was equally prevalent in whites (6%) and in blacks (5%) age ≥40 years.[26] This comparison must be made cautiously, as only seven eyes were legally blind.

2-3-2 Age and Duration of Diabetes

The 4-year incidence of blindness and doubling of the visual angle increased with increasing age in all of the WESDR diabetic groups and increased with increasing duration only in the younger- and older-onset groups taking insulin (Tables 2-5 and 2-6, Figures 2-6 and 2-7).[18] The relationship of the 10-year incidence of blindness and doubling of visual angle to age and duration of diabetes at baseline was similar to the 4-year incidence rates (data not shown).[24] Others have also reported similar relationships between longer duration of diabetes and impaired vision.[15–17,19]

TABLE 2-5

*Four-Year Incidence of Blindness in Diabetic Patients, by Age at Baseline Exam,
WESDR 1980–1986*

Age (Years)	Younger-Onset		Older-Onset Taking Insulin		Older-Onset Not Taking Insulin	
	No.	%	No.	%	No.	%
0–9	25	0				
10–19	222	0				
20–29	282	1.8				
30–44	242	2.1	26	0	19	0
45–54	97†	3.1†	86	1.2	52	1.9
55–64			137	1.5	148	2.7
65–74			160	3.1	177	0
≥75			56	12.5	94	8.5
P∗	<0.025		<0.001		0.051	

∗Based on test for trend. †Sample size and rate for age ≥45 years.

Source: *Moss SE, Klein R, Klein BEK: The incidence of vision loss in a diabetic population.* Ophthalmology *1988;95:
1340–1348.*

TABLE 2-6

*Four-Year Incidence of Blindness in Diabetic Patients, by Duration of Diabetes at Baseline Exam,
WESDR 1980–1986*

Duration (Years)	Younger-Onset		Older-Onset Taking Insulin		Older-Onset Not Taking Insulin	
	No.	%	No.	%	No.	%
0–4	157	0	78	0	204	2.9
5–9	232	0	83	3.6	151	2.0
10–14	162	1.2	78	2.6	54	1.9
15–19	117	5.1	106	3.8	54	5.6
20–24	73	2.7	75	2.7	27†	0†
25–29	61	4.9	28	10.7		
≥30	66	0	17	5.9		
P∗	<0.005		0.056		0.93	

∗Based on test for trend. †Sample size and rate for duration of diabetes ≥20 years.

Source: *Moss SE, Klein R, Klein BEK: The incidence of vision loss in a diabetic population.* Ophthalmology *1988;95:
1340–1348.*

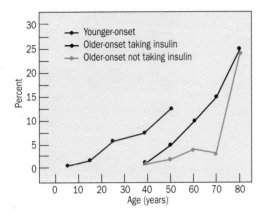

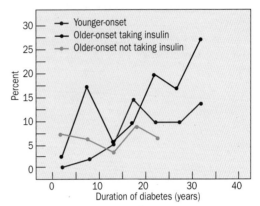

Figure 2-6 *Four-year incidence of doubling of visual angle in patients with diabetes, by age. Data are from WESDR 1980–1986.*

Moss SE, Klein R, Klein BEK: The incidence of vision loss in a diabetic population. Ophthalmology *1988;95: 1340–1348.*

Figure 2-7 *Four-year incidence of doubling of visual angle in patients with diabetes, by duration of diabetes. Data are from WESDR 1980–1986.*

Moss SE, Klein R, Klein BEK: The incidence of vision loss in a diabetic population. Ophthalmology *1988;95: 1340–1348.*

TABLE 2-7

Four-Year Incidence of Blindness in Right Eye of Diabetic Patients, by Retinopathy Level at Baseline Exam, WESDR 1980–1986

Retinopathy Level	Younger-Onset		Older-Onset Taking Insulin		Older-Onset Not Taking Insulin	
	No.	%	No.	%	No.	%
1	307	0.3	178	4.5	343	3.2
1.5–2	166	0.6	65	3.1	65	4.6
3	119	2.5	67	10.4	33	6.1
4–5	136	4.4	106	12.3	33	24.2
6	96	6.2	31	6.5	2	
7	21	23.8	4	0	1	
P*	<0.0001		<0.05		<0.001	

*Based on test for trend.

Source: *Moss SE, Klein R, Klein BEK: The incidence of vision loss in a diabetic population.* Ophthalmology *1988;95: 1340–1348.*

2-3-3 Severity of Retinopathy and Macular Edema

In the WESDR, the 4-year incidence of legal blindness increased with increasing severity of retinopathy (Table 2-7).[18] The 4-year relative risk of legal blindness in diabetic patients with retinopathy compared with the general population was estimated to be 29. Prior to the widespread use of panretinal photocoagulation, the risk of legal blindness associated with severe retinopathy was higher. Among 51 patients with type 1 diabetes with PDR observed in the Steno Hospital in Denmark, 50% had become legally blind after 5 years.[27] In the WESDR, the 4-year incidence of doubling of the visual angle was increased in the presence of macular edema at baseline; the risk was highest in the older-onset, non–insulin-taking subgroup.[18]

2-3-4 Other Risk Factors

Other factors increasing the risk of incidence of visual-angle doubling included glycosylated hemoglobin and gross proteinuria.[18] In the WESDR, at the 4-year follow-up, diabetic retinopathy was found to be the sole or contributing cause of impaired vision in 69% of eyes of younger-onset patients, 42% of eyes of older-onset patients taking insulin, and 26% of eyes of older-onset patients not taking insulin.[18]

2-4

REHABILITATION AND ECONOMIC COSTS OF BLINDNESS

Few data describe the socioeconomic and psychosocial characteristics of diabetic patients who have impaired vision and who need rehabilitative services. In the WESDR, younger-onset men age ≥25 years who had PDR and who were employed at baseline were more likely to become unemployed 4 years later.[28] Younger-onset women who were married and had impaired vision at baseline had an increased 4-year incidence of divorce. Data from two English studies suggest that diabetic patients have a greater disadvantage than patients with other diseases when seeking work.[29,30]

Psychological distress in diabetic patients with either stable or fluctuating decreases in vision, even when mild, has been thought to be a result of physical inactivity and inability to manage their diabetes.[31,32] Rehabilitation programs consisting of education concerning diabetes self-management skills, nutrition counseling, and exercise programs have been shown to lead to significant improvements in psychological profiles in diabetic patients with fluctuating vision or loss of vision.[33]

Some studies have provided estimates of costs associated with blindness due to diabetes. A minimum cost to the federal government of $12,769 was estimated for a person-year of blindness for a working-age American who becomes blind in adulthood; for those age ≥65 years, it was $823.[34] These estimates did not include reduced productivity, output loss, societal burdens of rehabilitation, and other local expenses. Based on the WESDR estimates of prevalence of blindness among patients with diagnosed diabetes in the US in 1980–1982, the annual cost is estimated to be about $500 million.[34]

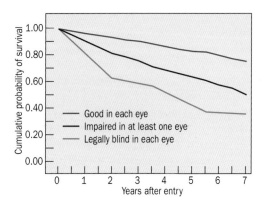

Figure 2-8 *Survival for insulin-taking patients with diabetes diagnosed at age <50 years, according to visual acuity. Patients were from a Wisconsin clinic. Visual acuity was determined at entry to study.*

Davis MD, Hiller R, Magli YL, et al: Prognosis for life in patients with diabetes: relation to severity of retinopathy. Trans Am Ophthalmol Soc *1979;77:144–170.*

Three studies[35–37] have estimated the cost-effectiveness of strategies for detecting diabetic retinopathy. Data from these analyses suggest that screening for diabetic retinopathy and obtaining ophthalmologic care result in significant savings in patients with younger-onset diabetes. One analysis[37] predicted an annual savings of an estimated $240.5 million and 138,390 person-years of sight for 60% screening and treatment rate implementation level. If all patients were to receive appropriate eye care, the predicted savings would exceed $400 million and savings of 230,000 person-years of sight in younger-onset patients. Another analysis[35] also found that targeting the younger-onset cohort and the older-onset cohort taking insulin could achieve cost savings. Conversely, the incremental number of sight-years to be gained in the older-onset population not taking insulin, even by annual ophthalmologic examination with fundus photography, was reported to be small. However, macular edema, an important cause of vision loss, was not included in the analyses.

2-5

VISUAL ACUITY AS PREDICTOR OF DEATH

The relationship between visual acuity and the probability of survival in insulin-taking diabetic patients seen in an eye clinic in Wisconsin is presented in Figure 2-8.[38] The probability of survival declined with decreasing levels of visual acuity. The observed 5-year survival was about 40% in persons who were legally blind.

In the WESDR, after adjusting for age and sex, younger-onset patients with visual

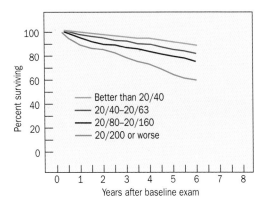

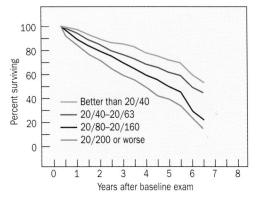

Figure 2-9 *Survival in patients diagnosed with diabetes at age <30 years, according to visual acuity. Visual acuity status was determined at baseline exam (1980–1982) in WESDR. Data are age- and sex-adjusted.*

Klein R, Moss SE, Klein BEK, DeMets DL: Relation of ocular and systemic factors to survival in diabetes. Arch Intern Med *1989;149:266–272.*

Figure 2-10 *Survival in patients diagnosed with diabetes at age ≥30 years, according to visual acuity. Visual acuity status was determined at baseline exam (1980–1982) in WESDR. Data are age- and sex-adjusted.*

Klein R, Moss SE, Klein BEK, DeMets DL: Relation of ocular and systemic factors to survival in diabetes. Arch Intern Med *1989;149:266–272.*

acuity of 20/200 or poorer in their better eye at baseline had a 6-year survival rate of 57.9%, compared with 89.9% in patients whose visual acuity was better than 20/40 in the better eye (Figure 2-9).[39] Poor 6-year survival was also seen in the older-onset group with poorer visual acuity at baseline (Figure 2-10). Those with visual acuity of 20/200 or worse in the better eye at baseline had a 6-year survival rate of 18.4%, compared with 56.2% for those whose visual acuity was better than 20/40 in the better eye.

The relationship between survival and visual acuity remained after controlling for other factors associated with mortality, such as increased age, longer duration of diabetes, higher blood pressure, higher glycosylated hemoglobin, history of cardiovascular disease, and male gender. These data suggest that patients with diabetes and poor visual acuity should be examined frequently by their primary care physicians to detect and possibly treat early renal disease, elevated blood pressure, and cardiovascular disease to minimize their effects.

2-6

PREVALENCE OF RETINOPATHY IN WESDR

In the WESDR, stereoscopic fundus photographs of seven standard photographic fields were taken of each eye.[10] Objective grading of retinopathy by standard protocols was used to assure reproducible assessment and classification of the severity of retinopathy.[40–42] In the WESDR, 71% of younger-onset patients had retinopathy, 23% had PDR, and 6% had clinically significant macular edema (CSME).[10,43] In older-onset patients in the WESDR, 39% of those who did not take insulin, and 70% of those who did, had retinopathy; 3% of the former and 14% of the latter had PDR; 4% of the former and 11% of the latter had CSME.[11,43]

Using WESDR estimates of prevalence of retinopathy, 1990 US Census estimates, and 1989 NHIS estimates of diabetes, the National Society to Prevent Blindness (NSPB) has developed estimates of 4 to 6 million diabetic patients with retinopathy in the US. The NSPB also provides state-specific estimates of retinopathy. Based on the WESDR data and an estimate in 1980–1982 of 5.8 million Americans known to have diabetes, 700,000 had PDR and 325,000 had CSME.

2-7

PREVALENCE OF RETINOPATHY IN OTHER STUDIES

Prevalence data have been reported in other population-based studies (Table 2-8).[14,19,44–67] Comparisons among studies must be made cautiously because there are a number of possible reasons for differences among them:

1. Definitions of diabetes and its component complications differ.

2. Methods used to detect and classify retinopathy may vary from study to study.

3. There are often age, sociodemographic, and genetic differences among groups under study.

Standardized protocols for detecting and classifying diabetic retinopathy have been developed. The use of photographic documentation of diabetic retinopathy and photographic standards for grading severity of retinal lesions has facilitated comparisons among some studies.[10,42,57,59]

The frequencies of retinopathy in the WESDR are higher than those previously reported from other large population-based studies using ophthalmoscopy to detect retinopathy.[10,11,44–47,67] Without adjusting for duration of diabetes, age, level of glycemia, and other factors associated with the prevalence of retinopathy, comparisons among populations are of limited usefulness, even when fundus photography and grading have been used to detect retinopathy.

TABLE 2-8

Selected Population-Based Studies Describing Prevalence and Incidence of Diabetic Retinopathy

References	Site	Type of Diabetes	No. Studied	Duration of Diabetes (Years)	Retinopathy Detection*	Crude Prevalence (%)	Crude Incidence (Years)
44	Pima Indians, AZ	2	399	0–10+	O	18	
45,67	Pima Indians, AZ	2	279		O		4 = 2.6%
46	Framingham, MA	2	229		O	18	
47,65,66	Oklahoma Indians	2	973	0–20+	O,P	24	10–16 = 72.3%
14	Poole, England	1 2	714	0–30+	O,P	Severe reti-nopathy 8.3	
48	Nauru, Central Pacific	2	343	0–10+	O	24	
19	Rochester, MN	1	75				45.8/1000 person-years
49	Rochester, MN	2	1060		O		15.6/1000 person-years
50	Iceland	1	212	0–20+	P	34	
51 52	Perth, Australia	1 2	179 904	0–20+ 0–20+	O,P O,P	33 27	
53	County of Fynn, Denmark	1	718	0–30+	O	48	
54,55	Falster, Denmark	1 2	215 333	0–58 0–42	P P	66 41	1 = 3.7% 1 = 3.7%
56	Switzerland	1 2	105 94	0–30+	O	51 9	8 = 39% 8 = 15%
57	San Antonio, TX	2	257	0–10+	O,P	45	
58	Gotland, Sweden	1 2	160 140	0–20+ 0–20+	P	56–65 17	
59	San Luis Valley, CO (Hispanics)	2	166	0–5+ 15+	P	19 88	
60	Leicester, England	1	350	0–30+	O,P	41	
10,11,40,68	South-Central, WI	1 2	996 1370	0–30+ 0–30+	O,P O,P	71 39	4 = 59% 4 = 34%
61,62	Allegheny County, PA	1	657	6–38	O,P	86	2 = 33%
63	Seattle, WA (2nd-generation Japanese American men)	1 2	78	0–10+	O,P	11.5	
64†	Alberta, Canada	1 2	2300 1346	0–60+ 0–35+	O,P O,P	59.9 29.9	

*O = ophthalmoscopy. P = photography.   †Unpublished data.

Source: *Klein R, Klein BEK, Moss S: The Wisconsin Epidemiologic Study of Diabetic Retinopathy: a review.* Diabetes Metab Rev *1989;5:559–570.*

TABLE 2-9

Four-Year Incidences of Any Retinopathy, Improvement or Progression of Retinopathy, and Progression to PDR in Younger-Onset Diabetic Patients, by Sex, WESDR 1980–1986

	Males			Females			Total		
Retinopathy	No. at Risk	%	95% CI	No. at Risk	%	95% CI	No. at Risk	%	95% CI
Any retinopathy	143	55.9	47.8,64.0	128	62.5	54.1,70.9	271	59.0	53.1,64.9
Improvement	181	4.4	1.4,7.4	195	9.2	5.1,13.3	376	6.9	4.3,9.5
No change	354	54.5	49.3,59.7	359	55.7	50.6,60.8	713	55.1	51.4,58.8
Progression	354	43.2	38.0,48.4	359	39.3	34.2,44.4	713	41.2	37.6,44.8
Progression to PDR	354	11.3	8.0,14.6	359	9.8	6.7,12.9	713	10.5	8.2,12.8

Note: *Number at risk for incidence of any retinopathy refers to group that had no retinopathy (level 10/10) at baseline exam and were at risk of developing retinopathy at followup exam. Number at risk for improvement in retinopathy refers to those with retinopathy levels of 21/21 to 51/51 at baseline exam who could have decrease in their retinopathy severity by at least two steps or more at followup exam. Number at risk for no change, progression, or progression to PDR refers to those with retinopathy levels of 10/10 to 51/51 who either did not change by two or more steps or progressed by two or more steps.*

Source: *Klein R, Klein BEK, Moss SE, et al: The Wisconsin Epidemiologic Study of Diabetic Retinopathy, IX: four-year incidence and progression of diabetic retinopathy when age at diagnosis is less than 30 years. Arch Ophthalmol 1989; 107:237–243.*

2-8

INCIDENCE AND PROGRESSION OF RETINOPATHY

The incidence of retinopathy in a 4-year interval in the entire WESDR population was 40.3%.[40,68] The 4-year incidence and progression of diabetic retinopathy in the WESDR are presented in Tables 2-9 and 2-10. The younger-onset group taking insulin had the highest 4-year incidence, rate of progression, and progression to PDR, while the older-onset group not taking insulin had the lowest rates, but the older-onset group taking insulin had the highest 4-year incidence of macular edema (Table 2-11).[69]

Based on WESDR data, it is estimated that, of the approximately 7.8 million Americans with known diabetes in 1993, 84,000 will develop PDR each year and 40,000 will develop PDR with Diabetic Retinopothy Study (DRS) high-risk characteristics for severe loss of vision. Each year, 95,000 patients with diabetes are estimated to develop macular edema.

The 10-year incidences of retinopathy (89%, 79%, and 67%), progression of retinopathy (76%, 69%, and 53%), and progression to PDR (30%, 24%, and 10%) were highest in the group diagnosed before age

TABLE 2-10

*Four-Year Incidences of Any Retinopathy, Improvement or Progression of Retinopathy,
and Progression to PDR in Older-Onset Diabetic Patients, by Sex, WESDR 1980–1986*

	Males			Females			Total		
Retinopathy	No. at Risk	%	95% CI	No. at Risk	%	95% CI	No. at Risk	%	95% CI
Taking Insulin									
Any retinopathy	62	46.8	34.4,59.2	92	47.8	37.6,58.0	154	47.4	39.5,55.3
Improvement	107	10.3	4.5,16.1	108	20.4	12.8,28.0	215	15.3	10.5,20.1
No change	193	62.2	55.4,69.0	225	54.7	48.2,61.2	418	58.1	53.4,62.8
Progression	193	32.1	25.5,38.7	225	35.6	29.3,41.9	418	34.0	29.5,38.5
Progression to PDR	193	7.3	3.6,11.0	225	7.6	4.1,11.1	418	7.4	4.9,9.9
Not Taking Insulin									
Any retinopathy	151	32.5	25.0,40.0	169	36.1	28.9,43.3	320	34.4	29.2,39.6
Improvement	35	11.4	0.9,21.9	69	24.2	13.9,34.5	101	19.8	12.0,27.6
No change	216	72.7	66.8,78.6	270	69.6	64.1,75.1	486	71.0	67.0,75.0
Progression	216	25.5	19.7,31.3	270	24.4	19.3,29.5	486	24.9	21.1,28.7
Progression to PDR	216	2.8	0.6,5.0	270	1.9	0.3,3.5	486	2.3	1.0,3.6

Note: *See Table 2-9.*

Source: *Klein R, Klein BEK, Moss SE, et al: The Wisconsin Epidemiologic Study of Diabetic Retinopathy, X: four-year incidence and progression of diabetic retinopathy when age at diagnosis is 30 years or more.* Arch Ophthalmol *1989; 107:244–249.*

30 years, intermediate in the insulin-taking group diagnosed at age 30 years or older, and lowest in the non–insulin-taking group, respectively.[23]

In the WESDR, the estimated annual incidences and rates of progression of retinopathy for the first 4 years of the study were compared with the next 6 years of the study.[23] There were few differences in the estimated annual incidence or rates of progression between these two periods. In the WESDR, the 14-year rate of progression of retinopathy in the younger-onset group

was 86%, progression to PDR was 37%, and incidence of macular edema was 26%.[70] These data suggest that incidence and progression of retinopathy remained unchanged or worsened despite improvements in glycemic control in patients taking insulin over the first 4 years of the study.

TABLE 2-11

Four-Year Incidences of Macular Edema and CSME, by Diabetes Group, WESDR 1980–1986

Group	No. of Patients	No. With Macular Edema	Incidence (%)	No. With CSME	Incidence (%)
Younger-Onset	610	50	8.2	26	4.3
Older-Onset	652	34	5.2	19	2.9
Taking insulin	273	23	8.4	14	5.1
Not taking insulin	379	11	2.9	5	1.3
Oral hypogly-cemic agents	243	9	3.7	4	1.6
Diet only	102	1	1.0	1	1.0
None	34	1	2.9	0	0

Source: *Klein R, Moss SE, Klein BEK, et al: The Wisconsin Epidemiologic Study of Diabetic Retinopathy, XI: the incidence of macular edema.* Ophthalmology *1989;96:1501–1510.*

2-9

RISK FACTORS FOR RETINOPATHY

2-9-1 Sex

In the WESDR, higher frequencies of PDR were present in younger-onset males compared with females,[10] but there was no significant difference in the 10-year incidence or progression of diabetic retinopathy.[23] There were no significant differences in the prevalence, incidence, or rates of progression to PDR between the sexes in patients with older-onset diabetes in the WESDR.[11,23,68]

2-9-2 Race

Pima and Oklahoma Indians with type 2 diabetes appear to be at increased risk of developing PDR compared with whites with type 2 diabetes.[66,67] However, the prevalence and severity of retinopathy appear to vary among different Indian groups.[44,47,64–67] This may reflect different levels of the same risk factors, different relative importance of those risk factors, or genetic differences.

Using similar protocols to measure risk factors and to detect diabetic retinopathy, after controlling for all measured risk factors, the frequency of retinopathy in Mexican Americans in San Antonio, Texas, was 2.4 times as high as the frequency of retinopathy in non-Hispanic whites studied in the WESDR.[57] The NHANES III found retinopathy to be more prevalent in Mexican Americans compared with non-Hispanic whites age ≥40 years (Figure 2-11),[71] controlling for glycemic control, but there was no difference in the San Luis Valley Diabetes Study.[59]

At present, there are limited epidemiologic data available on the prevalence of retinopathy and macular edema in black populations living in the US. The NHANES III found retinopathy more prevalent in non-Hispanic black men than in non-Hispanic white men age 40 years or older (no difference in women) to be explained by differences in glycemic control.[71] Similarly, after correction for glycemia and other risk factors, no difference was reported in the frequency of nonproliferative diabetic retinopathy (NPDR), as detected by direct ophthalmoscopy, in black Jamaicans with type 2 diabetes compared with whites with type 2 diabetes.[72] In a clinic-based cohort in St Louis, Missouri, after controlling for other risk factors, African Americans with type 1 diabetes, despite higher frequencies of hyperglycemia and hypertension, had a lower rate of progression of retinopathy than did a group of non-Hispanic whites.[73]

2-9-3 Genetics

The relationships between genetic factors and the prevalence and incidence of retinopathy have been inconsistent.[74–78] Clinical studies have reported a positive association between retinopathy severity and the presence of HLA-B8, HLA-B15, or HLA-DR4 antigens in patients with type 1 diabetes. In a case-control study of Joslin Clinic patients with type 1 diabetes, the patients with DR 3/0, 4/0, and X/X were more likely to have PDR than were patients with 3/X, 4/X, or 3/4.[76] However, antigens of the BF locus, located on chromosome 6, have not been found by others to be related to PDR.[77]

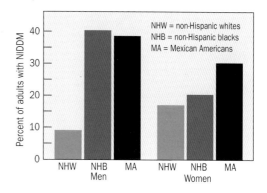

Figure 2-11 *Prevalence of diabetic retinopathy in patients with non–insulin-dependent diabetes mellitus (NIDDM) age ≥40 years, by sex and race/ethnic group. Data are from NHANES III, 1988–1991.*
Harris MI, Klein R, Cowie CC, et al: Is the risk of diabetic retinopathy greater in non-Hispanic blacks and Mexican Americans than in non-Hispanic whites with type 2 diabetes? A U.S. population study. Diabetes Care *1998;21: 1230–1235.*

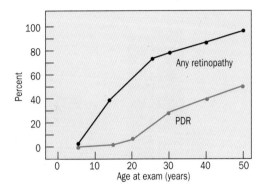

Figure 2-12 *Prevalence of any retinopathy and of PDR in insulin-taking patients diagnosed with diabetes at age <30 years, by age.*
Klein R: WESDR 1980–1982, unpublished data.

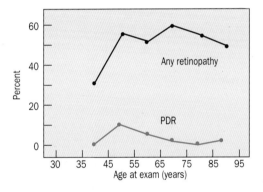

Figure 2-13 *Prevalence of any retinopathy and of PDR in patients diagnosed with diabetes at age ≥30 years, by age.*
Klein R: WESDR 1980–1982, unpublished data.

In a subset of the WESDR younger-onset group, after adjusting for factors associated with PDR, the presence of DR4 and the absence of DR3 were associated with a 5.4 times increase in the odds of having PDR compared with the absence of both DR4 and DR3.[78] No other genetic factors were statistically significantly associated with the presence of PDR. However, based on analyses of the 10-year followup data from this study, DR4 appeared to have a statistically significant protective effect for the incidence of PDR.[79] This might be explained, in part, by the higher mortality experienced by DR4+ individuals (7.6%) compared with DR4– individuals (4.7%). However, the protective effect was found even in patients with shorter durations of diabetes, where mortality was low, suggesting that selective mortality did not completely explain this relationship.

The reasons that specific HLA-DR antigens would change the risk of developing more severe retinopathy are not apparent. Study of specific genetic factors associated with the hypothesized pathogenetic factors for retinopathy, such as glycosylation, aldose reductase activity, collagen formation, and platelet adhesiveness and aggregation, may yield a better understanding of the possible causal relationships between genetic factors and diabetic retinopathy.

2-9-4 Age

The prevalence and severity of diabetic retinopathy increased with increasing age in younger-onset patients (Figure 2-12).[10] Prior to age 13 years, diabetic retinopathy was infrequent, irrespective of the duration of diabetes. In older-onset patients, preva-

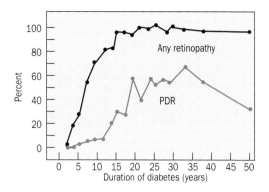

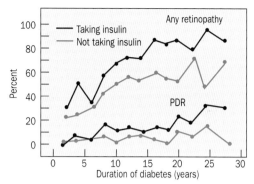

Figure 2-14 *Prevalence of any retinopathy and of PDR in insulin-taking patients diagnosed with diabetes at age <30 years, by duration of diabetes. Data are from WESDR 1980–1982.*

Klein R, Klein BEK, Moss SE: The epidemiology of ocular problems in diabetes mellitus. In: Ferman SS, ed: Ocular Problems in Diabetes Mellitus. *Boston: Blackwell; 1992:1–53.*

Figure 2-15 *Prevalence of any retinopathy and of PDR in patients diagnosed with diabetes at age ≥30 years, by duration of diabetes. Data are from WESDR 1980–1982.*

Klein R, Klein BEK, Moss SE: The epidemiology of ocular problems in diabetes mellitus. In: Ferman SS, ed: Ocular Problems in Diabetes Mellitus. *Boston: Blackwell; 1992:1–53.*

lence rates of retinopathy did not increase consistently with age (Figure 2-13).[11]

For younger-onset patients taking insulin, the 4-year incidence of retinopathy and progression of retinopathy increased with increasing age. In older-onset patients, for those taking insulin, the 4-year incidence of any retinopathy and progression of retinopathy had a tendency to decrease with increasing age. These findings are consistent with data from other population-based studies.[20,49,56,62,66]

2-9-5 Duration of Diabetes

For younger-onset patients, both the frequency and the severity of retinopathy increased with increasing duration of diabetes (Figure 2-14).[10,11] After diagnosis of diabetes, retinopathy was more frequent in the older-onset group compared with the younger-onset group (Figure 2-15). However, after 20 years or more of diabetes, fewer older-onset patients not taking insulin had any retinopathy (60% versus 99%) or PDR (5% versus 53%) than did younger-onset patients.

The 4-year incidence of diabetic retinopathy increased with increasing duration of diabetes at baseline (Tables 2-12 and 2-13).[40,68] The 4-year incidence of PDR increased from 0% during the first 3 years after diagnosis of diabetes to 27.9% in younger-onset patients with 13 to 14 years of diabetes. Thereafter, the incidence of PDR remained stable. In the older-onset groups, 2.0% of those with <5 years' duration who were not taking insulin at baseline developed signs of PDR at the 4-year followup (see Table 2-13).

TABLE 2-12

Four-Year Incidences of Any Retinopathy, Improvement or Progression of Retinopathy, and Progression to PDR in Younger-Onset Diabetic Patients, by Duration of Diabetes at Baseline Exam, WESDR 1980–1986

Duration (Years)	Any Retinopathy		Improvement		No. at Risk	No Change (%)	Progression (%)	Progression to PDR (%)
	No. at Risk	%	No. at Risk	%				
0–2	69	37.7	4		75	80.0	18.7	0
3–4	68	61.8	5		84	64.3	34.5	1.2
5–6	60	65.0	30	3.3	103	54.4	44.7	3.9
7–8	32	68.8	37	5.4	85	40.0	57.6	8.2
9–10	23	73.9	53	5.7	84	54.8	41.7	11.9
≥11	19	73.7						
11–12			43	0	54	44.4	55.6	22.2
13–14			38	7.9	43	30.2	62.8	27.9
15–19			68	2.9	79	55.7	41.8	16.5
20–24			39	15.4	42	57.1	28.6	14.3
25–29			32	9.4	34	61.8	29.4	14.7
≥30			27	14.8	30	56.7	30.0	16.7

Source: *Klein R, Klein BEK, Moss SE, et al: The Wisconsin Epidemiologic Study of Diabetic Retinopathy, IX: four-year incidence and progression of diabetic retinopathy when age at diagnosis is less than 30 years.* Arch Ophthalmol *1989; 107:237–243.*

2-9-6 Age at Diagnosis

In the WESDR, after controlling for duration of diabetes, age at diagnosis was not related to the 4-year incidence or progression of diabetic retinopathy in any of the diabetic groups studied.[40,68] In contrast, after controlling for other risk factors in a cohort with type 2 diabetes in Rochester, Minnesota, the development of retinopathy was significantly associated with younger age at diagnosis.[49]

2-9-7 Puberty

After controlling for other factors, such as diastolic blood pressure and duration of diabetes, younger-onset subjects who were postmenarchal in the WESDR were 3.2 times as likely to have diabetic retinopathy as those who were premenarchal.[80] Duration of diabetes after menarche conferred

TABLE 2-13

Four-Year Incidences of Any Retinopathy, Improvement or Progression of Retinopathy, and Progression to PDR in Older-Onset Diabetic Patients, by Duration of Diabetes at Baseline Exam, WESDR 1980–1986

Duration (Years)	Any Retinopathy		Improvement		No. at Risk	No Change (%)	Progression (%)	Progression to PDR (%)
	No. at Risk	%	No. at Risk	%				
Taking Insulin								
0–4	48	27.1	19	15.8	77	77.9	18.2	0
5–9	48	70.8	19	10.5	78	47.4	50.0	5.1
10–14	24	54.2	38	21.1	73	50.7	38.4	5.5
≥15	34	38.2	139	14.4	190	57.4	32.1	12.1
*P**	0.22		0.73			0.10	0.68	<0.001
Not Taking Insulin								
0–4	155	31.0	24	16.7	201	79.1	18.9	2.0
5–9	99	32.3	29	27.6	152	69.1	25.7	2.0
10–14	29	37.9	15	6.7	52	63.5	34.6	0
≥15	37	51.4	33	21.2	81	59.3	32.1	4.9
*P**	0.06		0.99			<0.001	<0.01	0.43

*Based on test for trend.

Source: *Klein R, Klein BEK, Moss SE, et al: The Wisconsin Epidemiologic Study of Diabetic Retinopathy, X: four-year incidence and progression of diabetic retinopathy when age at diagnosis is 30 years or more. Arch Ophthalmol 1989; 107:244–249.*

an increased risk of having any retinopathy compared with duration before menarche. The incidence of any retinopathy or of PDR over the following 4-year period was higher in those who were postmenarchal at baseline compared with those who were premenarchal. This has been reported by others.[81,82] Changes occurring at puberty, such as increases in insulin-like growth factor I, growth hormone, sex hormones, blood pressure, and poorer glycemic control (secondary to increased insulin resistance, poorer compliance, and inadequate insulin dosage), have been suggested as resulting in an increased risk.[83–89]

2-9-8 Hyperglycemia

A growing body of epidemiologic studies demonstrates a strong relationship between hyperglycemia and the development or progression of diabetic retinopathy.[10,11,40–44,52,53,56–59,61,62,64,65,90–92] In the WESDR, the glycosylated hemoglobin level at baseline was found to be a significant predictor of the 4- and 10-year incidence of retinopathy, progression, progression to PDR (Table 2-14), and incidence of macular edema in all three diabetic groups studied.[69,91,92] These relationships remained after controlling for duration of diabetes, severity of retinopathy, and other risk factors measured at baseline. In addition, a decrease in glycosylated hemoglobin between baseline and the 4-year followup examination was associated with a significant decrease in the progression of retinopathy and in the incidence of PDR in most of the WESDR diabetic groups.[92]

The WESDR data also suggest that, at any duration of diabetes prior to the development of severe NPDR or of PDR, there was no "point of no return" with regard to the glycosylated hemoglobin–retinopathy relationship. Rather, the relationship between level of glycemia and risk of retinopathy extended across the whole range of levels of glycemia, with no evidence of a threshold.

Most of the earlier clinical trials failed to demonstrate a beneficial effect of glycemic control in preventing the development or progression of diabetic retinopathy in patients with type 1 diabetes.[93–99] These trials were limited by their small size, relatively short followup times, and inclusion of patients with diabetes who had moderately severe NPDR at study entry. Initial worsening of retinopathy, manifest by the appearance of soft exudates and intraretinal microvascular abnormalities, was consistently found in the experimental tightly controlled groups in patients who had minimal or no retinopathy at baseline in these clinical trials.

A meta-analysis[100] of 16 published randomized clinical trials showed that the risk of retinopathy progression was insignificantly higher at 6 to 12 months of intensive glycemic control. However, after ≥2 years of intensive glycemic control, the risk was significantly lower. In addition, the incidence of severe hypoglycemia increased by 9.1 episodes per 100 person-years of followup in the intensively controlled patients. In the University Group Diabetes Program (UGDP), metabolic control was not related to the incidence or progression of retinopathy in patients with type 2 diabetes.[101]

The Diabetes Control and Complications Trial (DCCT), a large, randomized, controlled clinical trial of 1441 patients with type 1 diabetes, demonstrated that intensive glycemic control was associated with a reduced risk of incidence and progression of retinopathy, progression to NPDR and PDR, and incidence of macular edema, as well as a reduced need for panretinal photocoagulation compared with conventional insulin treatment (Tables 2-15 and 2-16).[102,103]

The United Kingdom Prospective Diabetes Study (UKPDS) was a randomized, controlled clinical trial involving 3867 newly diagnosed patients with type 2 diabetes.[104] After 3 months of diet treatment,

TABLE 2-14

Ten-Year Incidence and Progression of Retinopathy Rates for Diabetic Patients With NPDR at Baseline Exam, by Glycosylated Hemoglobin Quartile, WESDR 1980–1992

Glycosylated Hemoglobin Quartile	Any Retinopathy				Progression of Retinopathy				Progression to PDR		
	No. at Risk	%	RR	95% CI	No. at Risk	%	RR	95% CI	%	RR	95% CI
Younger-Onset											
1st	85	80.0	1.0		187	58.0	1.0		8.7	1.0	
2nd	53	95.3	1.5	1.2,1.9	153	73.6	1.5	1.2,1.9	22.7	2.6	1.5,4.6
3rd	54	92.2	1.5	1.2,1.9	174	85.6	2.1	1.7,2.5	41.3	5.5	3.5,8.8
4th	56	98.2	1.9	1.5,2.4	168	92.0	2.9	2.3,3.5	49.8	7.1	4.6,11.1
Older-Onset Taking Insulin											
1st	44	70.4	1.0		101	54.9	1.0		12.3	1.0	
2nd	43	80.6	1.1	0.7,1.7	92	59.3	1.1	0.8,1.6	18.5	1.2	0.5,2.9
3rd	25	79.6	1.1	0.7,1.8	99	72.7	1.4	1.0,1.9	24.2	2.0	1.0,4.3
4th	23	100.0	1.9	1.3,2.9	87	86.6	2.1	1.6,2.8	37.9	3.1	1.5,6.1
Older-Onset Not Taking Insulin											
1st	91	47.0	1.0		125	30.7	1.0		2.0	1.0	
2nd	71	57.2	1.4	0.9,2.2	114	45.7	1.8	1.2,2.7	2.4	1.2	0.2,8.3
3rd	69	83.9	2.5	1.7,3.5	110	66.8	2.8	1.9,4.2	9.6	4.0	1.0,16.6
4th	50	89.7	2.7	1.9,4.0	106	80.5	4.3	3.0,6.2	30.0	13.8	4.8,39.5

Note: *RR = relative risk. Values of glycosylated hemoglobin (%) for younger-onset group are 5.6–9.4, 9.5–10.5, 10.6–12.0, and 12.1–19.5; for older-onset group taking insulin, 5.9–8.8, 8.9–10.2, 10.3–11.5, and 11.6–17.0; and for the older-onset group not taking insulin, 5.4–7.6, 7.7–8.6, 8.7–10, and 10.1–20.8.*

Source: *Klein R, Klein BEK, Moss SE, Cruickshanks KJ: Relationship of hyperglycemia to the long-term incidence and progression of diabetic retinopathy.* Arch Intern Med *1994;154:2169–2178.*

TABLE 2-15

Risk Reduction in Incidence and Progression of Retinopathy, DCCT Primary Prevention Group

	Risk Reduction, Intensive vs Conventional Treatment Group	
	%	95% CI
≥1 microaneurysm	27	11–40
≥3-step progression	60	47–70
≥Sustained 3-step progression	76	62–85

Note: *Only 6 subjects developed PDR; 5 developed macular edema; 4 needed laser treatment.*

Source: *Diabetes Control and Complications Trial Research Group: The effect of intensive treatment of diabetes on the development and progression of long-term complications in insulin-dependent diabetes mellitus.* N Engl J Med *1993; 329:977–986.*

TABLE 2-16

Risk Reduction in Incidence and Progression of Retinopathy, DCCT Secondary Intervention Group

	Risk Reduction, Intensive vs Conventional Treatment Group	
	%	95% CI
≥3-step progression	34	18–46
≥Sustained 3-step progression	54	38–65
Incidence of NPDR or PDR	47	13–67
Incidence of macular edema	22	15–47
Laser treatment	54	23–74

Source: *Diabetes Control and Complications Trial Research Group: The effect of intensive treatment of diabetes on the development and progression of long-term complications in insulin-dependent diabetes mellitus.* N Engl J Med *1993; 329:977–986.*

patients with a mean of two fasting plasma glucose concentrations of 6.1 to 15.0 mmol/L were randomly assigned to an intensive glycemic control group with either a sulfonylurea (chlorpropamide, glibenclamide, or glipizide) or with insulin or a conventional glycemic control group with diet.

After 10 years of followup, hemoglobin A_{1c} was 7.0% in the intensive group and 7.9% in the conventional group. Compared with the conventional group, the risk reduction for progression of diabetic retinopathy—defined as two or more steps on the severity scale developed by the Early Treatment

Diabetic Retinopathy Study (ETDRS)—over a 12-year period in the intensive group was 21%. In addition, there was a 29% reduction in the need for retinal photocoagulation in the intensive group compared to the conventional group. These data conclusively showed that intensive treatment with either a sulfonylurea or insulin significantly reduced the risk of progression of retinopathy in patients with type 2 diabetes.

2-9-9 C-Peptide Status

The relationship of endogenous insulin secretion to diabetic retinopathy, independent of glycemic control, is not certain.[105–108] Some studies suggest a protective effect of remaining endogenous insulin secretion, whereas others do not. In the WESDR, the highest frequencies and most severe retinopathy were found in insulin-taking individuals with undetectable or low plasma C-peptide (<0.3 nM), whereas the lowest frequencies of retinopathy were found in older-onset, overweight individuals not taking insulin.[109] Older- and younger-onset individuals who were taking insulin and who had no detectable C-peptide had similar frequencies of PDR. After controlling for characteristics associated with retinopathy in older-onset patients with type 2 diabetes, there was no relationship between higher levels of C-peptide and lower frequency of less severe retinopathy. These findings suggest that the level of glycemia, not the level of endogenous C-peptide, is more important in determining the presence and severity of retinopathy in individuals with type 2 diabetes.

2-9-10 Exogenous Insulin

Exogenous insulin has been suggested as a possible cause of atherosclerosis and retinopathy in patients with type 2 diabetes.[110] In the WESDR, there was no association between the amount or type of exogenous insulin used and the presence and severity of retinopathy in the older-onset group taking insulin whose C-peptide was ≥0.3 nM.[109] These data suggest that exogenous insulin itself is probably not causally related to retinopathy in diabetic patients with normal C-peptide.

2-9-11 Blood Pressure

Anecdotal observations from clinical studies suggest a relationship between hypertension and the severity of diabetic retinopathy.[111] Increased blood pressure, through an effect on blood flow, has been hypothesized to damage the retinal capillary endothelial cells, resulting in development and progression of retinopathy.[112] Epidemiologic data from cross-sectional studies suggest a positive relationship between prevalence of retinopathy and hypertension, but data from cohort studies regarding the relationship between high blood pressure or hypertension and development and progression of retinopathy have not yielded consistent findings.[10,11,14,44,45,47–49,52,53,56,57,59–62,64,66,70] Some of the earlier studies were limited by small sample size, selection of patients, failure to control for possible confounders, selective dropout of patients, and insensitive measures of detecting retinopathy.

In the WESDR, diastolic blood pressure was a significant predictor of the 14-year progression of diabetic retinopathy and incidence of PDR in patients with younger-onset type 1 diabetes (Table 2-17).[70] After controlling for other risk factors, such as retinopathy severity, glycosylated hemoglobin, and duration of diabetes at baseline, the relationships between blood pressure and the incidence or progression of retinopathy remained. There was no relationship of either systolic or diastolic blood pressure to the incidence or progression of diabetic retinopathy in patients with older-onset diabetes in the WESDR.

The UKPDS also sought to determine whether tight control of blood pressure with either a beta blocker or an angiotensin-converting enzyme (ACE) inhibitor was beneficial in reducing macrovascular and microvascular complications associated with type 2 diabetes.[113] The study group randomized 1148 patients with hypertension

TABLE 2-17

Fourteen-Year Progression of Retinopathy for Younger-Onset Diabetic Patients With No Retinopathy or With NPDR at Baseline Exam, by Blood Pressure Quartile, WESDR 1980–1995

Blood Pressure Quartile	Range, mm Hg	No. at Risk	Progression of Retinopathy			Progression to PDR		
			%	RR	95% CI	%	RR	95% CI
Systolic								
1st	78–110	200	87.7	1.0		29.6	1.0	
2nd	111–120	215	85.6	1.0	0.9,1.2	31.4	1.1	0.8,1.6
3rd	121–134	192	85.4	1.0	0.9,1.2	42.8	1.6	1.1,2.2
4th	135–221	100	80.9	1.0	0.8,1.2	52.0	2.1	1.4,3.0
Test of trend			$P = 0.94$			$P < 0.001$		
Diastolic								
1st	42–71	207	82.4	1.0		25.7	1.0	
2nd	72–78	188	87.0	1.1	1.0,1.3	34.5	1.5	1.0,2.1
3rd	79–85	170	86.7	1.2	1.1,1.4	40.5	1.7	1.2,2.4
4th	86–117	140	87.0	1.2	1.0,1.4	52.8	2.6	1.8,3.6
Test of trend			$P < 0.05$			$P < 0.001$		

Note: *RR = relative risk.*
Source: *Klein R, Klein BEK, Moss SE, Cruickshanks KJ: The Wisconsin Epidemiologic Study of Diabetic Retinopathy, XVII: the 14-year incidence and progression of diabetic retinopathy and associated risk factors in type 1 diabetes.* Ophthalmology *1998;105:1801–1815.*

(mean blood pressure 160/94 mm Hg) to a regimen of tight control with either captopril or atenolol and another 390 patients to less tight control of their blood pressure. Tight blood pressure control resulted in a 35% reduction in retinal photocoagulation compared to conventional control.

After 7.5 years of followup, there was a 34% reduction in the rate of progression of retinopathy by two or more steps using the modified ETDRS severity scale and a 47% reduction in the deterioration of vi-sual acuity by three lines or more using the ETDRS charts (for example, going from 20/20 or 20/40 or worse on a Snellen chart). The effect was largely due to a reduction in the incidence of diabetic macular edema. Atenolol and captopril were equally effective in reducing the risk of developing these microvascular complications. The effects of blood pressure control were independent of those of glycemic control. These findings strongly support tight blood pressure control in patients with type 2 diabetes as a means of preventing visual loss due to the progression of diabetic retinopathy.

While beta blockers and ACE inhibitors were equally effective in reducing the risk of progression of retinopathy in newly diagnosed persons with type 2 diabetes in the UKPDS study, epidemiologic data from another, smaller clinical trial suggest that the type of antihypertensive drug chosen to control blood pressure may be important in persons with type 1 diabetes.[114] Recently, data from the EURODIAB Controlled Trial of Lisinopril in Insulin-Dependent Diabetes Mellitus (EUCLID) Study showed a 50% reduction in the progression of retinopathy, after adjustment for glycemic control in nonhypertensive or mildly hypertensive patients in the lisinopril treatment group compared to the placebo group.[115] Data from the WESDR and the Joslin Clinic suggest that the use of diuretics may be associated with poorer long-term survival, even while controlling for other risk factors.[39,116,117]

2-9-12 Proteinuria and Nephropathy

Rheologic, lipid, and platelet abnormalities associated with nephropathy may be involved in the pathogenesis of retinopathy. Data from most studies suggest an association between the prevalence of diabetic nephropathy, as manifest by microalbuminuria or gross proteinuria, and retinopathy.[10,11,47,52,57,58,60,62,118,119] In the WESDR, after controlling for other risk variables, the relationship was of borderline statistical significance ($P = 0.052$) in the younger-onset group with no retinopathy or early NPDR at baseline. Data from these studies suggest that patients with type 1 diabetes and microalbuminuria or gross proteinuria might benefit from having regular ophthalmologic evaluation.

2-9-13 Serum Lipids

Epidemiologic data suggest a relationship between serum lipids and the presence, development, or progression of diabetic retinopathy.[47,52,59,61,62,66,120] In the WESDR, higher total serum cholesterol was associated with higher prevalence of retinal hard exudates in both the younger- and the older-onset groups taking insulin.[120] In the ETDRS, higher levels of serum lipids—triglycerides, low-density lipoproteins (LDLs), and very-low-density lipoproteins (VLDLs)—were associated with increased risk of developing hard exudates in the macula; elevated triglycerides were associated with increased progression of retinopathy.[121]

2-9-14 Cigarette Smoking

Smoking is known to cause tissue hypoxia by increasing blood carbon monoxide levels,[122] and may lead to increased platelet aggregation and adhesiveness.[123,124] Both effects may explain, in part, the association of cigarette smoking with development of myocardial infarction and peripheral vascular disease, but most epidemiologic data show no relationship between cigarette smoking and diabetic retinopathy.[40,47,49,58,61,65,66,68,124,125] In the WESDR, cigarette smoking was not associated with the 4-year incidence or progression of diabetic retinopathy.[125] Despite the lack of an association, diabetic patients should be advised not to smoke because of an increased risk of cardiovascular and respiratory disease as well as cancer. In the

WESDR, after controlling for other risk factors, younger-onset patients who smoked were 2.4 times as likely to die as those who did not smoke, and older-onset patients were 1.6 times as likely.[39]

2-9-15 Alcohol

There are few epidemiologic studies on the relationship between alcohol consumption and diabetic retinopathy.[126–128] A possible protective effect of alcohol might be anticipated as a result of decreased platelet aggregation and adhesiveness,[129] but results have been conflicting.[126,127] In the WESDR, alcohol consumption was associated with a lower frequency of PDR in the younger-onset group.[128] However, there was no relationship between alcohol consumption at the 4-year examination and the incidence and progression of retinopathy in either the younger- or the older-onset groups at the 10-year followup.

2-9-16 Body Mass Index

There has been no consistency in the relationship between diabetic retinopathy and body mass index among various studies investigating this.[10,47,49,67,130,131] In the WESDR, body mass was inversely related to the presence or severity of diabetic retinopathy only in the older-onset patients not taking insulin. However, it was not predictive of the 4-year incidence or progression of retinopathy.

2-9-17 Physical Activity

Few epidemiologic data are available describing the relationship between diabetic retinopathy and physical activity.[131,132] An earlier study suggested no relationship between participation in team sports in high school and college and a history of laser treatment or blindness in patients with type 1 diabetes.[131] In the WESDR, in women diagnosed to have diabetes at age <14 years, those who participated in team sports were less likely to have PDR than those who did not. There was no association between physical activity or leisure-time energy expenditure and the presence and severity of diabetic retinopathy in men.[132]

2-9-18 Socioeconomic Status

Inconsistent relationships between socioeconomic status and retinopathy severity have been reported.[47,133,134] A significant correlation was found between PDR and occupational status (working class) or a lower income in a case-control study of 49 patients with type 1 diabetes.[133] However, there was no relationship between lower socioeconomic status, measured using a combination of the Duncan Socioeconomic Index, educational attainment, and income, and more severe retinopathy in 343 Mexican Americans and 79 non-Hispanic whites with type 2 diabetes in San Antonio, Texas.[134] Neither was a relationship observed between retinopathy severity and education level in a population of Oklahoma Indians with type 2 diabetes.[47]

In the WESDR, with the exception of a positive association of lower incidence of PDR with more education in younger-onset women age ≥25 years, socioeconomic status (education level and Duncan Socioeconomic Index score) was not associated with increased risk of developing PDR.[28] The reason for not finding a relationship of socioeconomic status with retinopathy severity in these studies may be because hyperglycemia, which may be causally related to retinopathy, was not related to socioeconomic status in the WESDR.

2-9-19 Pregnancy

Data from epidemiologic studies suggest that pregnancy is a significant predictor of progression of diabetic retinopathy.[135] In a case-control study of women with type 1 diabetes, the frequency of progression to PDR was higher in those who were pregnant compared with those who were not (7.3% versus 3.7%).[136] Women in this study were similar in age, duration of diabetes, and retinopathy status at baseline. Pregnancy remained a significant predictor of the progression of diabetic retinopathy after controlling for glycosylated hemoglobin and diastolic blood pressure. Severe retinopathy is also a risk indicator for higher risk of congenital abnormalities in children born of mothers with type 1 diabetes.[137]

2-10

RETINOPATHY, COMORBIDITY, AND MORTALITY

In the WESDR, the risk of heart attack, stroke, diabetic nephropathy, and amputation was higher in those with PDR compared with those with no retinopathy or minimal NPDR at baseline.[138] This finding is consistent with the association of severe retinopathy with cardiovascular disease risk factors, such as increased fibrinogen, increased platelet aggregation, hyperglycemia, and hypertension.

The ETDRS demonstrated that aspirin, when ingested for the prevention of myocardial infarction or stroke, does not increase the risk of vitreous hemorrhage or loss of vision in patients with PDR.[139] In both the ETDRS and the WESDR,[139,140] aspirin was not found to prevent the progression of retinopathy.

In the WESDR, increasing severity of retinopathy at baseline was associated with decreased survival over a 6-year period in both younger- and older-onset groups (Figures 2-16 and 2-17).[39] This finding had been reported by others[38] and is consistent with the association of severe retinopathy with the incidence of cardiovascular disease and diabetic nephropathy described above.

2-11

CATARACT

Cataract was one of the most common causes of decreased visual acuity in older-onset subjects in the WESDR.[7] It was responsible for more decrease in vision than was diabetic retinopathy in older-onset patients. Cataract is more common in diabetic subjects, but increases with increasing age in all persons (Figure 2-18 and Table 2-18).[7,141]

Lens opacities of any sort are often referred to as cataract, despite the fact that different anatomic locations in the lens may be involved. Cortical opacities were significantly more common among patients with older-onset diabetes compared with the rest of the Beaver Dam population, even after

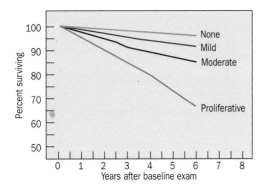

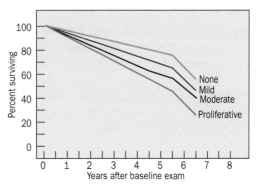

Figure 2-16 *Survival in patients diagnosed with diabetes at age <30 years, by retinopathy status at baseline exam. Survival is age- and sex-adjusted. Data are from WESDR 1980–1986.*

Klein R, Moss SE, Klein BEK, DeMets DL: Relation of ocular and systemic factors to survival in diabetes. Arch Intern Med *1989;149:266–272.*

Figure 2-17 *Survival in patients diagnosed with diabetes at age ≥30 years, by retinopathy status at baseline exam. Survival is age- and sex-adjusted. Data are from WESDR 1980–1986.*

Klein R, Moss SE, Klein BEK, DeMets DL: Relation of ocular and systemic factors to survival in diabetes. Arch Intern Med *1989;149:266–272.*

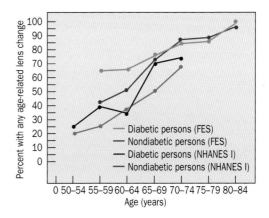

Figure 2-18 *Prevalence of age-related lens changes in diabetic and nondiabetic persons, according to age.*

Ederer F, Hiller R, Taylor HR: Senile lens changes and diabetes in two population studies. Am J Ophthalmol *1981;91:381–395.*

adjusting for age and sex.[142] Posterior subcapsular cataract was also more common in patients with diabetes, but the increase was not significant in all age groups.

With regard to risk factors for cataract in patients with diabetes in the WESDR, multivariate analyses indicated that age and duration of diabetes were the most important risk factors,[143] with the severity of diabetic retinopathy associated with a small but significant further increase in risk. In younger-onset patients, diuretic use and glycosylated hemoglobin were also associated with increased risk. In older-onset patients, diuretic use, intraocular pressure, smoking status (current and former), and diastolic blood pressure were associated with increased risk of cataract.

In prevalence data from the WESDR, 3.6% of younger-onset patients and 8.7% of older-onset patients had cataract extraction (Tables 2-19 and 2-20).[143] Prevalence and incidence increased with current age.[144] Past cataract surgery frequencies were also higher in diabetic patients in each age group in the Beaver Dam Eye Study.[142]

Multivariate analyses of risk factors for incidence of cataract surgery were performed on data from the WESDR.[144] For younger-onset patients, older age, past history of laser therapy, presence of proteinuria, higher glycosylated hemoglobin, and daily aspirin ingestion were associated with increased risk of cataract surgery. For older-onset patients, aside from older age, only use of insulin was associated with increased risk of cataract surgery.

In summary, there is evidence of increased risk of cataract or lens opacities and of cataract surgery in patients with diabetes. Although some data suggest a relationship

TABLE 2-18

Prevalence of Cataract* for Diabetic Patients, by Sex and Age, WESDR 1980–1982

Age (Years)	Females %	Females No.	Males %	Males No.
Younger-Onset				
0–19	4.8	6/126	2.1	3/140
20–29	15.2	22/145	13.4	20/149
30–44	39.4	54/137	29.4	42/143
≥45	87.1	61/70	92.4	61/66
Total	29.9	143/478	25.3	126/498
Older-Onset				
30–54	60.8	62/102	56.7	59/104
55–64	86.9	159/183	76.3	132/173
65–74	94.7	233/246	94.0	202/215
≥75	98.5	192/195	97.8	133/136
Total	89.0	646/726	83.8	526/628

*Includes surgical aphakia.

Source: *Klein BEK, Klein R, Moss SE: Prevalence of cataracts in a population-based study of persons with diabetes mellitus.* Ophthalmology *1985;92:1191–1196.*

TABLE 2-19

Prevalence of Surgical Aphakia in Either Eye of Diabetic Patients, by Age and Sex, WESDR 1980–1982

Sex	Age (Years) 0–19		20–29		30–34		≥45		Total	
	%	No.	%	No.	%	No.	%	No.	%	No.
Younger-Onset										
Females	1.6	2/126	0.7	1/149	5.0	7/139	17.1	12/70	4.5	22/484
Males	0	0/146	1.3	2/152	3.4	5/146	10.4	7/67	2.7	14/511
Total	0.7	2/272	1.0	3/301	4.2	12/285	13.9	19/137	3.6	36/995

	30–54		55–64		65–74		≥75		Total	
	%	No.	%	No.	%	No.	%	No.	%	No.
Older-Onset										
Females	1.9	2/106	6.0	11/184	10.4	26/249	14.7	29/197	9.2	68/736
Males	3.8	4/104	4.0	7/174	11.0	24/219	11.7	16/137	8.0	51/634
Total	2.9	6/210	5.0	18/358	10.7	50/468	13.5	45/334	8.7	119/1370

Source: *Klein BEK, Klein R, Moss SE: Prevalence of cataracts in a population-based study of persons with diabetes mellitus.* Ophthalmology *1985;92:1191–1196.*

TABLE 2-20

Ten-Year Incidence of Cataract Surgery in Diabetic Patients, by Age, WESDR 1980–1992

Age (Years)	No.	Incidence (%)	Age (Years)	No.	Incidence (%)
Younger-Onset			*Older-Onset*		
18–24	218	3.7	30–54	184	14.7
25–34	262	6.1	55–64	283	21.0
35–44	113	9.7	65–74	309	31.7
≥45	92	27.6	≥75	149	44.3

Note: *Test for trend with age. P <0.0005.*
Source: *Klein BEK, Klein R, Moss SE: Incidence of cataract surgery in the Wisconsin Epidemiologic Study of Diabetic Retinopathy.* Am J Ophthalmol *1995;119:295–300.*

between level of glucose control and risk of cataract surgery, it is unlikely that, even if tighter glycemic control were feasible, risk would be reduced to the usual age-related rates. Thus, it is necessary for health care planners to be mindful of the costs and services associated with increased rates of cataract surgery and postsurgical rehabilitation (for example, postoperative recovery time and new spectacles) in patients with diabetes.

2-12

GLAUCOMA

Data from the NHANES II and the 1989 NHIS indicate that diabetic patients age ≥35 years reported substantially higher rates of glaucoma than did the nondiabetic US population; rates increased with age in both groups. In the Beaver Dam Eye Study, diabetes was associated with a modest increase in risk of definite and probable glaucoma that was statistically significant only for definite glaucoma, controlling for age and sex (Table 2-21, on next page).[115]

In the WESDR, self-reported incidence of glaucoma was evaluated in both younger- and older-onset diabetes. The 10-year incidence of glaucoma varied with age and duration of diabetes (Figures 2-19 and 2-20). In older- as well as younger-onset patients, rates increased with age, although only in the latter group was the relationship significant. The decrease noted at the oldest age in older-onset patients may be the result of mortality in these patients.[146]

In summary, these data suggest an increased risk of open-angle glaucoma associated with diabetes. In addition, among pa-

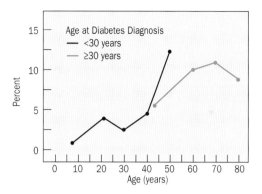

Figure 2-19 *Ten-year incidence of history of glaucoma in patients with diabetes diagnosed at age <30 or ≥30 years, by age. Test for trend: P <0.005, age <30 years; P = 0.88, age ≥30 years.*

Klein BEK, Klein R, Moss SE: Incidence of self-reported glaucoma in people with diabetes mellitus. Br J Ophthalmol *1997; 81:743–747.*

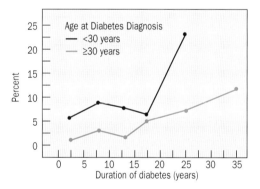

Figure 2-20 *Ten-year incidence of history of glaucoma in patients with diabetes diagnosed at age <30 or ≥30 years, by duration of diabetes. Test for trend: P <0.001, age <30 years; P <0.005, age ≥30 years.*

Klein BEK, Klein R, Moss SE: Incidence of self-reported glaucoma in people with diabetes mellitus. Br J Ophthalmol *1997; 81:743–747.*

TABLE 2-21

Frequency of Glaucoma in Older-Onset Diabetic Patients and Nondiabetic Persons, by Sex and Age, Beaver Dam Eye Study 1988–1990

Sex and Age	No. at Risk	Definite Glaucoma %	P	Probable Glaucoma %	P	Combined %	P
Both Sexes							
With diabetes	426	4.2		3.5		7.8	
Without diabetes	4420	2.0	0.004	1.9	0.031	3.9	0.0005
Women							
With diabetes	240	5.0		4.2		9.2	
Without diabetes	2480	2.0	0.009	2.5	0.133	4.4	0.002
Men							
With diabetes	186	3.2		2.7		5.9	
Without diabetes	1940	1.9	0.266	1.2	0.091	3.1	0.052
Both Sexes							
43–54 years							
With diabetes	57	1.8		0.0		1.8	
Without diabetes	1443	1.0	0.44	0.2	1.00	1.2	0.504
55–64 years							
With diabetes	124	0.8		2.4		3.2	
Without diabetes	1171	1.4	1.00	1.3	0.244	2.7	0.768
65–74 years							
With diabetes	149	6.0		4.7		10.7	
Without diabetes	1108	2.3	0.014	2.4	0.110	4.7	0.005
≥75 years							
With diabetes	96	7.3		5.2		12.5	
Without diabetes	698	4.4	0.207	5.6	1.00	10.0	0.474

Multiple Logistic Analyses of Glaucoma and Diabetes	OR	95% CI	P	OR	95% CI	P	OR	95% CI	P
Diabetes	1.84	1.09,3.11	0.02	1.47	0.83,2.59	0.184	1.68	1.14,2.50	0.01

Note: *Univariate significance tested by chi-square test. Multivariate analysis controlled for age and sex. OR = odds ratio.*

Source: *Klein BEK, Klein R, Jensen SC: Open-angle glaucoma and older-onset diabetes: the Beaver Dam Eye Study.* Ophthalmology *1994;101:1173–1177.*

tients with older-onset diabetes, increasing duration is associated with increased risk. Although some of this excess may be related to greater surveillance of patients with diabetes, it is unlikely to be the entire explanation.

HEALTH CARE DELIVERY

In the 1973 NHIS, participants age >40 years were asked, "How long has it been since you had a test for glaucoma?" No distinction was made between care by an ophthalmologist and care by an optometrist. Diabetic patients were more likely to have had a glaucoma test than were nondiabetic persons. More than 32% of diabetic patients stated that they had never had an eye pressure test.

In the 1989 NHIS, participants age ≥18 years were asked if they had had a dilated eye examination in the past year. Only 49% (57% of patients with type 1 diabetes, 55% of insulin-treated patients with type 2 diabetes, and 44% of patients with type 2 diabetes not treated with insulin) reported a dilated eye examination within 1 year of the interview (Table 2-22).[5] Patients with type 2 diabetes were more likely to have had a dilated eye examination if they were older, had a higher socioeconomic status, and had attended a diabetes education class. Receiving a dilated eye examination was not related to race, duration of diabetes, frequency of physician visits for diabetes, or health insurance.

In the 1989 NHIS, 69% of patients with type 1 diabetes and 61% of patients with type 2 diabetes reported that they had had an eye examination within 1 year of the survey. Of all adults with diabetes, 45% reported that they had seen an ophthalmologist in the past 12 months.

In the WESDR, participants were queried as to whether they had been seen by an ophthalmologist and, if so, when they were last seen.[147] Those who were never seen by an ophthalmologist were asked if they had received optometric care. About 63% of younger-onset and 50% of older-onset diabetic patients had seen an ophthalmologist within the past 2 years; 25% of younger- and 36% of older-onset patients had never had an ophthalmologic examination. Approximately 90% of younger-onset and 93% of older-onset patients with DRS high-risk characteristics for visual loss had been examined in the 2 years prior to the survey.

Because PDR is usually initially asymptomatic and may require treatment to prevent severe visual loss, it must be diagnosed correctly. Internists, diabetologists, and senior medical residents were found to correctly diagnose the presence of PDR in 49% of cases they examined, whereas ophthalmologists and retinal specialists correctly diagnosed its presence in 96% of cases.[148] Using direct and indirect ophthalmoscopy, well-trained nonophthalmologists and ophthalmologists specializing in retinal diseases were found to have a high rate of detecting PDR.[149]

TABLE 2-22

Frequency of Ophthalmic Care in Diabetic Patients, US 1989

Frequency of Test	Age (Years)	All Patients With Diabetes		Type 1 Diabetes		Type 2 Diabetes	
		No.	%	No.	%	No.	%
Ever had photos taken of retina	≥18	2121	27.53	115	40.07	1996	26.68
	18–44	317	25.75	93	34.96	220	21.43
	45–64	881	25.68	19	61.59	858	24.73
	≥65	923	29.90	3		918	29.74
Ever had laser treatment	≥18	2296	6.57	122	19.22	2164	5.67
	18–44	348	8.08	100	18.50	244	3.00
	45–64	946	6.75	19	20.80	923	6.25
	≥65	1002	5.88	3		997	5.80
Saw ophthalmologist in past 12 months	≥18	2386	44.72	123	54.35	2253	44.14
	18–44	352	40.94	101	55.08	247	34.71
	45–64	973	41.83	19	58.04	950	41.44
	≥65	1061	48.63	3		1056	48.76
Dilated Eye Exam							
≤12 months	≥18	2282	48.51	120	56.93	2153	47.96
	18–44	346	45.06	98	57.38	244	39.52
	45–64	935	45.81	19	62.63	913	45.38
	≥65	1001	52.23	3		996	52.38
13–24 months	≥18	2282	17.41	120	22.51	2153	17.17
	18–44	346	16.87	98	23.87	244	14.05
	45–64	935	20.59	19	13.73	913	20.82
	≥65	1001	14.68	3		996	14.66
≥24 months	≥18	2282	20.91	120	13.26	2153	21.30
	18–44	346	20.84	98	14.61	244	24.26
	45–64	935	18.42	19	14.13	913	18.45
	≥65	1001	23.21	3		996	23.13

TABLE 2-22 *(cont.)*

Frequency of Ophthalmic Care in Diabetic Patients, US 1989

Frequency of Test	Age (Years)	All Patients With Diabetes		Type 1 Diabetes		Type 2 Diabetes	
		No.	%	No.	%	No.	%
Any Eye Exam							
≤12 months	≥18	2399	61.39	124	68.93	2265	60.97
	18–44	355	57.29	102	68.44	249	52.34
	45–64	977	60.73	19	81.68	954	60.33
	≥65	1067	63.39	3		1062	63.59
13–24 months	≥18	2388	17.96	123	21.03	2255	17.84
	18–44	353	20.06	101	21.08	248	19.77
	45–64	974	19.40	19	13.97	951	19.59
	≥65	1067	15.94	3		1062	15.84
≥24 months	≥18	2388	20.38	123	9.48	2255	20.93
	18–44	353	22.35	101	9.81	248	27.70
	45–64	974	19.69	19	4.35	951	19.90
	≥65	1061	20.32	3		1062	20.22

Source: *Brechner RJ, Cowie CC, Howie LJ, et al: Ophthalmic examination among adults with diagnosed diabetes mellitus.* J Am Med Assoc *1993;270:1714–1718.*

The accuracy of detection of retinopathy by (1) well-trained diabetologists and endocrinology fellows using ophthalmoscopy through an undilated pupil, (2) ophthalmologists using ophthalmoscopy through a dilated pupil, and (3) grading of nonmydriatic photographs was compared with detection of retinopathy by grading of seven field stereoscopic fundus photographs.[150] Nonophthalmologists missed all cases of macular edema and most cases of PDR; however, they did detect other lesions that accompany severe retinopathy. Detection by nonmydriatic photography was similar to that by direct ophthalmoscopy.

In both this study and another,[151] the most sensitive method for detection of retinopathy was fundus photography. For this reason, it was suggested that, if any signs of retinopathy were detected or if visual acuity was worse than 20/30, referral to an ophthalmologist should be required.[150] Data from a number of studies suggest that, in the absence of trained ophthalmoscopists or ophthalmologists, nonmydriatic cameras may provide an alternative screening approach for detection of retinopathy in patients with diabetes.[149,152] Current guidelines for detection of diabetic retinopathy are presented in Table 2-23.

TABLE 2-23

*Recommendations for Eye Care
for Diabetic Patients*

Primary-care physician informs patient at time of diagnosis of diabetes that:

- Ocular complications are associated with diabetes and may threaten sight

- Timely detection and treatment may reduce risk of decreased vision

Referral to eye doctor competent in ophthalmoscopy:

- Patients age 10–30 years with diabetes duration ≥5 years: annual referral

- Patients diagnosed at age ≥30 years: referral at time of diagnosis or shortly thereafter

Referral to ophthalmologist:

- All women with IDDM planning pregnancy within 12 months, in first trimester, and thereafter at discretion of ophthalmologist

- Patients found to have reduced corrected visual acuity, elevated intraocular pressure, or any other vision-threatening ocular abnormalities

Sources: *Klein R, Klein BEK, Moss S: The Wisconsin Epidemiologic Study of Diabetic Retinopathy: a review.* Diabetes Metab Rev *1989;5:559–570.*

Eye Care for People with Diabetes Mellitus. *Information Statement. San Francisco: American Academy of Ophthalmology; 1999.*

Prevalence rates of reported photocoagulation in the WESDR are presented in Tables 2-24 and 2-25.[153,154] In younger-onset patients, the rates of photocoagulation treatment increased with increasing current age and were higher in males than in females. In older-onset patients, the reported rate for the group was 3.8%.

2-14

CONCLUSION

The successful implementation of guidelines for achieving tight glycemic control and screening for diabetic retinopathy will result in a reduction in visual loss in patients with diabetes. However, implementation of these guidelines has been difficult. Achieving the recommended levels of glycemic control, as recommended by the DCCT, is associated with severe hypoglycemia.[103]

Other medical approaches to preventing or reducing the progression of retinopathy, such as control of hypertension and dyslipidemia, and development of new medical interventions may be of benefit in reducing the incidence of microvascular and macrovascular complications. Currently, clinical trials are under way to study the efficacy of control of hypertension and dyslipidemia.

In addition, randomized clinical trials are under way to study the efficacy of ACE inhibitors and of new drugs such as protein kinase C inhibitors and antivascular endothelial growth factors, which may play a role in the pathogenesis of diabetic retinopathy. Clinical trials have also been suggested to examine the benefits of vitamin E to prevent the incidence of retinopathy. If genetic susceptibility factors are found that explain variations in incidence and progres-

TABLE 2-24

History of Photocoagulation Treatment in Insulin-Taking, Younger-Onset Diabetic Patients, by Sex, WESDR 1980–1982

Age (Years)	Males			Females		
	Number	No	Yes	Number	No	Yes
<15	61	100.0	0	52	100.0	0
15–44	384	83.3	16.7	362	87.6	12.2
≥45	66	68.2	31.8	70	78.6	21.4
Total	511	83.4	16.6	484	87.6	12.2

Note: *History of photocoagulation was uncertain in 0.2% of females.*
Source: *Klein R: WESDR 1980–1982, unpublished data.*

sion of retinopathy, then new treatments targeted to specific mechanisms and administered at a specific stage in the natural history of the retinopathy may provide a complementary approach to glycemic control in preventing the progression of retinopathy.

Implementing educational programs for both physicians and patients, such as those developed by the National Eye Health and Education Program, overcoming economic barriers to care, and developing cost-effective approaches using newer computer-assisted approaches for detecting retinopathy in patients at risk for developing retinopathy will likely result in a decline in diabetic retinopathy as an important cause of loss of visual acuity.

Epidemiologic data show that the presence of more severe retinopathy or visual impairment in diabetic patients is an important indicator for increased risk of death from ischemic heart disease.[155] Because vascular disease is involved in most deaths of people with diabetes, a public health benefit should accrue from identifying such individuals and monitoring them for heart disease.

TABLE 2-25

History of Photocoagulation Treatment in Older-Onset Diabetic Patients, WESDR 1980–1982

Age (Years)	Number	No	Yes
30–44	49	98.1	1.9
45–64	519	94.4	5.1
65–84	738	96.6	2.8
≥85	64	91.8	5.8
Total	1370	95.6	3.8

Note: *History of photocoagulation treatment was uncertain in 0.6% of patients.*
Source: *Klein R: WESDR 1980–1982, unpublished data.*

ACKNOWLEDGMENT

This research was supported by National Institutes of Health grants EYO3083 and EYO6594 (R. Klein, B. E. K. Klein) and, in part, by Research to Prevent Blindness, New York, NY (R. Klein, Senior Scientific Investigator Award).

REFERENCES

1. *Vision Problems in the U.S.: A Statistical Analysis.* New York: National Society to Prevent Blindness; 1980.

2. Kahn HA, Moorhead HB: *Statistics on Blindness in the Model Reporting Area, 1969–70.* National Eye Institute. National Institutes of Health Publ. No. 73–427. Washington, DC: US Govt Printing Office; 1973.

3. US Department of Health, Education and Welfare (US DHEW): *Model Reporting Area—Proceedings of the 2nd Annual Conference of the Model Reporting Area for Blindness Statistics.* Public Health Service Publ. No. 1135. Washington, DC: US Govt Printing Office; 1963.

4. Kahn HA, Hiller R: Blindness caused by diabetic retinopathy. *Am J Ophthalmol* 1974;78:58–67.

5. Brechner RJ, Cowie CC, Howie LJ, et al: Ophthalmic examination among adults with diagnosed diabetes mellitus. *J Am Med Assoc* 1993;270:1714–1718.

6. Hiller R, Krueger DE: Validity of a survey question as a measure of visual acuity impairment. *Am J Public Health* 1983;73:93–96.

7. Klein R, Klein BEK, Moss SE: Visual impairment in diabetes. *Ophthalmology* 1984;91:1–9.

8. Ferris FL III, Kassoff A, Bresnick GH, Bailey I: New visual acuity charts for clinical research. *Am J Ophthalmol* 1982;94:91–96.

9. Klein R, Klein BEK, Moss SE, et al: Prevalence of diabetes mellitus in southern Wisconsin. *Am J Epidemiol* 1984;119:54–61.

10. Klein R, Klein BEK, Moss SE, et al: The Wisconsin Epidemiologic Study of Diabetic Retinopathy, II: prevalence and risk of diabetic retinopathy when age at diagnosis is less than 30 years. *Arch Ophthalmol* 1984;102:520–526.

11. Klein R, Klein BEK, Moss SE, et al: The Wisconsin Epidemiologic Study of Diabetic Retinopathy, III: prevalence and risk of diabetic retinopathy when age at diagnosis is 30 or more years. *Arch Ophthalmol* 1984;102:527–532.

12. Roberts J: *Monocular Visual Acuity of Persons 4 to 74 Years, United States, 1971–72.* Vital and Health Statistics Series 11, No. 201. Rockville, MD: National Center for Health Statistics; 1977.

13. Leibowitz HM, Krueger DE, Maunder LR, et al: The Framingham Eye Study monograph: an ophthalmological and epidemiological study of cataract, glaucoma, diabetic retinopathy, macular degeneration, and visual acuity in a general population of 2,631 adults, 1973–1975. *Surv Ophthalmol* 1980;24(suppl):335–610.

14. Houston A: Retinopathy in the Poole area: an epidemiological inquiry. In: Eschwege E, ed: *Advances in Diabetes Epidemiology.* Amsterdam: Elsevier; 1982:199–206.

15. Cohen DL, Neil HA, Thorogood M, Mann JI: A population-based study of the incidence of complications associated with type 2 diabetes in the elderly. *Diabet Med* 1991;8:928–933.

16. Sjollie AK, Greene A: Blindness in insulin-treated diabetic patients with age at onset <30 years. *J Chron Dis* 1987;40:215–220.

17. Caird FI, Pirie A, Ramsell TG: *Diabetes and the Eye.* Oxford and Edinburgh: Blackwell Scientific; 1969.

18. Moss SE, Klein R, Klein BEK: The incidence of vision loss in a diabetic population. *Ophthalmology* 1988;95:1340–1348.

19. Dwyer MS, Melton LJ III, Ballard DJ, et al: Incidence of diabetic retinopathy and blindness: a population-based study in Rochester, Minnesota. *Diabetes Care* 1985;8:316–322.

20. Grey RH, Burns-Cox CJ, Hughes A: Blind and partial sight registration in Avon. *Br J Ophthalmol* 1989;73:88–94.

21. Thompson JR, Du L, Rosenthal AR: Recent trends in the registration of blindness and partial sight in Leicestershire. *Br J Ophthalmol* 1989;73: 95–99.

22. Sorsby A: *The Incidence and Causes of Blindness in England and Wales 1963–1968.* Reports on Public Health and Medical Subjects. No. 128. London: HMSO; 1972.

23. Klein R, Klein BEK, Moss SE, Cruickshanks KJ: The Wisconsin Epidemiologic Study of Diabetic Retinopathy, XIV: ten-year incidence and progression of diabetic retinopathy. *Arch Ophthalmol* 1994;112:1217–1228.

24. Moss SE, Klein R, Klein BEK: Ten-year incidence of visual loss in a diabetic population. *Ophthalmology* 1994;101:1061–1070.

25. Moss SE, Klein R, Klein BEK: The 14-year incidence of visual loss in a diabetic population. *Ophthalmology* 1998;105:998–1003.

26. Sommer A, Tielsch JM, Katz J, et al: Racial differences in the cause-specific prevalence of blindness in east Baltimore. *N Engl J Med* 1991; 325:1412–1417.

27. Deckert T, Simonsen SE, Poulsen JE: Prognosis of proliferative retinopathy in juvenile diabetics. *Diabetes* 1967;16:728–733.

28. Klein R, Klein BEK, Jensen SC, Moss SE: The relation of socioeconomic factors to the incidence of proliferative diabetic retinopathy and loss of vision. *Ophthalmology* 1994;101:68–76.

29. Robinson N: Disability and diabetes. *Int Disabil Stud* 1990;12:28–31.

30. Kuh D, Lawrence C, Tripp J, Creber G: Work and work alternative for disabled young people. *Disabil, Handicap Soc* 1988;3:3–26.

31. Wulsin LR, Jacobson AM, Rand LI: Psychosocial correlates of mild visual loss. *Psychosom Med* 1991;53:109–117.

32. Wulsin LR, Jacobson AM, Rand LI: Psychosocial adjustment to advanced proliferative diabetic retinopathy. *Diabetes Care* 1993;16: 1061–1066.

33. Bernbaum M, Albert SG, Duckro PN: Psychosocial profiles in patients with visual impairment due to diabetic retinopathy. *Diabetes Care* 1988;11:551–557.

34. Chiang YP, Bassi LJ, Javitt JC: Federal budgetary costs of blindness. *Milbank Q* 1992; 70:319–340.

35. Dasbach EJ, Fryback DG, Newcomb PA, et al: Cost-effectiveness of strategies for detecting diabetic retinopathy. *Med Care* 1991;29:20–39.

36. Javitt JC, Canner JK, Frank RG, et al: Detecting and treating retinopathy in patients with type I diabetes mellitus: a health policy model. *Ophthalmology* 1990;97:483–494; discussion 494–495.

37. Javitt JC, Aiello LP, Bassi LJ, et al: Detecting and treating retinopathy in patients with type I diabetes mellitus: savings associated with improved implementation of current guidelines. American Academy of Ophthalmology. *Ophthalmology* 1991;98:1565–1573; discussion 1574.

38. Davis MD, Hiller R, Magli YL, et al: Prognosis for life in patients with diabetes: relation to severity of retinopathy. *Trans Am Ophthalmol Soc* 1979;77:144–170.

39. Klein R, Moss SE, Klein BEK, DeMets DL: Relation of ocular and systemic factors to survival in diabetes. *Arch Intern Med* 1989;149: 266–272.

40. Klein R, Klein BEK, Moss SE, et al: The Wisconsin Epidemiologic Study of Diabetic Retinopathy, IX: four-year incidence and progression of diabetic retinopathy when age at diagnosis is less than 30 years. *Arch Ophthalmol* 1989;107:237–243.

41. Klein BEK, Davis MD, Segal P, et al: Diabetic retinopathy: assessment of severity and progression. *Ophthalmology* 1984;91:10–17.

42. Early Treatment Diabetic Retinopathy Study Research Group: Grading diabetic retinopathy from stereoscopic color fundus photographs: an extension of the modified Airlie House classification. ETDRS Report Number 10. *Ophthalmology* 1991;98:786–806.

43. Klein R, Klein BEK, Moss SE, et al: The Wisconsin Epidemiologic Study of Diabetic Retinopathy, IV: diabetic macular edema. *Ophthalmology* 1984;91:1464–1474.

44. Dorf A, Ballintine EJ, Bennett PH, Miller M: Retinopathy in Pima Indians: relationships to glucose level, duration of diabetes, age at diagnosis of diabetes, and age at examination in a population with a high prevalence of diabetes mellitus. *Diabetes* 1976;25:554–560.

45. Bennett PH, Rushforth NB, Miller M, LeCompte PM: Epidemiologic studies of diabetes in the Pima Indians. *Recent Prog Horm Res* 1976;32:333–376.

46. Kahn HA, Leibowitz HM, Ganley JP, et al: The Framingham Eye Study, I: outline and major prevalence findings. *Am J Epidemiol* 1977; 106:17–32.

47. West KM, Erdreich LJ, Stober JA: A detailed study of risk factors for retinopathy and nephropathy in diabetes. *Diabetes* 1980;29:501–508.

48. King H, Balkau B, Zimmet P, et al: Diabetic retinopathy in Nauruans. *Am J Epidemiol* 1983; 117:659–667.

49. Ballard DJ, Melton LJ III, Dwyer MS, et al: Risk factors for diabetic retinopathy: a population-based study in Rochester, Minnesota. *Diabetes Care* 1986;9:334–342.

50. Danielsen R, Jonasson F, Helgason T: Prevalence of retinopathy and proteinuria in type I diabetics in Iceland. *Acta Med Scand* 1982;212: 277–280.

51. Constable IJ, Knuiman MW, Welborn TA, et al: Assessing the risk of diabetic retinopathy. *Am J Ophthalmol* 1984;97:53–61.

52. Knuiman MW, Welborn TA, McCann VJ, et al: Prevalence of diabetic complications in relation to risk factors. *Diabetes* 1986;35:1332–1339.

53. Sjolie AK: Ocular complications in insulin treated diabetes mellitus: an epidemiological study. *Acta Ophthalmol* 1985;172(suppl):1–77.

54. Nielsen NV: Diabetic retinopathy, II: the course of retinopathy in diabetics treated with oral hypoglycaemic agents and diet regimen alone. A one year epidemiological cohort study of diabetes mellitus. The Island of Falster, Denmark. *Acta Ophthalmol* 1984;62:266–273.

55. Nielsen NV: Diabetic retinopathy, I: the course of retinopathy in insulin-treated diabetics. A one year epidemiological cohort study of diabetes mellitus. The Island of Falster, Denmark. *Acta Ophthalmol* 1984;62:256–265.

56. Teuscher A, Schnell H, Wilson PW: Incidence of diabetic retinopathy and relationship to baseline plasma glucose and blood pressure. *Diabetes Care* 1988;11:246–251.

57. Haffner SM, Fong D, Stern MP, et al: Diabetic retinopathy in Mexican Americans and non-Hispanic whites. *Diabetes* 1988;37:878–884.

58. Jerneld B: Prevalence of diabetic retinopathy: a population study from the Swedish island of Gotland. *Acta Ophthalmol* 1988;188(suppl): 3–32.

59. Hamman RF, Mayer EJ, Moo-Young GA, et al: Prevalence and risk factors of diabetic retinopathy in non-Hispanic whites and Hispanics with NIDDM. San Luis Valley Diabetes Study. *Diabetes* 1989;38:1231–1237.

60. McLeod BK, Thompson JR, Rosenthal AR: The prevalence of retinopathy in the insulin-requiring diabetic patients of an English county town. *Eye* 1988;2:424–430.

61. Kostraba JN, Klein R, Dorman JS, et al: The epidemiology of diabetes complications study, IV: correlates of diabetic background and proliferative retinopathy. *Am J Epidemiol* 1991;133: 381–391.

62. Lloyd CE, Klein R, Maser RE: The progression of retinopathy over two years: the Pittsburgh Epidemiology of Diabetes Complications (EDC) Study. *J Diabetes Complications* 1995;9: 140–148.

63. Fujimoto W, Fukuda M: Natural history of diabetic retinopathy and its treatment in Japan. In: Baba S, Goto Y, Fukui I, eds: *Diabetes Mellitus in Asia.* Amsterdam: Excerpta Medica; 1976: 225–231.

64. Ross SA, Huchcroft SA: Hyperlipidemia and vascular risk factors among diabetics in southern Alberta. *Clin Invest Med* 1989;12:B25.

65. Lee ET, Lee VS, Lu M, Russell D: Development of proliferative retinopathy in NIDDM: a follow-up study of American Indians in Oklahoma. *Diabetes* 1992;41:359–367.

66. Lee ET, Lee VS, Kingsley RM, et al: Diabetic retinopathy in Oklahoma Indians with NIDDM: incidence and risk factors. *Diabetes Care* 1992;15:1620–1627.

67. Nelson RG, Newman JM, Knowler WC, et al: Incidence of end-stage renal disease in type 2 (non–insulin-dependent) diabetes mellitus in Pima Indians. *Diabetologia* 1988;31:730–736.

68. Klein R, Klein BEK, Moss SE, et al: The Wisconsin Epidemiologic Study of Diabetic Retinopathy, X: four-year incidence and progression of diabetic retinopathy when age at diagnosis is 30 years or more. *Arch Ophthalmol* 1989;107: 244–249.

69. Klein R, Moss SE, Klein BEK, et al: The Wisconsin Epidemiologic Study of Diabetic Retinopathy, XI: the incidence of macular edema. *Ophthalmology* 1989;96:1501–1510.

70. Klein R, Klein BEK, Moss SE, Cruickshanks KJ: The Wisconsin Epidemiologic Study of Diabetic Retinopathy, XVII: the 14-year incidence and progression of diabetic retinopathy and associated risk factors in type 1 diabetes. *Ophthalmology* 1998;105:1801–1815.

71. Harris MI, Klein R, Cowie CC, et al: Is the risk of diabetic retinopathy greater in non-Hispanic blacks and Mexican Americans than in non-Hispanic whites with type 2 diabetes? A U.S. population study. *Diabetes Care* 1998;21: 1230–1235.

72. Cruickshank JK, Alleyne SA: Black West Indian and matched white diabetics in Britain compared with diabetics in Jamaica: body mass, blood pressure, and vascular disease. *Diabetes Care* 1987;10:170–179.

73. Arfken CL, Salicrup AE, Meuer SM, et al: Retinopathy in African Americans and whites with insulin-dependent diabetes mellitus. *Arch Intern Med* 1994;154:2597–2602.

74. Barbosa J, Ramsay RC, Knobloch WH, et al: Histocompatibility antigen frequencies in diabetic retinopathy. *Am J Ophthalmol* 1980;90: 148–153.

75. Dornan TL, Ting A, McPherson CK, et al: Genetic susceptibility to the development of retinopathy in insulin-dependent diabetics. *Diabetes* 1982;31:226–231.

76. Rand LI, Krolewski AS, Aiello LM, et al: Multiple factors in the prediction of risk of proliferative diabetic retinopathy. *N Engl J Med* 1985;313:1433–1438.

77. Jervell J, Solheim B: HLA-antigens in long standing insulin dependent diabetics with terminal nephropathy and retinopathy with and without loss of vision. *Diabetologia* 1979;17:391.

78. Cruickshanks KJ, Vadheim CM, Moss SE, et al: Genetic marker associations with proliferative retinopathy in persons diagnosed with diabetes before 30 years of age. *Diabetes* 1992;41:879–885.

79. Cruickshanks KJ, Klein R, Klein BEK, et al: HLA-DR4 and the incidence of proliferative retinopathy. *Diabetes* 1993;42:33A.

80. Klein BEK, Moss SE, Klein R: Is menarche associated with diabetic retinopathy? *Diabetes Care* 1990;13:1034–1038.

81. Murphy RP, Nanda M, Plotnick L, et al: The relationship of puberty to diabetic retinopathy. *Arch Ophthalmol* 1990;108:215–218.

82. Kostraba JN, Dorman JS, Orchard TJ, et al: Contribution of diabetes duration before puberty to development of microvascular complications in IDDM subjects. *Diabetes Care* 1989;12:686–693.

83. Dills DG, Moss SE, Klein R, et al: Is insulin-like growth factor I associated with diabetic retinopathy? *Diabetes* 1990;39:191–195.

84. Pieters GF, Smals AG, Kloppenborg PW: Defective suppression of growth hormone after oral glucose loading in adolescence. *J Clin Endocrinol Metab* 1980;51:265–270.

85. Klein R, Klein BEK, Moss SE, DeMets DL: Blood pressure and hypertension in diabetes. *Am J Epidemiol* 1985;122:75–89.

86. Blethen SL, Sargeant DT, Whitlow MG, Santiago JV: Effect of pubertal stage and recent blood glucose control on plasma somatomedin C in children with insulin-dependent diabetes mellitus. *Diabetes* 1981;30:868–872.

87. Allen C, Zaccaro DJ, Palta M, et al: Glycemic control in early IDDM. The Wisconsin Diabetes Registry. *Diabetes Care* 1992;15:980–987.

88. Sizonenko PC: Endocrinology in preadolescents and adolescents, I: hormonal changes during normal puberty. *Am J Dis Child* 1978;132:704–712.

89. Haffner SM, Klein R, Dunn JF, et al: Increased testosterone in type I diabetic subjects with severe retinopathy. *Ophthalmology* 1990;97:1270–1274.

90. Nilsson SV, Nilsson JE, Frostberg N, Emilsson T: The Kristianstad survey, II: studies in a representative adult diabetic population with special reference to comparison with an adequate control group. *Acta Med Scand* 1967;469 (suppl):1–42.

91. Klein R, Klein BEK, Moss SE, et al: Glycosylated hemoglobin predicts the incidence and progression of diabetic retinopathy. *J Am Med Assoc* 1988;260:2864–2871.

92. Klein R, Klein BEK, Moss SE, Cruickshanks KJ: Relationship of hyperglycemia to the long-term incidence and progression of diabetic retinopathy. *Arch Intern Med* 1994;154:2169–2178.

93. Kroc Collaborative Study Group: Blood glucose control and the evolution of diabetic retinopathy and albuminuria: a preliminary multicenter trial. *N Engl J Med* 1984;311:365–372.

94. Kroc Collaborative Study Group: Diabetic retinopathy after two years of intensified insulin treatment: follow-up of the Kroc Collaborative Study. *J Am Med Assoc* 1988;260:37–41.

95. Lauritzen T, Frost-Larsen K, Larsen HW, Deckert T: Effect of 1 year of near-normal blood glucose levels on retinopathy in insulin-dependent diabetics. *Lancet* 1983;1:200–204.

96. Lauritzen T, Frost-Larsen K, Larsen HW, Deckert T: Two-year experience with continuous subcutaneous insulin infusion in relation to retinopathy and neuropathy. *Diabetes* 1985;34 (suppl 3):74–79.

97. Dahl-Jorgensen K, Brinchmann-Hansen O, Hanssen KF, et al: Rapid tightening of blood glucose control leads to transient deterioration of retinopathy in insulin dependent diabetes mellitus: the Oslo Study. *Br Med J* 1985;290:811–815.

98. Dahl-Jorgensen K, Brinchmann-Hansen O, Hanssen KF, et al: Effect of near normoglycaemia for two years on progression of early diabetic retinopathy, nephropathy, and neuropathy: the Oslo Study. *Br Med J* 1986;293:1195–1199.

99. Beck-Nielsen H, Richelsen B, Morgensen CE, et al: Effect of insulin pump treatment for one year on renal function and retinal morphology in patients with IDDM. *Diabetes Care* 1985; 8:585–589.

100. Wang PH, Lau J, Chalmers TC: Meta-analysis of effects of intensive blood-glucose control on late complications of type I diabetes. *Lancet* 1993;341:1306–1309.

101. University Group Diabetes Program: Effects of hypoglycemic agents on vascular complications in patients with adult-onset diabetes, VIII: evaluation of insulin therapy. *Diabetes* 1982; 31(suppl 5):1–81.

102. DCCT Research Group: Diabetes Control and Complications Trial (DCCT): results of feasibility study. *Diabetes Care* 1987;10:1–19.

103. Diabetes Control and Complications Trial Research Group: The effect of intensive treatment of diabetes on the development and progression of long-term complications in insulin-dependent diabetes mellitus. *N Engl J Med* 1993; 329:977–986.

104. UK Prospective Diabetes Study Group: Intensive blood-glucose control with sulphonylureas or insulin compared with conventional treatment and risk of complications in patients with type 2 diabetes. UKPDS 33. *Lancet* 1998; 352:837–853.

105. Smith RB, Pyke DA, Watkins PJ, et al: C-peptide response to glucagon in diabetics with and without complications. *N Z Med J* 1979;89: 304–306.

106. Sjoberg S, Gunnarsson R, Gjotterberg M, et al: Residual insulin production, glycaemic control and prevalence of microvascular lesions and polyneuropathy in long-term type I (insulin-dependent) diabetes mellitus. *Diabetologia* 1987; 30:208–213.

107. Sjoberg S, Gjotterberg M, Lefvert AK, et al: Significance of residual insulin production in long-term type I diabetes mellitus. *Transplant Proc* 1986;18:1498–1499.

108. Madsbad S, Lauritzen E, Faber OK, Binder C: The effect of residual beta-cell function on the development of diabetic retinopathy. *Diabet Med* 1986;3:42–45.

109. Klein R, Moss SE, Klein BEK, et al: Wisconsin Epidemiologic Study of Diabetic Retinopathy, XII: relationship of C-peptide and diabetic retinopathy. *Diabetes* 1990;39:1445–1450.

110. Serghieri G, Bartolomei G, Pettenello C, et al: Raised retinopathy prevalence rate in insulin-treated patients: a feature of obese type II diabetes. *Transplant Proc* 1986;18:1576–1577.

111. Davis MD: Diabetic retinopathy, diabetic control and blood pressure. *Transplant Proc* 1986; 18:1565–1568.

112. Kohner EM: Diabetic retinopathy. *Br Med Bull* 1989;45:148–173.

113. UK Prospective Diabetes Study Group: Tight blood pressure control and risk of macrovascular and microvascular complications in Type 2 diabetes. UKPDS 38. *Br Med J* 1998; 317:703–713.

114. Parving HH, Andersen AR, Hommel E, Smidt U: Effects of long-term antihypertensive treatment on kidney function in diabetic nephropathy. *Hypertension* 1985;7:114–117.

115. Chaturvedi N, Sjolie AK, Stephenson JM, et al: Effect of lisinopril on progression of retinopathy in normotensive people with type 1 diabetes: the EUCLID Study Group. EURODIAB Controlled Trial of Lisinopril in Insulin-Dependent Diabetes Mellitus. *Lancet* 1998;351:28–31.

116. Warram JH, Laffel LM, Valsania P, et al: Excess mortality associated with diuretic therapy in diabetes mellitus. *Arch Intern Med* 1991; 151:1350–1356.

117. Klein BEK, Moss SE, Klein R: Use of cardiovascular disease medications and mortality in people with older onset diabetes. *Am J Public Health* 1992;82:1142–1144.

118. Cruickshanks KJ, Ritter LL, Klein R, Moss SE: The association of microalbuminuria with diabetic retinopathy: the Wisconsin Epidemiologic Study of Diabetic Retinopathy. *Ophthalmology* 1993;100:862–867.

119. Klein R, Moss SE, Klein BEK: Is gross proteinuria a risk factor for the incidence of proliferative diabetic retinopathy? *Ophthalmology* 1993; 100:1140–1146.

120. Klein BEK, Moss SE, Klein R, Surawicz TS: The Wisconsin Epidemiologic Study of Diabetic Retinopathy, XIII: relationship of serum cholesterol to retinopathy and hard exudate. *Ophthalmology* 1991;98:1261–1265.

121. Chew EY, Klein ML, Ferris FL III, et al: Association of elevated serum lipid levels with retinal hard exudate in diabetic retinopathy. ETDRS Report Number 22. *Arch Ophthalmol* 1996;114:1079–1084.

122. Goldsmith JR, Landaw SA: Carbon monoxide and human health. *Science* 1968;162: 1352–1359.

123. Hawkins RI: Smoking, platelets and thrombosis. *Nature* 1972;236:450–452.

124. Klein R, Klein BEK, Davis MD: Is cigarette smoking associated with diabetic retinopathy? *Am J Epidemiol* 1983;118:228–238.

125. Moss SE, Klein R, Klein BEK: Association of cigarette smoking with diabetic retinopathy. *Diabetes Care* 1991;14:119–126.

126. Kingsley LA, Dorman JS, Doft BH, et al: An epidemiologic approach to the study of retinopathy: the Pittsburgh diabetic morbidity and retinopathy studies. *Diabetes Res Clin Pract* 1988;4:99–109.

127. Young RJ, McCulloch DK, Prescott RJ, Clarke BF: Alcohol: another risk factor for diabetic retinopathy? *Br Med J* 1984;288:1035–1037.

128. Moss SE, Klein R, Klein BEK: Alcohol consumption and the prevalence of diabetic retinopathy. *Ophthalmology* 1992;99:926–932.

129. Jakubowski JA, Vaillancourt R, Deykin D: Interaction of ethanol, prostacyclin, and aspirin in determining human platelet reactivity in vitro. *Arteriosclerosis* 1988;8:436–441.

130. Diabetes Drafting Group: Prevalence of small vessels and large vessel disease in diabetic patients from 14 centres: the World Health Organisation Multinational Study of Vascular Disease in Diabetics. *Diabetologia* 1985;28(suppl): 615–640.

131. LaPorte RE, Dorman JS, Tajima N, et al: Pittsburgh Insulin-Dependent Diabetes Mellitus Morbidity and Mortality Study: physical activity and diabetic complications. *Pediatrics* 1986; 78:1027–1033.

132. Cruickshanks KJ, Moss SE, Klein R, Klein BEK: Physical activity and proliferative retinopathy in people diagnosed with diabetes before age 30 yr. *Diabetes Care* 1992;15:1267–1272.

133. Hanna AK, Roy M, Zinman B, et al: An evaluation of factors associated with proliferative diabetic retinopathy. *Clin Invest Med* 1985; 8:109–116.

134. Haffner SM, Hazuda HP, Stern MP, et al: Effects of socioeconomic status on hyperglycemia and retinopathy levels in Mexican Americans with NIDDM. *Diabetes Care* 1989;12: 128–134.

135. Rodman HM, Singerman LJ, Aiello LM, Merkatz IR: Diabetic retinopathy and its relationship to pregnancy. In: Merkatz IR, Adams PAJ, eds: *The Diabetic Pregnancy: A Perinatal Perspective.* New York: Grune & Stratton; 1979; 73–91.

136. Klein BEK, Moss SE, Klein R: Effect of pregnancy on progression of diabetic retinopathy. *Diabetes Care* 1990;13:34–40.

137. Klein BEK, Klein R, Meuer SM, et al: Does the severity of diabetic retinopathy predict pregnancy outcome? *J Diabetes Complications* 1988;2: 179–184.

138. Klein R, Klein BEK, Moss SE: The epidemiology of proliferative diabetic retinopathy. *Diabetes Care* 1992;15:1875–1891.

139. Early Treatment Diabetic Retinopathy Study Research Group: Effects of aspirin treatment on diabetic retinopathy. ETDRS Report Number 8. *Ophthalmology* 1991;98(suppl): 757–765.

140. Klein BEK, Klein R, Moss SE: Is aspirin usage associated with diabetic retinopathy? *Diabetes Care* 1987;10:600–603.

141. Ederer F, Hiller R, Taylor HR: Senile lens changes and diabetes in two population studies. *Am J Ophthalmol* 1981;91:381–395.

142. Klein BEK, Klein R, Wang Q, Moss SE: Older-onset diabetes and lens opacities: The Beaver Dam Eye Study. *Ophthalmic Epidemiol* 1995;2:49–55.

143. Klein BEK, Klein R, Moss SE: Prevalence of cataracts in a population-based study of persons with diabetes mellitus. *Ophthalmology* 1985; 92:1191–1196.

144. Klein BEK, Klein R, Moss SE: Incidence of cataract surgery in the Wisconsin Epidemiologic Study of Diabetic Retinopathy. *Am J Ophthalmol* 1995;119:295–300.

145. Klein BEK, Klein R, Jensen SC: Open-angle glaucoma and older-onset diabetes: the Beaver Dam Eye Study. *Ophthalmology* 1994; 101:1173–1177.

146. Klein BEK, Klein R, Moss SE: Incidence of self-reported glaucoma in people with diabetes mellitus. *Br J Ophthalmol* 1997;81:743–747.

147. Witkin SR, Klein R: Ophthalmologic care for persons with diabetes. *J Am Med Assoc* 1984; 251:2534–2537.

148. Sussman EJ, Tsiaras WG, Soper KA: Diagnosis of diabetic eye disease. *J Am Med Assoc* 1982;247:3231–3234.

149. Moss SE, Klein R, Kessler SD, Richie KA: Comparison between ophthalmoscopy and fundus photography in determining severity of diabetic retinopathy. *Ophthalmology* 1985;92:62–67.

150. Nathan DM, Fogel HA, Godine JE, et al: Role of diabetologist in evaluating diabetic retinopathy. *Diabetes Care* 1991;14:26–33.

151. Valez R, Haffner S, Stern MP, VanHeuven WAJ: Ophthalmologist vs. retinal photographs in screening for diabetic retinopathy [abstract]. *Clin Res* 1987;35:363A.

152. Ryder RE, Vora JP, Atiea JA, et al: Possible new method to improve detection of diabetic retinopathy: Polaroid non-mydriatic retinal photography. *Br Med J* 1985;291:1256–1257.

153. Klein R, Klein BEK, Moss SE, et al: The Wisconsin Epidemiologic Study of Diabetic Retinopathy, VI: retinal photocoagulation. *Ophthalmology* 1987;94:747–753.

154. Klein R, Moss SE, Klein BEK, et al: The Wisconsin Epidemiologic Study of Diabetic Retinopathy, VIII: the incidence of retinal photocoagulation. *J Diabetes Complications* 1988;2: 79–87.

155. Klein R, Klein BEK, Moss SE, Cruickshanks KJ: Association of ocular disease and mortality in a diabetic population. *Arch Ophthalmol* 1999;117:1487–1498.

History of Evolving Treatments for Diabetic Retinopathy

George W. Blankenship, MD

The earliest known written record of diabetes was made by the Hindu physician Susruta, who described a condition of honey urine. Descriptions of diabetes also appear in early Egyptian records, and Greek physicians reported the melting away of flesh and limbs to urine. Other diabetic complications such as blindness undoubtedly occurred, but were probably rare because of the patients' relatively short life span following the development of diabetes.

Diabetic retinopathy was first described by Jaeger in 1855.[1] Initially, the fundus changes were thought to be the result of hypertension, which often coexisted with diabetes, or an inflammatory response to elevated albumin and urea levels, resulting in the descriptive term *diabetic retinitis*. Later, the specific relationship between diabetes and retinal vascular changes was appreciated.

3-1

BLOOD GLUCOSE AND RETINOPATHY

The discovery of insulin by Banting and Best[2] in 1921 revolutionized the treatment of diabetes and markedly extended the lives of people with this disease. The increased longevity provided more time for the development of late complications, such as retinopathy. Visual loss and blindness from diabetic retinopathy became an increasing problem without a reasonable means of treatment.

There was great debate about the relationship of blood sugar levels and diabetic retinopathy. Some argued that diabetes had a primary effect on the basement membrane of blood vessels, independent of blood sugar,[3] while others contended that tight glucose control would inhibit the progression of the vascular changes. Only when instruments were developed whereby patients could check their blood sugar levels repeatedly throughout the day, did truly "good control" become feasible. Later, the Diabetes Control and Complications Trial (DCCT), a large, multicenter clinical trial, settled the matter by demonstrating that good control of blood sugar was the single most important factor in preventing or slowing the progression of retinopathy.[4]

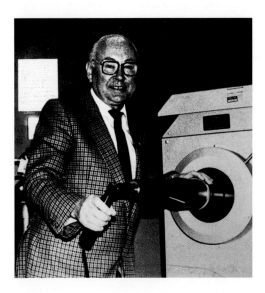

Figure 3-1 *Gerd Meyer-Schwickerath, father of photocoagulation, with xenon photocoagulator.*

3-2

LIGHT ENERGY FOR TREATMENT

The possibility of using light to treat retinal disease had been considered, and the risk of scotomas from retinal damage caused by looking at the sun had been known for centuries. Following a solar eclipse on July 10, 1945, Meyer-Schwickerath (Figure 3-1) became interested in the possible use of light energy to treat retinal diseases. He initially used reflected sunlight, but found this to be impractical and tried other sources of light before refining the use of a high-pressure xenon arc bulb. His results of treating retinal tears and small, suspected melanomas were first published in 1949.[5,6] Morón-Salas had been independently doing similar research and published his results shortly thereafter, in 1950.[7]

The initial results of treating specific diabetic retinopathy lesions with photocoagulation produced by xenon light were discouraging, but persistent efforts during the 1950s and 1960s by Wetzig,[8,9] Amalric,[10] Okun,[11–13] Wessing,[14] and numerous other ophthalmologists began to produce better visual results than those reported for the natural course of the disease by Caird[15] and Beetham.[16] The early concepts of photocoagulation treatment of diabetic retinopathy were unclear. Treatment strategies ranged from "hitting everything that was red" (that is, every hemorrhage or microaneurysm), through producing a line of coagulation along either side of the major veins, to directing confluent treatment of each area of neovascularization.

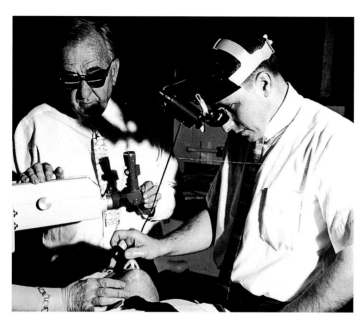

Figure 3-2 *In 1960s, William P. Beetham (left) and Lloyd M. Aiello pioneered panretinal laser photocoagulation. Later, Dr Aiello spearheaded studies demonstrating laser's value in reducing vision loss. In this photograph, Dr Beetham is holding original ruby laser, while Dr Aiello is performing indirect ophthalmoscopy to evaluate retina of patient treated with laser. In late 1970s, Dr Aiello was selected to direct Early Treatment Diabetic Retinopathy Study Group.* Courtesy Lloyd Paul Aiello, MD, PhD.

3-3

LASER PHOTOCOAGULATION

During this time, there was increasing interest in research to adapt laser wavelengths for photocoagulation. Campbell[17,18] and Zweng[19] independently used ruby laser wavelengths with limited success in the early 1960s, but Beetham[20] and Aiello[21] had much better success treating diabetic retinopathy a few years later. Using the ruby laser, Beetham and Aiello recognized the positive treatment potential of panretinal photocoagulation (Figure 3-2).

In the late 1960s, the potential value of laser wavelengths produced by argon gas was recognized. Independent research by L'Esperance[22,23] and by Little and Zweng[24,25] resulted in instruments and technology to adapt argon laser wavelengths with delivery systems for successful photocoagulation.

The successful treatment of diabetic retinopathy with argon laser wavelengths was reported by Patz[26] and numerous others. When the argon laser was developed, it was hoped that the absorption of argon green by hemoglobin would allow direct treatment of elevated disc neovascularization. After a great deal of effort treating the "feeder" arteriolar vessels of the elevated neovascular frond, and often re-treating several times within a few days, this technique was abandoned because it often led to vitreous hemorrhage. Unless the stimulus for the neovascularization was reduced, the treated new vessels simply reopened and continued to grow.

The studies by Davis[27,28] on the natural history of diabetic retinopathy had made it clear that some cases evolved into a state of spontaneous fibrosis and resolution of the neovascular process. This led to the attempt to increase the incidence of such spontaneous resolution by a standardized pattern of panretinal photocoagulation (PRP) that would spare the macula, but somehow reduce the stimulus for neovascular proliferation. The efficacy of this treatment method was demonstrated by the multicenter Diabetic Retinopathy Study (DRS).[29] While this study proved the value of a standardized PRP pattern in inducing regression of proliferative retinopathy, it remained for a later multicenter study, the Early Treatment of Diabetic Retinopathy Study (ETDRS),[30] to show that laser treatment of the posterior fundus was of value in preventing visual loss from macular edema.

3-4

MECHANISM OF ACTION OF PHOTOCOAGULATION

Although the DRS and the ETDRS proved that laser treatment was effective, they did not answer the question of "how" or "why" it was effective. The lack of understanding of the mechanism underlying the beneficial effect of laser photocoagulation has led to ongoing debate about treatment technique, especially in regard to macular edema. The experimental work of Landers[31] with a primate model showed that the hypoxia surrounding an area of ischemic retina could be eliminated by a "checkerboard" pattern of PRP. Thus, it seemed that PRP might function by turning off the hypoxic stimulus for neovascular growth, including such proliferative factors as vascular endothelial growth factor (VEGF). The explanation of the beneficial effect of laser treatment for macular edema is less certain, allowing for disagreement between those who believe they are doing the most good by focal, direct treatment of each leaking microaneurysm and those who feel they should just lightly treat the retinal pigment epithelium with a grid pattern.

Regression of diabetic retinopathy and preservation of vision had also been observed following loss of pituitary function, and therapeutic roles of pituitary ablation were also studied.[32] Various surgical and irradiation procedures were developed,[33–35] but this form of therapy was abandoned with the development of photocoagulation, which was much simpler to perform, had fewer systemic side effects, and produced better results.

3-5

VITREOUS SURGERY FOR COMPLICATIONS OF RETINOPATHY

Coincidental with the development of photocoagulation treatment of diabetic retinopathy, radical new concepts and revolutionary surgery for the management of diseases and disorders affecting the vitreous were being developed at the Bascom Palmer Eye Institute of the University of Miami School of Medicine. David Kasner, MD, had suc-

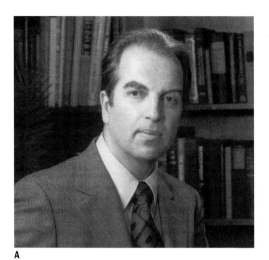

A

cessfully preserved vision in a severely injured eye by removing a large portion of the opaque, formed vitreous. He was achieving good results with similar aggressive techniques while teaching ophthalmology residents how to manage loss of vitreous during cataract surgery at the Miami Veterans Administration Hospital. The important role of vitreous traction in the progression of proliferative diabetic retinopathy had also been noted by Davis.[36]

Robert Machemer, MD, also at Bascom Palmer, was intrigued with Dr Kasner's experience and began a research program to better understand the pathophysiology of vitreous diseases and how they might be successfully treated. With the support and encouragement of Edward W. D. Norton, MD, Director of Bascom Palmer, Dr Machemer and coworkers developed microsurgical instruments and procedures with which the contents of the vitreous cavity could be safely removed through the pars plana while maintaining intraocular pressure and a formed globe (Figure 3-3).[37–40]

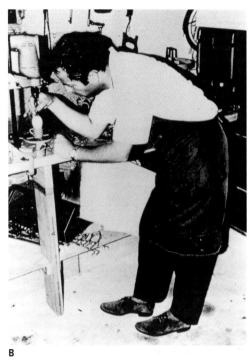

B

Figure 3-3 *(A) Robert Machemer, father of pars plana vitrectomy surgery. (B) Dr Machemer in his garage using drill to extract contents of an egg. Continued experiments led to modern vitrectomy instruments and procedures.*

Dr Machemer performed the first pars plana vitrectomy in 1970 and soon realized the potential value of removing not only opaque vitreous hemorrhages but also proliferative membranes. By releasing vitreous traction, this new form of surgery also repaired retinal detachments and enabled the restoration of sight in people who had become blind from diabetic retinopathy.

The initial vitrectomies were done with just the coaxial light of the operating microscope. Visualization of the vitreous was soon improved by adaptation of a nearly coaxial slit beam to the operating microscope and then by introduction of fiberoptic light sources into the eye. At this stage, the vitrectomy instruments consisted of a suction cutter, an infusing tube, and a light pipe, all in concentric sleeves.[38] O'Malley[41,42] stressed the value of decreasing the diameter of the instrument used in the eye by separating the functions. He introduced the guillotine type of cutter and the three-port system used by most surgeons today, separating the suction cutter from the infusion tube and light source. Aaberg,[43–45] Charles,[46,47] Douvas,[48] Klöti,[49,50] Michels,[51,52] Parel,[53,54] Peyman,[55] Ryan,[56] Tolentino,[57,58] and many others expanded and clarified the indications for vitrectomy and made important contributions to instrumentation and surgical techniques.

3-6

CLINICAL TRIALS

In the late 1960s, major questions remained about the treatment of diabetic retinopathy, despite the availability of retinal photocoagulation with light wavelengths produced from either xenon arc or argon laser and despite the development of pars plana vitrectomy to restore sight in people who had been blinded by retinopathy. Additional information was needed on the natural history of patients with diabetic retinopathy whose disease was managed without photocoagulation or vitreous surgery, the specific indications for surgery, the best surgical techniques, the risks and side effects of surgery, and the long-term results. The value of good control of diabetes and normalization of blood sugar with intensive therapy was also questioned. The importance of resolving these issues was heightened by the growing number of people with diabetes surviving long enough to develop retinopathy.

In 1968, these issues were addressed at the Symposium on the Treatment of Diabetic Retinopathy, developed by Morton F. Goldberg, MD, and Stuart L. Fine, MD, and held at the Airlie House in Warrenton, Virginia, from September 29 to October 1 for the United States Department of Health, Education, and Welfare (Figure 3-4). Following the symposium, the National Eye Institute (NEI) of the National Institutes of Health (NIH) funded several large, multicenter, prospective clinical trials with randomization of the treatments being evaluated. The NEI asked Matthew D. Davis, MD (Figure 3-5), of the Department of Ophthalmology at the University of Wisconsin School of Medicine, to be the direc-

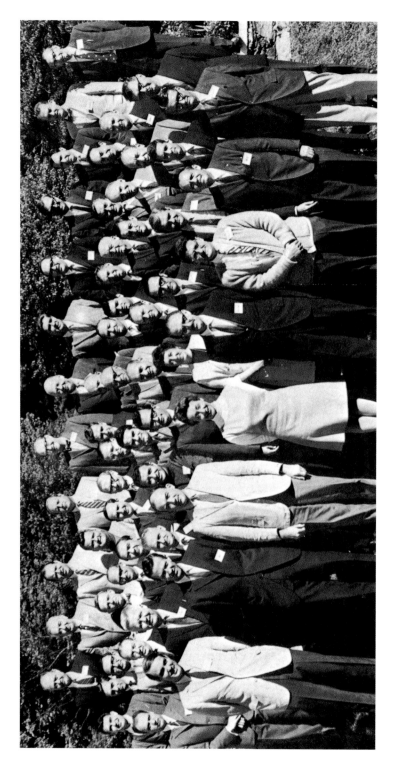

Figure 3-4 *Attendees at Symposium on Treatment of Diabetic Retinopathy. **Row 1 (front):** S. L. Fine, M. D. Davis, N. Oakley, E. Kohner, M. Balodimos, H. Spalter, J. Linfoot, T. Duane. **Row 2:** A. Wessing, R. Kjellberg, W. Sweet, N. Zervas, E. Finkelstein, E. Hallworth, L. Jagerman, E. W. D. Norton, H. Lester. **Row 3:** B. Ray, J. Hardy, A. Panisset, E. Okun, B. Straatsma, G. Cleasby, O. Pearson, J. W. McMeel. **Row 4:** F. Myers, M. Goldberg, H.-W. Larsen, R. Blach, T. R. Fraser, W. van Heuven, R. Feinberg, K. Gabbay, G. McDonald, J. Dobree, R. Schimek. **Row 5:** R. Packman, R. Bradley, P. Jahnke, F. Caird, P. Thornfeldt, C. Mortimer, G. Harris, K. Lundbaek, H. Keen. **Row 6:** P. Wetzig, W. Beetham, W. Peretz, J. Glaser, M. Rubin, J. Ferre, Se. Simonsen, N. Roth, H. C. Zweng, L. Aiello, E. Greenberg, G. Joplin.*

Reproduced from Goldberg MF, Fine SL, eds: Symposium on the Treatment of Diabetic Retinopathy. (Airlie House, 1968) Public Health Service Publ. No. 1980. Washington, DC: US Govt Printing Office; 1969.

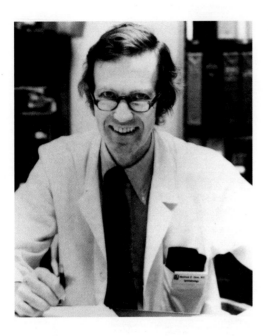

Figure 3-5 *Matthew D. Davis, MD, selected to direct newly organized Diabetic Retinopathy Study in 1971 and Diabetic Retinopathy Vitrectomy Study in 1976.*

tor of both the DRS[29,59] and the Diabetic Retinopathy Vitrectomy Study (DRVS)[60,61] and Lloyd M. Aiello, MD, of the Joslin Institute, to be the director of the ETDRS.[30,62] All three of these NEI studies and the subsequent DCCT[4] were very successful and are extensively discussed in other chapters of this monograph.

The American Academy of Ophthalmology recognized the importance of using the findings of these clinical trials in the care of people with diabetes. In 1989, with the support of the Academy, Arnall Patz, MD, initiated the Diabetes 2000® project, an educational program to increase the awareness and knowledge of ophthalmologists, other physicians, and other caregivers involved in the care of people with diabetes about the clinical trials' findings and recommendations.

3-7

CONCLUSION

The current history of the treatment for diabetic retinopathy encompasses almost 150 years. It is composed of many important observations, creative new concepts, elaborate laboratory and clinical research projects, development and refinement of revolutionary instruments and procedures, sophisticated evaluations confirming the benefits of good control of blood sugar levels, and appropriate photocoagulation and vitreous surgery. A large number of people have made important contributions to the current level of knowledge and treatment abilities, and the future is even more encouraging for additional discoveries that will further enhance the ability to preserve and regain vision for people with diabetes.

REFERENCES

1. von Jaeger E: *Beitrage zur Pathologie des Augen.* Wien: K. K. Hof- und Staatsdruckerei; 1855.

2. Banting FG, Best CH: The internal secretion of the pancreas. *J Lab Clin Med* 1922;7:251–266.

3. Hutton WL, Snyder WB, Vaiser A, Siperstein MD: Retinal microangiopathy without associated glucose intolerance. *Trans Am Acad Ophthalmol Otolaryngol* 1972:76:968–980.

4. Diabetes Control and Complications Trial Research Group: The effect of intensive treatment of diabetes on the development and progression of long-term complications in insulin-dependent diabetes mellitus. *New Engl J Med* 1993;329: 977–986.

5. Meyer-Schwickerath G: Koagulation der Netzhaut mit Sonnenlicht. *Ber Dtsch Ophthalmol Ges* 1950;55:256–259.

6. Meyer-Schwickerath G: *Light Coagulation.* Drance SM, trans. St Louis: CV Mosby Co; 1960.

7. Morón-Salas J: Obliteración de los desgarros retinianos por quemadura con luz. *Arch Soc Oftalmol Hisp-Am* 1950;10:566–578.

8. Wetzig PC, Worlton JT: Treatment of diabetic retinopathy by light-coagulation: a preliminary study. *Br J Ophthalmol* 1963;47:539–541.

9. Wetzig PC, Jepson CN: Treatment of diabetic retinopathy by light coagulation. *Am J Ophthalmol* 1966;62:459–465.

10. Amalric MP: [Trial of treatment of exudative diabetic retinopathy.] *Bull Soc Ophtalmol Fr* 1960; 6:359–363.

11. Okun E, Cibis P: The role of photocoagulation in the therapy of proliferative diabetic retinopathy. *Arch Ophthalmol* 1966;75:337–352.

12. Okun E: The effectiveness of photocoagulation in the therapy of proliferative diabetic retinopathy (PDR): a controlled study in 50 patients. *Trans Am Acad Ophthalmol Otolaryngol* 1968;72: 246–252.

13. Okun E, Johnston GP, Boniuk I: *Management of Diabetic Retinopathy: A Stereoscopic Presentation.* St Louis: CV Mosby Co; 1971.

14. Wessing AK, Meyer-Schwickerath G: Results of photocoagulation in diabetic retinopathy. In: Goldberg MF, Fine SL, eds: *Symposium on the Treatment of Diabetic Retinopathy.* (Airlie House, 1968) Public Health Service Publ. No. 1980. Washington, DC: US Govt Printing Office; 1969:569–592.

15. Caird FI, Garrett CJ: Prognosis for vision in diabetic retinopathy. *Diabetes* 1963;12:389–397.

16. Beetham WP: Visual prognosis of proliferating diabetic retinopathy. *Br J Ophthalmol* 1963; 47:611–619.

17. Campbell CJ, Rittler MC, Koester CJ: The optical maser as a retinal coagulator: an evaluation. *Trans Am Acad Ophthalmol Otolaryngol* 1963; 67:58–67.

18. Campbell CJ, Koester CJ, Curtice V, et al: Clinical studies in laser photocoagulation. *Arch Ophthalmol* 1965;74:57–65.

19. Zweng HC, Flocks M, Kapany NS, et al: Experimental laser photocoagulation. *Am J Ophthalmol* 1964;58:353–362.

20. Beetham WP, Aiello LM, Balodimos MC, Koncz L: Ruby laser photocoagulation of early diabetic neovascular retinopathy: preliminary report of a long-term controlled study. *Arch Ophthalmol* 1970;83:261–272.

21. Aiello LM, Beetham WP, Balodimos MC, et al: Ruby laser photocoagulation in treatment of diabetic proliferating retinopathy: preliminary report. In: Goldberg MF, Fine SL, eds: *Symposium on the Treatment of Diabetic Retinopathy.* (Airlie House, 1968) Public Health Service Publ. No. 1980. Washington, DC: US Govt Printing Office; 1969:437–463.

22. L'Esperance FA Jr: An ophthalmic argon laser photocoagulation system: design, construction, and laboratory investigations. *Trans Am Ophthalmol Soc* 1968;66:827–904.

23. L'Esperance FA Jr: Argon laser photocoagulation of diabetic retinal neovascularization: a five-year appraisal. *Trans Am Acad Ophthalmol Otolaryngol* 1973;77:OP6–OP24.

24. Little HL, Zweng HC, Peabody RR: Argon laser slit-lamp retinal photocoagulation. *Trans Am Acad Ophthalmol Otolaryngol* 1970;74:85–97.

25. Zweng HC, Little HL, Peabody RR: Further observations on argon laser photocoagulation of diabetic retinopathy. *Trans Am Acad Ophthalmol Otolaryngol* 1972;76:990–1004.

26. Patz A, Maumenee AE, Ryan SJ: Argon laser photocoagulation: advantages and limitations. *Trans Am Acad Ophthalmol Otolaryngol* 1971;75:569–579.

27. Davis MD: Natural course of diabetic retinopathy. In: Kimura SJ, Caygill WM, eds: *Vascular Complications of Diabetes Mellitus with Special Emphasis on Microangiopathy of the Eye.* St Louis: CV Mosby Co; 1967:139–169.

28. Davis MD: The natural course of diabetic retinopathy. *Trans Am Acad Ophthalmol Otolaryngol* 1968;72:237–240.

29. Diabetic Retinopathy Study Research Group: Preliminary report on effects of photocoagulation therapy. *Am J Ophthalmol* 1976;81:383–396.

30. Early Treatment Diabetic Retinopathy Study Research Group: Photocoagulation for diabetic macular edema. ETDRS Report Number 1. *Arch Ophthalmol* 1985;103:1796–1806.

31. Landers MB III, Stefansson E, Wolbarsht ML: Panretinal photocoagulation and retinal oxygenation. *Retina* 1982;2:167–175.

32. Luft R, et al: Hypophysectomy in man: further experiences in severe diabetes mellitus. *Br Med J* 1955;2:752–756.

33. Bradley RF, Rees SB: Surgical pituitary ablation for diabetic retinopathy. In: Goldberg MF, Fine SL, eds: *Symposium on the Treatment of Diabetic Retinopathy.* (Airlie House, 1968) Public Health Service Publ. No. 1980. Washington, DC: US Govt Printing Office; 1969:171–191.

34. Field RA, McMeel JW, Sweet WH, Schepens CL: Hypophyseal stalk section for angiopathic diabetic retinopathy. In: Goldberg MF, Fine SL, eds: *Symposium on the Treatment of Diabetic Retinopathy.* (Airlie House, 1968) Public Health Service Publ. No. 1980. Washington, DC: US Govt Printing Office; 1969:213–225.

35. Oakley NW, Joplin GF, Kohner EM, et al: The treatment of diabetic retinopathy by pituitary implantation of radioactive yttrium. In: Goldberg MF, Fine SL, eds: *Symposium on the Treatment of Diabetic Retinopathy.* (Airlie House, 1968) Public Health Service Publ. No. 1980. Washington, DC: US Govt Printing Office; 1969:317–329.

36. Davis MD: Vitreous contraction in proliferative diabetic retinopathy. *Arch Ophthalmol* 1965;74:741–751.

37. Machemer R, Buettner H, Norton EW, Parel JM: Vitrectomy: a pars plana approach. *Trans Am Acad Ophthalmol Otolaryngol* 1971;75:813–820.

38. Machemer R, Parel JM, Buettner H: A new concept for vitreous surgery, I: instrumentation. *Am J Ophthalmol* 1972;73:1–7.

39. Machemer R: A new concept for vitreous surgery, 7: two instrument techniques in pars plana vitrectomy. *Arch Ophthalmol* 1974;92:407–412.

40. Machemer R: Vitrectomy in diabetic retinopathy; removal of preretinal proliferations. *Trans Am Acad Ophthalmol Otolaryngol* 1975;79:OP394–OP395.

41. O'Malley C, Heintz RM: Vitrectomy via the pars plana: a new instrument system. *Trans Pac Coast Otoophthalmol Soc Annu Meet* 1972;50:121–137.

42. O'Malley C, Heintz RM Sr: Vitrectomy with an alternative instrument system. *Ann Ophthalmol* 1975;7:585–588, 591–594.

43. Aaberg TM: Clinical results in vitrectomy for diabetic traction retinal detachment. *Am J Ophthalmol* 1979;88:246–253.

44. Aaberg TM: Pars plana vitrectomy for diabetic traction retinal detachment. *Ophthalmology* 1981;88:639–642.

45. Aaberg TM, Abrams GW: Changing indications and techniques for vitrectomy in management of complications of diabetic retinopathy. *Ophthalmology* 1987;94:775–779.

46. Charles S: Endophotocoagulation. *Retina* 1981;1:117–120.

47. Charles S: *Vitreous Microsurgery*. 2nd ed. Baltimore: Williams & Wilkins; 1987.

48. Douvas NG: Microsurgical roto-extractor instrument for vitrectomy. *Mod Probl Ophthalmol* 1975;15:253–260.

49. Klöti R: Vitrektomie, I: ein neues Instrument für die hintere Vitrektomie. *Graefes Arch Klin Exp Ophthalmol* 1973;187:161–170.

50. Klöti R: Indications for vitrectomy and results in 115 cases. In: McPherson A, ed: *New and Controversial Aspects of Vitreoretinal Surgery*. St Louis: CV Mosby Co; 1977:237–244.

51. Michels RG: Vitrectomy for complications of diabetic retinopathy. *Arch Ophthalmol* 1978;96:237–246.

52. Michels RG: *Vitreous Surgery*. St Louis: CV Mosby Co; 1981.

53. Parel JM, Machemer R, Aumayr W: A new concept for vitreous surgery, 4: improvements in instrumentation and illumination. *Am J Ophthalmol* 1974;77:6–12.

54. Parel JM, Machemer R, Aumayr W: A new concept for vitreous surgery, 5: an automated operating microscope. *Am J Ophthalmol* 1974;77:161–168.

55. Peyman GA, Dodich NA: Experimental vitrectomy: instrumentation and surgical technique. *Arch Ophthalmol* 1971;86:548–551.

56. Ryan SJ, Michels RG: Pars plana vitrectomy: indications and results in 100 cases. In: McPherson A, ed: *New and Controversial Aspects of Vitreoretinal Surgery*. St Louis: CV Mosby Co; 1977:250–256.

57. Tolentino FI, Banko A, Schepens CL, et al: Vitreous surgery, XII: new instrumentation for vitrectomy. *Arch Ophthalmol* 1975;93:667–672.

58. Tolentino FI, Freeman HM, Tolentino FL: Closed vitrectomy in the management of diabetic traction retinal detachment. *Ophthalmology* 1980;87:1078–1089.

59. Diabetic Retinopathy Study Research Group: Four risk factors for severe visual loss in diabetic retinopathy: the third report from the Diabetic Retinopathy Study. *Arch Ophthalmol* 1979;97:654–655.

60. Diabetic Retinopathy Vitrectomy Study Research Group: Early vitrectomy for severe vitreous hemorrhage in diabetic retinopathy: two-year results of a randomized trial. DRVS Report Number 2. *Arch Ophthalmol* 1985;103:1644–1652.

61. Diabetic Retinopathy Vitrectomy Study Research Group: Early vitrectomy for severe proliferative diabetic retinopathy in eyes with useful vision: results of a randomized trial. DRVS Report Number 3. *Ophthalmology* 1988;95:1307–1320.

62. Early Treatment Diabetic Retinopathy Study Research Group: Early photocoagulation for diabetic retinopathy. ETDRS Report Number 9. *Ophthalmology* 1991;98(suppl):766–785.

CHAPTER 4

Clinical Studies on Treatment for Diabetic Retinopathy

Frederick L. Ferris III, MD

Matthew D. Davis, MD

Lloyd M. Aiello, MD

Emily Y. Chew, MD

Diabetic retinopathy has been, and probably remains, one of the four major causes of blindness in the United States.[1,2] Without treatment, eyes that develop proliferative diabetic retinopathy (PDR) have at least a 50% chance of becoming blind within 5 years.[3-5] Appropriate application of treatments that have been developed in the last three decades can reduce this risk of blindness to less than 5%.[6] Medical treatments designed to maximize blood glucose control and prevent the development of retinopathy can further reduce the risk of blindness.[7] This chapter discusses the treatments available, the evidence that the treatments are effective, and whether the treatments are widely used.

4-1

PHOTOCOAGULATION

Blindness from PDR was a growing public health problem in the 1960s. Although a number of possible treatments were tried, there was general uncertainty as to the best approach for treating diabetic retinopathy.[8]

Introduced by Meyer-Schwickerath, photocoagulation was initially used to coagulate patches of new vessels on the surface of the retina.[9] During the 1960s, it became apparent that extensive retinal photocoagulation seemed to have a beneficial, but unexplained, indirect effect on both neovascularization and macular edema.[10] By the early 1970s, a few small clinical trials had indicated that photocoagulation might be an effective treatment.[11]

4-1-1 Diabetic Retinopathy Study, 1971–1978

Because of the public health importance of the disease and the collective doubt as to its treatment, the Diabetic Retinopathy Study (DRS) was organized in 1971 to test the effect of photocoagulation on diabetic retinopathy (Table 4-1). This was the first randomized, multicenter, collaborative clinical trial sponsored by the newly formed National Eye Institute of the National Institutes of Health. The DRS enrolled 1742 patients with severe nonproliferative or pro-

TABLE 4-1

Diabetic Retinopathy Study

Study Question

Is photocoagulation (argon or xenon) effective for treating diabetic retinopathy?

Eligibility

Proliferative diabetic retinopathy or bilateral severe nonproliferative diabetic retinopathy, with visual acuity 20/100 or better in each eye

Randomization

1742 participants: one eye randomly assigned to photocoagulation (argon or xenon), and one eye assigned to no photocoagulation

Outcome Variable

Visual acuity less than 5/200 for at least 4 months

Result

Photocoagulation (argon or xenon) reduces risk of severe visual loss compared to no treatment

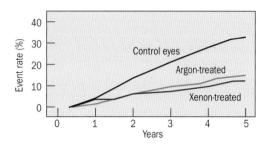

Figure 4-1 *DRS results: Cumulative incidence of severe visual loss (visual acuity worse than 5/200 at two consecutive 4-month followup visits) for untreated eyes (N = 1681), argon-treated eyes (N = 835), and xenon-treated eyes (N = 847). P <0.001 for both treated groups versus control group.*

liferative diabetic retinopathy and visual acuity of 20/100 or better in each eye.[12] The age distribution of the population was bimodal, with 23% in the 20 to 29 years age group and 27% in the 50 to 59 group. The majority of DRS patients were male (56%) and white (94%).

One eye of each patient was randomly assigned to receive photocoagulation, and the fellow eye was observed without treatment. One of two photocoagulation techniques, using either the xenon arc or the newly developed argon laser, was randomly selected. All treated eyes received both direct and scatter photocoagulation, and the treatment techniques, using either photocoagulation modality, were similar.

Direct treatment involved the placement of photocoagulation burns over abnormal new vessels. All neovascularization elsewhere (NVE) was treated directly with either modality, but neovascularization of the disc (NVD) was treated directly only with the argon laser. Direct treatment was also applied to microaneurysms or other lesions thought to be causing macular edema. Scatter photocoagulation consisted of photocoagulation burns placed throughout the midperipheral retina, with each burn separated from its neighbors by one burn width. This resulted in a polka-dot pattern of burns in the retina that extended from the temporal vascular arcades to beyond the equator. In general, the argon laser burns were smaller and less intense than the xenon arc burns.

Analysis of followup data from that study demonstrated a 50% reduction in severe visual loss in eyes that had received photocoagulation (Figure 4-1).[13] Severe visual loss was defined as visual acuity <5/200 at two or more consecutively completed followup visits, which were scheduled at 4-month intervals. In addition to demonstrating that photocoagulation was effective, the DRS identified retinopathy features associated with a particularly high risk of severe visual loss.[14–17] Treatment was recommended for eyes with these high-risk characteristics, which can be summarized as either neovascularization accompanied by vitreous hemorrhage or obvious neovascularization on or near the optic disc (Figure 4-2), even in the absence of vitreous hemorrhage.

After 24 months of followup in the DRS, the rates of severe visual loss for eyes with high-risk characteristics in the control group and treated group were 26% and 11%, respectively. Eyes with PDR but without high-risk characteristics had a much lower risk of developing severe visual loss by 2 years in both the control group and the treated group (7% and 3%, respectively). These rates were even lower for the eyes with nonproliferative diabetic retinopathy (NDPR).

Harmful effects of treatment were greater in the xenon group, as shown in Table 4-2. Of the xenon-treated eyes, 25%

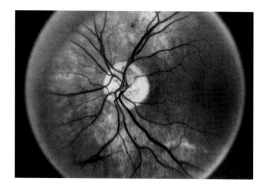

Figure 4-2 *DRS standard photograph 10A demonstrating definite disc neovascularization.*

Published with permission from Diabetic Retinopathy Study Research Group: Photocoagulation treatment of proliferative diabetic retinopathy: the second report of Diabetic Retinopathy Study findings. Ophthalmology *1978;85:82–106.*

TABLE 4-2

Estimated Percentages of Eyes With Harmful Effects Attributable to Treatment in Diabetic Retinopathy Study

Constriction of Visual Field (Goldmann IVe4) to Average of	Argon	Xenon
#45° but >30° per meridian	5%	25%
#30° per meridian	0%	25%
Decrease in Visual Acuity	**Argon**	**Xenon**
1 line	11%	19%
≥2 lines	3%	11%

TABLE 4-3

Early Treatment Diabetic Retinopathy Study

Study Questions

1. Is photocoagulation effective for treating diabetic macular edema?

2. Is early photocoagulation effective for treating diabetic retinopathy?

3. Is aspirin effective for preventing progression of diabetic retinopathy?

Eligibility

Mild nonproliferative diabetic retinopathy through early proliferative diabetic retinopathy, with visual acuity 20/200 or better in each eye

Randomization

3711 participants: one eye randomly assigned to photocoagulation (scatter and/or focal), and one eye assigned to no photocoagulation; patients randomly assigned to 650 mg/d aspirin or placebo

Outcome Variables

Visual acuity less than 5/200 for at least 4 months; visual acuity worsening by doubling of initial visual angle (for example, 20/40 to 20/80); retinopathy progression

suffered a modest loss of visual field, and an additional 25% suffered a more severe loss. Loss of visual field was much less in the argon-treated group, with only 5% of eyes suffering a modest loss as measured using the largest test object (Goldmann IVe4). About 19% of xenon-treated eyes had a persistent visual acuity decrease of one line, which was probably due to treatment, and an additional 11% had a persistent decrease of two or more lines. Comparable estimates for the argon-treated group were 11% and 3%, respectively. Subjectively, many patients noticed difficulties with dark adaptation and driving at night after either argon or xenon scatter photocoagulation.

Based on DRS results and clinical experience, argon laser is recommended, rather than xenon arc, because of similar benefits but fewer side effects. Direct treatment of neovascularization, although part of the original DRS protocol, has generally been discontinued based on the comparison of xenon and argon treatment in eyes with NVD. In the DRS, the argon treatment included direct photocoagulation of NVD, whereas this was not possible with xenon. There was no increase in regression of NVD in the argon group, but there was an increased risk of hemorrhage at the time of focal treatment.

4-1-2 Early Treatment Diabetic Retinopathy Study, 1980–1989

Although scatter photocoagulation was shown by the DRS to be beneficial for patients with high-risk retinopathy, the question remained as to whether treatment at an earlier stage would be more helpful. The

Early Treatment Diabetic Retinopathy Study (ETDRS) was designed to address this question, as well as questions related to the treatment of diabetic macular edema and the use of aspirin (Table 4-3).[18,19] The 3711 ETDRS patients had mild-to-severe NPDR or early PDR, with or without diabetic macular edema. Compared with patients in the DRS, patients in the ETDRS were somewhat older (70% classified as type 2 and 52% over age 50), were less predominantly white (76%), and were equally likely to be male (56%).

All ETDRS patients were randomly assigned to 650 mg aspirin per day or placebo to assess whether the antiplatelet effects of aspirin would affect the microcirculation of the retina and slow the development of PDR.[20–24] One eye of each patient was randomly assigned to immediate photocoagulation, while the fellow eye was assigned to deferral of photocoagulation, that is, careful followup and prompt scatter photocoagulation if high-risk retinopathy developed. If the eye assigned to immediate photocoagulation had macular edema, photocoagulation to areas of edema was also initiated, including direct (focal) treatment of leaking microaneurysms and grid treatment to areas of diffuse leakage.

Aspirin use did not affect the progression of retinopathy (Table 4-4 and Figure 4-3), nor did it affect the risk of visual loss. Perhaps surprisingly, aspirin use did not increase the risk of vitreous hemorrhage in patients with PDR.[25] In addition, aspirin use was associated with a 17% reduction in morbidity and mortality from cardiovascular disease.[26] Therefore, aspirin use should be considered for persons with diabetes, not because of any effect on their diabetic reti-

TABLE 4-4

Early Treatment Diabetic Retinopathy Study: Aspirin Use Results

1. Aspirin use did not alter progression of diabetic retinopathy.

2. Aspirin use did not increase risk of vitreous hemorrhage.

3. Aspirin use did not affect visual acuity.

4. Aspirin use reduced risk of cardiovascular morbidity and mortality.

5. Aspirin use did not increase rates of vitrectomy.

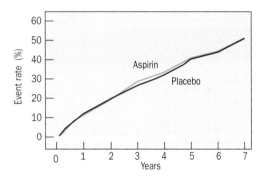

Figure 4-3 *ETDRS results: Cumulative incidence of development of high-risk PDR for eyes assigned to deferral of photocoagulation in patients given placebo (N = 1855) and in aspirin-treated patients (N = 1856). P = 0.58.*

TABLE 4-5

Early Treatment Diabetic Retinopathy Study: Early Scatter Photocoagulation Results

1. Early scatter photocoagulation resulted in small reduction in risk of severe visual loss (<5/200 for at least 4 months).

2. Early scatter photocoagulation is not indicated for eyes with mild-to-moderate diabetic retinopathy.

3. Early scatter photocoagulation may be most effective in patients with type 2 diabetes.

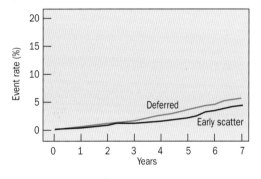

Figure 4-4 *ETDRS results: Cumulative incidence of severe visual loss (<5/200 for at least 4 months) for eyes assigned to early scatter photocoagulation (N = 3711) and eyes assigned to deferral of treatment (N = 3711). P <0.01.*

nopathy, but because of their increased risk of cardiovascular disease. The presence of PDR should not be considered a contraindication to aspirin use.

The ETDRS utilized a factorial study design of aspirin (persons randomized) and photocoagulation (eyes randomized). Because aspirin use had little if any effect on any of the ETDRS ocular outcome variables and aspirin use was not associated with any statistically significant interactions with photocoagulation treatment, all randomized comparisons of photocoagulation treatment versus control combined the aspirin and placebo groups.

The comparison of early photocoagulation versus deferral in the ETDRS revealed a small reduction in the incidence of severe visual loss in the early-treated eyes (Table 4-5 and Figure 4-4), but 5-year rates were low in both the early-treatment group and the deferral group (2.6% and 3.7%, respectively).[27] For eyes with only mild-to-moderate NPDR, rates of progression to severe vision loss were even lower; early photocoagulation benefits were not sufficient to compensate for the unwanted side effects. However, with very severe nonproliferative or early proliferative stages (Figure 4-5), the risk–benefit ratio was more favorable and consideration of initiating scatter photocoagulation before the development of high-risk PDR is suggested.

Recent analyses of ETDRS data suggest that early scatter treatment for eyes with severe NPDR or early PDR is especially effective in reducing severe visual loss in patients with type 2 diabetes (Figure 4-6).[28] These data provide an additional reason to recommend early scatter photocoagulation in older patients with very severe NPDR or early PDR.

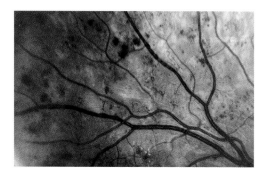

Figure 4-5 *Red-free photograph of eye with severe NPDR.*

The ETDRS results also provide clinically important information to guide the treatment of diabetic macular edema.[29–32] In the ETDRS, focal/grid photocoagulation reduced the risk of moderate visual acuity loss for eyes with diabetic macular edema by about 50% (Table 4-6 and Figure 4-7). Moderate visual acuity loss was defined as a doubling of the visual angle from baseline to followup, for example, 20/20 to 20/40 or 20/50 to 20/100. However, not all eyes with macular edema need immediate treatment. Eyes with edema that either involves or threatens the center of the macula benefit from photocoagulation, but treatment may be deferred when edema is farther from the macular center. Side effects of treatment include scotomas related to the focal laser burns, although there was limited documentation of this using the visual fields as measured in the ETDRS. Careful followup with intervention only when retinal thickening or lipid deposits threaten or involve the center of the macula can reduce the risk of visual loss and limit the number of patients needing treatment.

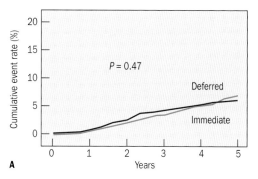

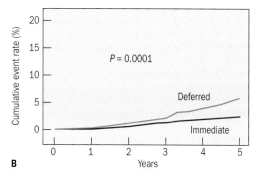

Figure 4-6 *ETDRS results: Cumulative incidence of severe visual loss (<5/200 for at least 4 months) for eyes with (A) severe NPDR or (B) early PDR in patients with type 2 diabetes assigned to early scatter photocoagulation (N = 557) or deferral of photocoagulation (N = 584). P <0.01 for interaction of diabetes type and treatment effect.*

TABLE 4-6

Early Treatment Diabetic Retinopathy Study: Macular Edema Results

1. Focal photocoagulation for diabetic macular edema decreased risk of moderate visual loss (doubling of initial visual angle).

2. Focal photocoagulation for diabetic macular edema increased chance of moderate visual gain (halving of initial visual angle).

3. Focal photocoagulation for diabetic macular edema reduced retinal thickening.

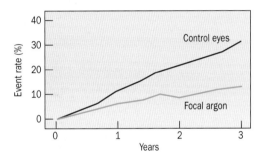

Figure 4-7 *ETDRS results: Proportion of eyes with mild-to-moderate NPDR and macular edema involving center of macula that had loss of three lines of visual acuity from baseline (doubling of initial visual angle, for example, 20/20 to 20/40) for eyes assigned to no treatment (N = 607) or to immediate focal treatment for macular edema (N = 292). P <0.01 for each visit after 4 months.*

4-2

VITRECTOMY

While photocoagulation treatment was being developed, another major advance was added to the practice of ophthalmology. New instrumentation and techniques made it possible to remove the vitreous gel and operate in the posterior aspect of the eye. This vitreous surgery offered hope of dramatic visual improvement in patients with severe vitreous hemorrhage.[33–35]

4-2-1 Diabetic Retinopathy Vitrectomy Study, 1976–1983

The Diabetic Retinopathy Vitrectomy Study (DRVS) provides randomized clinical trial data demonstrating the benefits and risks of vitrectomy in eyes with severe vitreous hemorrhage or very severe neovascularization even in the absence of severe hemorrhage (Table 4-7).[36–40] Results from the DRVS showed that conventional management—deferring vitrectomy for 1 year in patients with severe vitreous hemorrhage or until tractional retinal detachment involved the macula—reduced the chance of obtaining good vision compared to doing early (<6 months) vitrectomy. After 2 years of followup, 25% of the early-vitrectomy group had visual acuity of 20/40 or better, compared with 15% in the deferral group (P = 0.01). For patients with type 1 diabetes, who were on the average younger and had more severe PDR, this difference at 2 years was even greater (36% versus 12% , P = 0.001).

Early vitrectomy was also effective in saving good visual acuity in patients without severe vitreous hemorrhage, but with severe or very severe PDR. The early-treated group had a higher percentage of eyes with 20/40 or better visual acuity at each of the 6-month visits during the 4 years of follow-up. About one third of treated eyes with more severe retinopathy had good vision at these 6-month visits, compared to less than 20% of the deferral eyes ($P <0.05$ at every visit except the 6- and 24-month visits).

In both trials, the proportion of eyes with no light perception vision reached about 20% to 25% at 4 years in both the treated and the control groups, but there were more patients with no light perception in the treated group during the first several years of followup, especially in those eyes with the least severe retinopathy. Complications during followup included phthisis, endophthalmitis or uveitis, and corneal epithelial problems or neovascular glaucoma. Up to one third of treated eyes had at least one of these complications.[37-40]

Vitrectomy techniques have progressed considerably since this clinical trial. Instrumentation is markedly improved and photocoagulation can be done at the time of vitrectomy. Side effects have been reduced.[41-44] These clinical trial data, supported by additional case series, document the value of vitrectomy in eyes with very severe PDR or severe vitreous hemorrhage.

4-3

MEDICAL APPROACHES

Although photocoagulation, in combination with vitrectomy when necessary, is markedly effective in reducing the risk of blindness in persons with diabetic retinopathy, prevention of the development of retinopathy would be even more effective in preserving vision.

TABLE 4-7

Diabetic Retinopathy Vitrectomy Study

Study Questions

Is early vitrectomy preferable to deferral of vitrectomy in eyes with:

1. Severe vitreous hemorrhage from proliferative diabetic retinopathy?

2. Very severe proliferative diabetic retinopathy?

Eligibility

Recent severe vitreous hemorrhage from proliferative diabetic retinopathy (616 eyes); advanced, active, severe proliferative diabetic retinopathy (370 eyes, 240 with prior scatter photocoagulation)

Randomization

Early vitrectomy versus conventional management

Outcome Variable

Visual acuity 20/40 or better

Results

Visual acuity 20/40 or better was more frequent in early-vitrectomy groups (1 to 6 months from baseline); benefit of early vitrectomy was seen only in eyes with most severe proliferative diabetic retinopathy

TABLE 4-8

Diabetes Control and Complications Trial

Study Questions

1. Primary prevention study: Will intensive control of blood glucose slow development and subsequent progression of diabetic retinopathy?

2. Secondary prevention study: Will intensive control of blood glucose slow progression of diabetic retinopathy?

Eligibility

1. 726 patients with insulin-dependent diabetes mellitus (1 to 5 years' duration) and no diabetic retinopathy

2. 715 patients with insulin-dependent diabetes mellitus (1 to 15 years' duration) and mild-to-moderate diabetic retinopathy

Randomization

Intensive control of blood glucose (multiple daily insulin injections or insulin pump) versus conventional management

Outcome Variables

Development of diabetic retinopathy or progression of retinopathy by three steps using modified Airlie House classification scale; neuropathy, nephropathy, and cardiovascular outcomes were also assessed

Results

Intensive control reduced risk of developing retinopathy by 76% and slowed progression of retinopathy by 54%; intensive control also reduced risk of clinical neuropathy by 60% and albuminuria by 54%

4-3-1 Blood Glucose Control

For years, there was debate as to whether improved control of blood glucose would reduce the chronic complications of diabetes, including diabetic retinopathy.

4-3-1-1 Diabetes Control and Complications Trial, 1983–1989

The Diabetes Control and Complications Trial (DCCT) was initiated to address this important clinical and scientific question.[45] The DCCT enrolled 1441 patients with type 1 diabetes (726 with no retinopathy and 715 with mild-to-moderate NPDR at baseline). These patients were randomly assigned to either intensive or conventional insulin therapy. Not only was there a remarkable reduction in the rate of development or progression of retinopathy in those patients assigned to intensive treatment (Table 4-8 and Figure 4-8), there was also a reduction in the progression of diabetic nephropathy and neuropathy.[46–48]

A smaller randomized clinical trial of 102 patients with type 1 diabetes, observed for more than 7 years, also found that intensified insulin treatment reduced all three of the major microvascular complications of diabetes.[49] These consistent clinical trial results, combined with the strong observational study results,[50] directly implicate elevated blood glucose in the development of the chronic microvascular complications of diabetes.

Evidence is accumulating to confirm the impression that microvascular complications are the result of chronic elevations of blood glucose. These complications take years to develop and are directly associated with long-term elevations of glycosylated hemoglobin. It also appears that it may take years to realize the benefits of effective interventions to lower blood glucose.

Early studies of the effect of intensified glucose control on retinopathy actually demonstrated an unanticipated and paradoxical worsening of retinopathy in patients whose blood glucose control was markedly improved.[51–57] However, in patients with mild-to-moderate NPDR, this early worsening is not usually associated with visual loss, and the long-term benefits of intensive insulin treatment greatly outweighed this risk in the DCCT.[58] When intensive insulin treatment is to be instituted in patients who have PDR or severe NPDR, ophthalmologic consultation is desirable because photocoagulation may be indicated.

The effect of glycemic control on the incidence and progression of diabetic microvascular complications, as assessed in observational studies, is similar in both type 1 and type 2 patients.[59] Randomized studies of the effect of intensive glucose control on type 2 patients in Japan and the United Kingdom have demonstrated benefits from reduced blood glucose similar to those found for type 1 patients by the DCCT.[60–62]

The clinical implications of the DCCT results have been extensively discussed, and the evidence is compelling that better blood glucose control lowers the risk of the chronic complications of diabetes. Data exist to suggest that avoiding prolonged blood glucose elevations may be useful for most patients with diabetes. Unfortunately, although the risk is significantly reduced with intensive effort, it is not yet eliminated for many patients. The search for additional methods of preventing and treating the chronic complications of diabetes, including retinopathy, therefore continues.

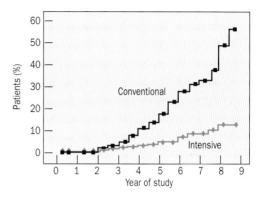

Figure 4-8 *DCCT results: Cumulative incidence of sustained worsening of retinopathy (three steps on modified Airlie House scale for at least 6 months) in patients with type 1 diabetes and no diabetic retinopathy at baseline receiving intensive (N = 342) or conventional (N = 375) insulin therapy. P <0.001.*

Redrawn with permission from Diabetes Control and Complications Trial Research Group: The effect of intensive treatment of diabetes on the development and progression of long-term complications in insulin-dependent diabetes mellitus. N Engl J Med 1993;329:977–986. Copyright © 1993, Massachusetts Medical Society. All rights reserved.

4-3-2 Serum Lipid Lowering

Some currently available treatments may be effective in slowing the progression of diabetic retinopathy or reducing its complications. Higher serum lipids are associated with a greater risk of developing high-risk PDR, as well as with a greater risk of developing vision loss from diabetic macular edema and associated retinal hard exudates. Therefore, in addition to reducing the risk of cardiovascular disease, lowering elevated serum lipids may also reduce the risk of vision loss from diabetic retinopathy.[63]

4-3-3 Blood Pressure Lowering

A randomized clinical trial of lisinopril, an inhibitor of angiotensin-converting enzyme (ACE), suggested that ACE inhibition or blood pressure lowering, even in normotensive persons, may slow the progression of diabetic retinopathy.[64]

4-3-3-1 United Kingdom Prospective Diabetes Study, 1981–1998 Data from another randomized clinical trial, the United Kingdom Prospective Diabetes Study (UKPDS), suggest that it may be the blood pressure lowering that is responsible for slowing the progression of retinopathy and not a specific retina–vascular response to ACE inhibition.[65,66] The UKPDS showed that both captopril, an ACE inhibitor, and atenolol, a beta blocker, were effective in slowing the progression of retinopathy compared with the control group and that there was no statistically significant difference between the two treatment groups.

4-3-4 Aldose-Reductase Inhibition

A medical approach for preventing the development of retinopathy that has been hypothesized for decades involves blocking the effects of aldose reductase.[67] This enzyme facilitates the conversion of glucose to sorbitol, which accumulates in cells during hyperglycemia and may result in cell death.[68,69] Animal experiments suggest that an aldose-reductase inhibitor could slow the development of diabetic retinopathy.[70,71] Unfortunately, clinical trials in patients with diabetes have not yet demonstrated any slowing of the progression of retinopathy.

4-3-4-1 Sorbinil Retinopathy Trial, 1983–1985 The Sorbinil Retinopathy Trial (SRT) enrolled 497 patients with type 1 diabetes and little or no retinopathy. After 3 to 4 years of followup, progression of diabetic retinopathy and neuropathy was apparently unaffected by administration of the drug sorbinil (Table 4-9 and Figure 4-9).[72,73] However, interest continues in developing more potent inhibitors, which may slow the progression of diabetic retinopathy or neuropathy.

4-3-5 Other Medical Investigations

Other medical approaches to reduce the secondary complications of diabetes are currently under evaluation. Drugs with antiangiogenic activity, such as inhibitors of vascular endothelial growth factor (VEGF), protein kinase C inhibitors, and growth hormone antagonists are in early clinical trials, as are inhibitors of advanced glycosylated end products.[74–77] Prevention will inevitably be more effective than treatment, and methods to prevent the development of diabetes and improved techniques for blood glucose control are also being tested.

TABLE 4-9

Sorbinil Retinopathy Study

Study Question

Does aldose-reductase inhibitor sorbinil reduce rate of progression of diabetic retinopathy?

Eligibility

Type 1 diabetes of 1 to 15 years' duration and no more than 5 microaneurysms in either eye

Randomization

497 patients randomly assigned to sorbinil (250 mg/d) or placebo

Outcome Variable

Progression of retinopathy

Result

No significant reduction in progression of retinopathy in treated eyes compared with placebo

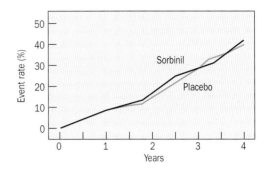

Figure 4-9 *SRT results: Cumulative incidence of sustained worsening of retinopathy (two steps on modified Airlie House scale for at least 6 months) in patients with type 1 diabetes with mild or no retinopathy at baseline receiving placebo or 250 mg/d sorbinil.*

4-4

CONCLUSION

The history of the development of treatments for diabetic retinopathy is one of the best examples of the use of evidence-based patient care. From developing methods of preventing retinopathy to treatment with photocoagulation or vitrectomy, there are clinical trial results that reveal which treatments are effective, who is most at risk, and who will benefit most from intervention.

Diabetic retinopathy is probably still the leading cause of visual loss in the United States among working-age Americans. This is surprising because, when diabetes is properly treated, the 5-year risk of blindness for patients with PDR is reduced by 90% and the risk of visual loss from mac-

TABLE 4-10

Recommended Eye Examination Schedule

Time of Onset of Diabetes	Recommended Time for First Examination	Routine Minimum Followup
<30 years of age	Just prior to, or soon after, conception	Yearly
≥30 years of age	5 years after onset or at puberty	Yearly
Prior to pregnancy	At time of diagnosis	Every 3 months or at discretion of ophthalmologist

ular edema is reduced by 50%. Unfortunately, only 50% of patients with diabetes receive regular dilated eye examinations and many patients go blind without treatment,[78–80] despite the fact that the value of screening eye examinations has been well documented.[81]

Many professional groups, including the American Diabetes Association, the American College of Physicians, the American Academy of Ophthalmology, and the American Optometric Association, have provided guidelines for their members as to when eye examinations should be performed, as summarized in Table 4-10. Emphasis on identifying patients at risk and new screening methods will hopefully reduce the number of patients who do not have regular eye examinations.

Improved patient education programs, such as the National Eye Health Education Program, can motivate patients to take better care of themselves.[82–84] Access to the educational materials and facilities that will enable patients to improve the control of their diabetes will lead to fewer secondary complications.

Prevention is cost-effective.[85–88] The record of carefully developing new treatments for diabetic retinopathy is a good one. With continued careful research, the risk of blindness from diabetic retinopathy can be further reduced.

ACKNOWLEDGMENT

This chapter has been adapted from Ferris FL, Davis MD, Aiello LM: Treatment of diabetic retinopathy. *New Engl J Med* 1999;341:667–678.

REFERENCES

1. Kahn HA, Hiller R: Blindness caused by diabetic retinopathy. *Am J Ophthalmol* 1974;78:58–67.

2. Kahn HA, Bradley RF: Prevalence of diabetic retinopathy: age, sex, and duration of diabetes. *Br J Ophthalmol* 1975;59:345–349.

3. Beetham WP: Visual prognosis of proliferating diabetic retinopathy. *Br J Ophthalmol* 1963;47:611–619.

4. Caird FI, Burditt AF, Draper GJ: Diabetic retinopathy: a further study of prognosis for vision. *Diabetes* 1968;17:121–123.

5. Deckert T, Simonsen SE, Poulson JE: Prognosis of proliferative retinopathy in juvenile diabetics. *Diabetes* 1967;16:728–733.

6. Ferris FL III: How effective are treatments for diabetic retinopathy? *J Am Med Assoc* 1993; 269:1290–1291.

7. Diabetes Control and Complications Trial Research Group: The effect of intensive treatment of diabetes on the development and progression of long-term complications in insulin-dependent diabetes mellitus. *N Engl J Med* 1993;329: 977–986.

8. Goldberg MF, Fine SL, eds: *Symposium on the Treatment of Diabetic Retinopathy.* (Airlie House, 1968) Public Health Service Publ. No. 1890. Washington, DC: US Govt Printing Office; 1969.

9. Meyer-Schwickerath G: *Light Coagulation.* Drance SM, trans. St Louis: CV Mosby Co; 1960.

10. Beetham WP, Aiello LM, Balodimos MC, Koncz L: Ruby-laser photocoagulation of early diabetic neovascular retinopathy: preliminary report of a long-term controlled study. *Trans Am Ophthalmol Soc* 1969;67:39–67.

11. Ederer F, Hiller R: Clinical trials, diabetic retinopathy and photocoagulation: a reanalysis of five studies. *Surv Ophthalmol* 1975;19:267–286.

12. Diabetic Retinopathy Study Research Group: Design, methods, and baseline results. DRS Report Number 6. *Invest Ophthalmol* 1981;21: 149–209.

13. Diabetic Retinopathy Study Research Group: Preliminary report on effects of photocoagulation therapy. *Am J Ophthalmol* 1976;81:383–396.

14. Diabetic Retinopathy Study Research Group: Photocoagulation treatment of proliferative diabetic retinopathy: clinical application of diabetic retinopathy study (DRS) findings. DRS Report Number 8. *Ophthalmology* 1981;88:583–600.

15. Diabetic Retinopathy Study Research Group: Photocoagulation treatment of proliferative diabetic retinopathy: the second report of Diabetic Retinopathy Study findings. *Ophthalmology* 1978; 85:82–106.

16. Diabetic Retinopathy Study Research Group: Four risk factors for severe visual loss in diabetic retinopathy: the third report from the Diabetic Retinopathy Study. *Arch Ophthalmol* 1979;97: 654–655.

17. Diabetic Retinopathy Study Research Group: Photocoagulation treatment of proliferative diabetic retinopathy: relationship of adverse treatment effects to retinopathy severity. DRS Report Number 5. *Dev Ophthalmol* 1981;2:248–261.

18. Early Treatment Diabetic Retinopathy Study Research Group: Early Treatment Diabetic Retinopathy Study design and baseline patient characteristics. ETDRS Report Number 7. *Ophthalmology* 1991;98(suppl):741–756.

19. Early Treatment Diabetic Retinopathy Study Research Group: Effects of aspirin treatment on diabetic retinopathy. ETDRS Report Number 8. *Ophthalmology* 1991;98(suppl):757–765.

20. Sagel J, Colwell JA, Crook L, Laimins M: Increased platelet aggregation in early diabetes mellitus. *Ann Intern Med* 1975;82:733–738.

21. Dobbie JG, Kwaan HC, Colwell JA, Suwanwela N: The role of platelets in pathogenesis of diabetic retinopathy. *Trans Am Acad Ophthalmol Otolaryngol* 1973;77:OP43–OP47.

22. Regnault F: [The role of platelets in the pathogenesis of diabetic retinopathy.] *Sem Hop* (Paris) 1972;48:893–902.

23. Powell ED, Field RA: Diabetic retinopathy and rheumatoid arthritis. *Lancet* 1964;42:17–18.

24. Carroll WW, Geeraets WJ: Diabetic retinopathy and salicylates. *Ann Ophthalmol* 1972;4:1019–1045.

25. Chew EY, Klein ML, Murphy RP, et al: Effects of aspirin on vitreous/preretinal hemorrhage in patients with diabetes mellitus. ETDRS Report Number 20. *Arch Ophthalmol* 1995;113:52–55.

26. Early Treatment Diabetic Retinopathy Study Research Group: Aspirin effects on mortality and morbidity in patients with diabetes mellitus. ETDRS Report Number 14. *J Am Med Assoc* 1992;268:1292–1300.

27. Early Treatment Diabetic Retinopathy Study Research Group: Early photocoagulation for diabetic retinopathy. ETDRS Report Number 9. *Ophthalmology* 1991;98(suppl):766–785.

28. Ferris F: Early photocoagulation in patients with either type I or type II diabetes. *Trans Am Ophthalmol Soc* 1996;94:505–537.

29. Early Treatment Diabetic Retinopathy Study Research Group: Photocoagulation for diabetic macular edema. ETDRS Report Number 1. *Arch Ophthalmol* 1985;103:1796–1806.

30. Early Treatment Diabetic Retinopathy Study Research Group: Treatment techniques and clinical guidelines for photocoagulation of diabetic macular edema. ETDRS Report Number 2. *Ophthalmology* 1987;94:761–774.

31. Early Treatment Diabetic Retinopathy Study Research Group: Techniques for scatter and local photocoagulation treatment of diabetic retinopathy. ETDRS Report Number 3. *Int Ophthalmol Clin* 1987;27:254–264.

32. Early Treatment Diabetic Retinopathy Study Research Group: Photocoagulation for diabetic macular edema. ETDRS Report Number 4. *Int Ophthalmol Clin* 1987;27:265–272.

33. Machemer R, Parel JM, Buettner H: A new concept for vitreous surgery, I: instrumentation. *Am J Ophthalmol* 1972;73:1–7.

34. Machemer R: A new concept for vitreous surgery, 2: surgical technique and complications. *Am J Ophthalmol* 1972;74:1022–1033.

35. Machemer R, Norton EW: A new concept for vitreous surgery, 3: indications and results. *Am J Ophthalmol* 1972;74:1034–1056.

36. Diabetic Retinopathy Vitrectomy Study Research Group: Two-year course of visual acuity in severe proliferative diabetic retinopathy with conventional management. DRVS Report Number 1. *Ophthalmology* 1985;92:492–502.

37. Diabetic Retinopathy Vitrectomy Study Research Group: Early vitrectomy for severe vitreous hemorrhage in diabetic retinopathy: two-year results of a randomized trial. DRVS Report Number 2. *Arch Ophthalmol* 1985;103:1644–1652.

38. Diabetic Retinopathy Vitrectomy Study Research Group: Early vitrectomy for severe proliferative diabetic retinopathy in eyes with useful vision: results of a randomized trial. DRVS Report Number 3. *Ophthalmology* 1988;95:1307–1320.

39. Diabetic Retinopathy Vitrectomy Study Research Group: Early vitrectomy for severe proliferative diabetic retinopathy in eyes with useful vision: clinical application of results of a randomized trial. DRVS Report Number 4. *Ophthalmology* 1988;95:1321–1334.

40. Diabetic Retinopathy Vitrectomy Study Research Group: Early vitrectomy for severe vitreous hemorrhage in diabetic retinopathy: four-year results of a randomized trial. DRVS Report Number 5. *Arch Ophthalmol* 1990;108:958–964.

41. Smiddy WE, Feuer W, Irvine WD, et al: Vitrectomy for complications of proliferative diabetic retinopathy: functional outcomes. *Ophthalmology* 1995;102:1688–1695.

42. Smiddy W: Vitrectomy for complications of diabetic retinopathy. *Int Ophthalmol Clin* 1998;38:155–167.

43. Early Treatment Diabetic Retinopathy Study Research Group: Pars plana vitrectomy in the Early Treatment Diabetic Retinopathy Study. ETDRS Report Number 17. *Ophthalmology* 1992;99:1351–1357.

44. Smiddy, WE, Flynn HW Jr: Vitrectomy in the management of diabetic retinopathy. *Surv Ophthalmol* 1999;43:491–507.

45. Diabetes Control and Complications Trial Research Group: The Diabetes Control and Complications Trial (DCCT): design and methodologic considerations for the feasibility phase. *Diabetes* 1986;35:530–545.

46. Diabetes Control and Complications Trial Research Group: The effect of intensive treatment of diabetes on the development and progression of long-term complications in insulin-dependent diabetes mellitus. *N Engl J Med* 1993;329:977–986.

47. Diabetes Control and Complications Trial Research Group: Effect of intensive therapy on the development and progression of diabetic nephropathy in the Diabetes Control and Complications Trial. *Kidney Int* 1995;47:1703–1720.

48. Diabetes Control and Complications Trial Research Group: Effect of intensive diabetes treatment on nerve conduction in the Diabetes Control and Complications Trial. *Ann Neurol* 1995;38:869–880.

49. Reichard P, Nilsson BY, Rosenqvist U: The effect of long-term intensified insulin treatment on the development of microvascular complications of diabetes mellitus. *N Engl J Med* 1993;329:304–309.

50. Klein R, Klein BE, Moss SE, et al: Glycosylated hemoglobin predicts the incidence and progression of diabetic retinopathy. *J Am Med Assoc* 1988;260:2864–2871.

51. Dahl-Jorgensen K, Brinchmann-Hansen O, Hanssen KF, et al: Rapid tightening of blood glucose control leads to transient deterioration of retinopathy in insulin dependent diabetes mellitus: the Oslo Study. *Br Med J* 1985;290:811–815.

52. Daneman D, Drash A, Lobes LA, et al: Progressive retinopathy with improved control in diabetic dwarfism (Mauriac's syndrome). *Diabetes Care* 1981;4:360–365.

53. Puklin JE, Tamborlane WV, Felig P, et al: Influence of long-term insulin infusion pump treatment of type I diabetes on diabetic retinopathy. *Ophthalmology* 1982;89:735–747.

54. Lauritzen T, Frost-Larsen K, Larsen HW, Deckert T: Effect of 1 year of near-normal blood glucose levels on retinopathy. *Lancet* 1983;1:200–204.

55. Lauritzen T, Frost-Larsen K, Larsen HW, Deckert T: Two-year experience with continuous subcutaneous insulin infusion in relation to retinopathy and neuropathy. *Diabetes* 1985;34 (suppl):74–79.

56. Kroc Collaborative Study Group: Blood glucose control and the evolution of diabetic retinopathy and albuminuria: a multicenter trial. *N Engl J Med* 1984;311:365–372.

57. Kroc Collaborative Study Group: Diabetic retinopathy after two years of intensified insulin treatment: follow-up of the Kroc Collaborative Study. *J Am Med Assoc* 1988;260:37–41.

58. Diabetes Control and Complications Trial Research Group: Early worsening of diabetic retinopathy in the Diabetes Control and Complications Trial. *Arch Ophthalmol* 1998;116: 874–886.

59. Klein R, Klein BE, Moss SE: Relation of glycemic control to diabetic microvascular complications in diabetes mellitus. *Ann Intern Med* 1996;124:90–96.

60. Ohkubo Y, Kishikawa H, Araki E, et al: Intensive insulin therapy prevents the progression of diabetic microvascular complications in Japanese patients with non–insulin-dependent diabetes mellitus: a randomized prospective 6-year study. *Diabetes Res Clin Pract* 1995;28:103–117.

61. United Kingdom Prospective Diabetes Study Group: Intensive blood-glucose control with sulphonylureas or insulin compared with conventional treatment and risk of complications in patients with type 2 diabetes. UKPDS 33. *Lancet* 1998;352:837–853.

62. United Kingdom Prospective Diabetes Study Group: Effect of intensive blood-glucose control with metformin on complications in overweight patients with type 2 diabetes. UKPDS 34. *Lancet* 1998;352:854–865.

63. Chew EY, Klein ML, Ferris FL III, et al: Association of elevated serum lipid levels with retinal hard exudate in diabetic retinopathy. ETDRS Report Number 22. *Arch Ophthalmol* 1996;114:1079–1084.

64. Chaturvedi N, Sjolie AK, Stephenson JM, et al: Effect of lisinopril on progression of retinopathy in normotensive people with type 1 diabetes. EUCLID Study Group. EURODIAB Controlled Trial of Lisinopril in Insulin-Dependent Diabetes Mellitus. *Lancet* 1998;351:28–31.

65. United Kingdom Prospective Diabetes Study Group: Tight blood pressure control and risk of macrovascular and microvascular complications in type 2 diabetes. UKPDS 38. *Br Med J* 1998; 317:703–713.

66. United Kingdom Prospective Diabetes Study Group: Efficacy of atenolol and captopril in reducing risk of macrovascular and microvascular complications in type 2 diabetes. UKPDS 39. *Br Med J* 1998;317:713–720.

67. Frank RN: The aldose reductase controversy. *Diabetes* 1994;43:169–172.

68. Kinoshita JH: Mechanisms initiating cataract formation. [Proctor Lecture] *Invest Ophthalmol* 1974;13:713–724.

69. Gabbay KH: Hyperglycemia, polyol metabolism, and complications of diabetes mellitus. *Ann Rev Med* 1975;26:521–536.

70. Kador PF, Akagi Y, Takahashi Y, et al: Prevention of retinal vessel changes associated with diabetic retinopathy in galactose-fed dogs by aldose reductase inhibitors. *Arch Ophthalmol* 1990; 108:1301–1309.

71. Robinson WG Jr, Laver NM, Jacot JL, et al: Diabetic-like retinopathy ameliorated with the aldose reductase inhibitor WAY-121,509. *Invest Ophthalmol Vis Sci* 1996;37:1149–1156.

72. Sorbinil Retinopathy Trial Research Group: A randomized trial of sorbinil, an aldose reductase inhibitor, in diabetic retinopathy. *Arch Ophthalmol* 1990;108:1234–1244.

73. Sorbinil Retinopathy Trial Research Group: The sorbinil retinopathy trial: neuropathy results. *Neurology* 1993;43:1141–1149.

74. Aiello LP, Pierce EA, Foley ED, et al: Suppression of retinal neovascularization in vivo by inhibition of vascular endothelial growth factor (VEGF) using soluble VEGF-receptor chimeric proteins. *Proc Natl Acad Sci USA* 1995; 92:10457–10461.

75. Smith LE, Kopchick JJ, Chen W, et al: Essential role of growth hormone in ischemia-induced retinal neovascularization. *Science* 1997; 276:1706–1709.

76. Brownlee M, Cerami A, Vlassara H: Advanced glycosylation end products in tissue and the biochemical basis of diabetic complications. *N Engl J Med* 1988;318:1315–1321.

77. Brownlee M, Vlassara H, Kooney A, et al: Aminoguanidine prevents diabetes-induced arterial wall protein cross-linking. *Science* 1986;232: 1629–1632.

78. Moss SE, Klein R, Klein BE: Factors associated with having eye examinations in persons with diabetes. *Arch Fam Med* 1995;4:529–534.

79. Sprafka JM, Fritsche TL, Baker R, et al: Prevalence of undiagnosed eye disease in high-risk diabetic individuals. *Arch Intern Med* 1990; 150:857–861.

80. Will JC, German RR, Schuman E, et al: Patient adherence to guidelines for diabetes eye care: results from the diabetic eye disease follow-up study. *Am J Public Health* 1994;84: 1669–1671.

81. Javitt JC, Canner JK, Sommer A: Cost effectiveness of current approaches to the control of retinopathy in type I diabetics. *Ophthalmology* 1989;96:255–264.

82. Kupfer C: The challenge of transferring research results into patient care. *Ophthalmology* 1989;96:737–738.

83. Klein R: Eye-care delivery for people with diabetes: an unmet need. *Diabetes Care* 1994; 17:614–615.

84. Klein R: Barriers to prevention of vision loss caused by diabetic retinopathy. *Arch Ophthalmol* 1997;115:1073–1075.

85. Diabetes Control and Complications Trial Research Group: Lifetime benefits and costs of intensive therapy as practiced in the Diabetes Control and Complications Trial. *J Am Med Assoc* 1996;276:1409–1415.

86. Ackerman SJ: Benefits of preventive programs in eye care are visible on the bottom line: a new nationwide effort to improve eye care for people with diabetes gets backing from a study on the cost-effectiveness of screening for retinopathy. *Diabetes Care* 1992;15:580–581.

87. Javitt JC, Aiello LP, Chiang Y, et al: Preventive eye care in people with diabetes is cost-saving to the federal government: implications for health-care reform. *Diabetes Care* 1994;17: 909–917.

88. Javitt JC, Aiello LP: Cost-effectiveness of detecting and treating diabetic retinopathy. *Ann Intern Med* 1996;124:164–169.

Photography, Angiography, and Ultrasonography in Diabetic Retinopathy

Gaurav K. Shah, MD
Gary C. Brown, MD

In addition to the clinical examination, color fundus photography, fluorescein angiography, and ultrasonography are important in the evaluation and management of diabetic retinopathy. This chapter reviews the clinical usefulness and indications for ancillary testing in the management of diabetic retinopathy.

5-1

COLOR FUNDUS PHOTOGRAPHY

Color fundus photography is an important tool that can be used to document retinal findings in diabetic patients.[1] It can be used for tracking the progression of the disease and also in some instances for the screening of diabetic retinopathy.[2] Photographs may be very helpful for following subtle changes in the posterior pole and for patients with evolving disease. For comparison purposes, it is essential that photographs be produced in a consistent, standardized manner, that is, similar exposure and field of view. Guidelines for the use of color fundus photography are given in Table 5-1; use must be individualized.

Color fundus photographs may be obtained in either stereoscopic or nonstereoscopic fashion, depending on the capabilities of the camera. They can be performed in the traditional seven stereoscopic 30° fields or wide-angle 60° fields. Both 30° and 60° have advantages and disadvantages, but in general the seven stereoscopic 30° fields provide the most complete coverage, and the 60° view is useful in more advanced proliferative disease with vitreous traction. In some instances, fundus photography can be used at the initial examination and may be repeated either to document significant progression of disease or to track responses to treatment.[3,4] Fundus photography may

TABLE 5-1

Uses of Color Fundus Photography in Diabetic Retinopathy

Situation	Yes	Occasionally	No
Before retinal surgery	X		
To document severe, changing disease	X		
When significant pathology is present		X	
At initial examination as baseline for subsequent examination		X	
After treatment		X	
To document minimal diabetic retinopathy			X
To document stable diabetic retinopathy			X

Source: Diabetic Retinopathy. *Preferred Practice Pattern. San Francisco: American Academy of Ophthalmology; 1998.*

be used to assess retinal thickening or to document the proximity to the foveal avascular zone.[5]

Ophthalmoscopy and fundus photography are best used in concert for screening. Indirect ophthalmoscopy allows examination of the peripheral fundus, provides stereopsis, and allows the viewer to look around media opacities.[6] Direct ophthalmoscopy, even in the hands of an experienced ophthalmologist, has a sensitivity as low as 65% for the detection of sight-threatening disease.[7] Fundus photography provides detailed, quality images for grading retinopathy. Fundus photographs may miss cases of proliferative disease that occur outside the area covered by the photographic field. If fundus photographs are used, they must be graded by a person trained in the

detection of diabetic retinopathy. Besides the documentation of diabetic retinopathy, the role of fundus photography is being investigated for telemedicine applications.

Digital retinal images are being increasingly used, instead of 35-mm color transparencies, for screening diabetic retinopathy in medically underserved populations.[8–12] As technology improves, telemedicine will become a more important part of the screening process and of tracking patients with diabetic retinopathy.

5-2

FLUORESCEIN ANGIOGRAPHY

In 1955, MacClean and Maumenee were the first to use intravenous fluorescein in humans to aid in the differential diagnosis of choroidal hemangiomas and choroidal melanomas.[13] Then, in 1960, Novotny and Alvis developed the present technique of

TABLE 5-2

Uses of Fluorescein Angiography in Diabetic Retinopathy

Situation	Yes	Occasionally	No
Guiding treatment of clinically significant macular edema	X		
Evaluating unexplained visual loss	X		
Determining extent of peripheral capillary nonperfusion		X	
Searching for subtle neovascularization		X	
Screening patient with no or minimal diabetic retinopathy			X

Source: Diabetic Retinopathy. *Preferred Practice Pattern. San Francisco: American Academy of Ophthalmology; 1998.*

fluorescein angiography.[14] While orally administered fluorescein has been attempted, intravenous administration is still the exclusive standard for acceptable resolution.

Sodium fluorescein, which is protein-bound to albumin, is the dye used in fluorescein angiography. It diffuses freely through the choriocapillaris, Bruch's membrane, optic nerve, and sclera. However, it does not diffuse through the tight junctions of the retinal endothelial cells, the retinal pigment epithelium, and the larger choroidal vessels. A physiologic inner blood–retina barrier exists at the level of the retinal capillaries due to the tight junctions (zonula occludens) within these vessels. If there is a disruption of the inner blood–retina barrier, dye leakage occurs. The tight junctions between the retinal pigment epithelial cells constitute the outer blood–retina barrier, which, under normal nonpathologic conditions, is also impermeable to fluorescein.

Understanding the external and internal retinal vascular barriers is the key to understanding and interpreting a fluorescein angiogram. Fluorescein angiographic quality depends on technique, filters, film, ocular media, and patient cooperation. Lenticular opacities, such as cataracts, scatter light, and the yellow lens absorbs the blue excitation light. Media opacities, such as vitreous hemorrhages, also impair the fluorescein test. By contrast, a remarkably normal study can be obtained through asteroid hyalosis.

Fluorescein angiography does not have a role in the screening of diabetic retinopathy. Guidelines for the use of fluorescein angiography are given in Table 5-2; use must be individualized. Although sodium fluorescein is generally safe, severe anaphylactic reactions can occur in some patients (1 in 200,000).[15,16]

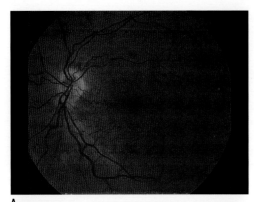

A

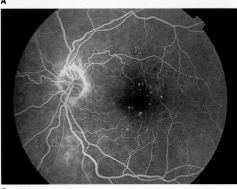

B

Figure 5-1 *Microaneurysms in perifoveal region.
(A) Color photograph. (B) Fluorescein angiogram.*

5-2-1 Mild Nonproliferative Retinopathy

In early stages of mild nonproliferative diabetic retinopathy (NPDR), there may be a few discrete microaneurysms (MAs), with normal vision (Figure 5-1). Although fluorescein angiography may show more MAs than are detected on clinical examination, it is usually not necessary for management or evaluating severity of retinopathy.[17] Fluorescein angiography has been reported to have greater sensitivity than do color stereoscopic fundus photographs for the detection of MAs.[18] Histologically proven MAs that are associated with definite abnormalities on fluorescein angiography could not be correlated with color photographs.[18,19]

Irregular or hyalinized MAs are difficult to find in photographs because the hyalinized vessel walls contrast poorly with the fundus background.[20] One report documented that 4 times as many MAs were detected with fluorescein angiography as with color or red-free photographs.[21] The Diabetes Control and Complications Trial (DCCT) and Friberg and associates noted similar changes.[22–24]

These results indicate that MAs detected with fluorescein angiography and photographs may reflect different structural alterations in the retina. It is possible that small red dots in color fundus photographs represent hemorrhages rather than MAs. In some cases, even fluorescein angiography did not demonstrate histologically proven MAs because some aneurysms become temporarily nonperfused at the time of angiography. A study by Kohner and Henkind[25] noted fluorescent spots that disappeared and reappeared in serial angiographic studies of diabetic patients. The authors attributed intermittent perfusion to reversible plugging of the neck of MAs with aggregated red blood cells.

Several histologic types of MAs have been identified.[25,26] The main types in one study were as follows:

1. Endothelium-lined MAs containing white blood cells

2. MAs devoid of endothelium containing viable red blood cells

3. Occluded MAs containing breakdown debris of red blood cells

4. Sclerosed, fibrotic MAs

The various types may have different appearance rates on angiography. If fluorescein angiography is used, it is important to concentrate on the area of greatest interest and yield. In early diabetic retinopathy, the macula and the area temporal to the macula are the fields most likely to show MAs. MAs in the retinal periphery are less frequent and, if present, are less numerous than in the macular region. The clinical correlates and significance of these types of MAs are not clearly defined.

5-2-2 Moderate Nonproliferative Retinopathy Without Macular Edema

Fluorescein angiography is generally not indicated for patients with moderate NPDR, unless the degree of visual loss seems to exceed the diabetic retinopathy. Color photographs may be helpful for baseline comparison, but are usually not necessary. If numerous flame-shaped or splinter hemorrhages are noted, the patient's blood pressure should be checked. The hemorrhages appear as hypofluorescent defects on the angiogram, while lipid exudates are generally not visible in the study. If the hemorrhages are pronounced and confluent, they can cause mild hypofluorescence due to blockage of the choroidal fluorescent pattern.

5-2-3 Moderate Nonproliferative Retinopathy With Macular Edema Not Clinically Significant

Patients with moderate NPDR and macular edema that is not clinically significant should be watched primarily with clinical examination. Fluorescein angiography or color photographs may also be helpful occasionally to track the amount of exudation or associated features, especially if visual acuity seems to decrease disproportionately to clinical findings.

5-2-4 Nonproliferative Retinopathy With Clinically Significant Macular Edema

Clinically significant macular edema (CSME), as defined by the Early Treatment Diabetic Retinopathy Study (ETDRS), includes the following[27,28]:

1. Thickening of the retina at or within 500 μm of the center of the macula

2. Hard exudates at or within 500 μm of the center of the macula if associated with thickening of the adjacent retina

3. A zone or zones of retinal thickening 1 disc diameter (DD) or larger, any part of which is within 1 DD of the center of the macula

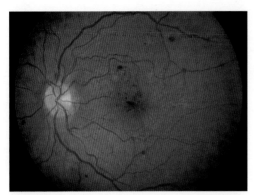

A

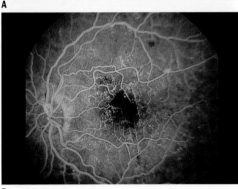

B

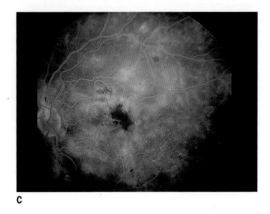

C

Figure 5-2 *(A) Macular edema along with microaneurysms in perifoveal region. (B) Fluorescein angiogram reveals macular ischemia with enlarged foveal avascular zone and diffuse leakage. (C) Patient was treated with grid laser photocoagulation.*

The diagnosis of CSME is by clinical examination and not by fluorescein angiography. Fluorescein angiography may be helpful in guiding treatment by identifying sites of leakage or by defining areas of capillary nonperfusion accounting for visual loss (Figure 5-2).[29,30] In focal diabetic maculopathy, there are MAs with areas of discrete leakage and adequate macular perfusion (Figure 5-3). If the areas of leakage are near the foveal avascular zone, edema of the macula in the form of hyperfluorescence may be seen. In diffuse diabetic maculopathy, diffusion due to hyperpermeability of the entire dilated perimacular capillary bed occurs due to the breakdown of the inner blood–retina barrier (Figure 5-4).[31] Besides the perimacular network, fluid dynamics in the retinal extracellular space and subretinal space may also affect the final visual outcome. Impairments in the pumping mechanism of the retinal pigment epithelium have been hypothesized as influencing these fluid dynamics.

The treatment outcomes in ischemic and diffuse types of macular edema are less favorable than those in focal diabetic macular edema. A fluorescein angiogram should be considered if CSME is still present 3 to

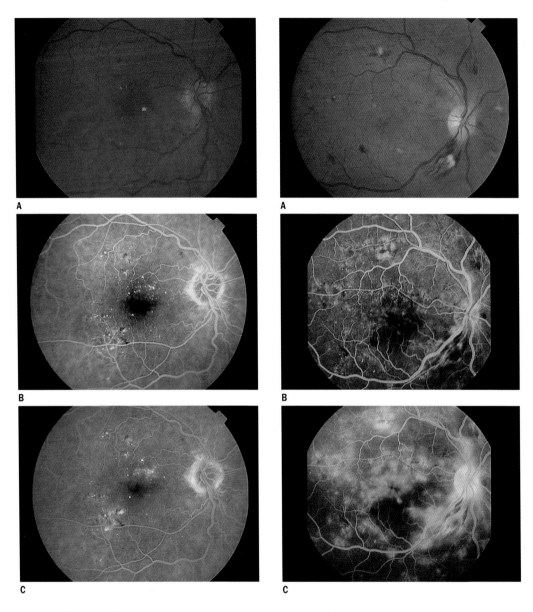

Figure 5-3 *(A) Focal diabetic macular edema noted superonasal to fovea. (B) Fluorescein angiography confirms presence of microaneurysms and leakage in corresponding region. (C) Patient was treated with focal laser photocoagulation.*

Figure 5-4 *(A) Diffuse cystoid macular edema is seen on color photograph. (B) Fluorescein angiogram confirms early hyperfluorescence with late leakage in perifoveal region. (C) Patient was treated with grid laser photocoagulation.*

4 months after treatment,[32] as angiographic features may factor into a decision for additional treatment.

5-2-5 Severe Nonproliferative Retinopathy

The risk of progression from very severe NPDR to high-risk proliferative diabetic retinopathy (PDR) is approximately 50% within 1 year.[33] Fluorescein angiographic features correlate well with the defining fundus lesions, such as hemorrhages, venous abnormalities, and intraretinal microvascular abnormalities (IRMAs). However, fluorescein angiography is not recommended for severe NPDR alone.

Peripheral capillary nonperfusion, as seen on wide-angle fluorescein angiography, has been shown to be associated with the progression of PDR.[34] It appears that the midperipheral and peripheral retina are the sites of initial capillary nonperfusion. A Japanese study attempted to quantify the progression of retinopathy with the distribution of nonperfusion.[34] The four types of characteristic nonperfusion seen were peripheral, midperipheral, central, and general. Color fundus photographs may also be useful to assess the extent of disease and facilitate evaluation of disease progression.[35]

5-3

FLUORESCEIN ANGIOSCOPY

Fluorescein angioscopy uses the indirect ophthalmoscope instead of a camera, requires less equipment and provides an immediate assessment of capillary leakage as well as large areas of nonperfusion and neovascularization. However, because no camera is used, a permanent record cannot be kept. This technique may be most useful as part of an examination under anesthesia if fluorescein angiography is not available in the operating room setting. In cases where the media are not clear but proliferative retinopathy or macular edema is suspected, this technique may be useful.

5-4

ULTRASONOGRAPHY

The use of ultrasound becomes important in the management of diabetic vitreoretinopathy when cataract develops or vitreous hemorrhage occurs.[36–38] Although vitreous hemorrhage secondary to the primary disease occurs, other causes, such as retinal tears, should also be considered (Figure 5-5). To obtain complete information, a thorough evaluation and a systemic approach are necessary. Examination can be done either through the eyelids or with the probe placed directly on the globe for improved resolution.

In eyes with diabetic vitreoretinopathy, the major pathologic processes that must be differentiated include the following[38]:

1. Hemorrhage in the vitreous cavity

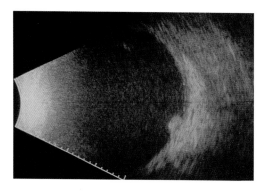

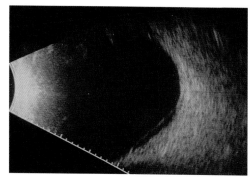

Figure 5-5 *Vitreous hemorrhage with frond of new vessels seen on ultrasound.*

Figure 5-6 *Fibrovascular membranes located between two epicenters of proliferation.*

2. Fibrovascular membranes, tufts, and stalks that arise from the PDR

3. Layered blood on the surface of the retina

4. Detached retina

5. Posterior vitreous detachment

Topography is an important feature of B-scan ultrasonography. Localized tractional retinal detachments, fibrovascular stalks or tufts, and localized areas of attachment of the posterior vitreous face in a posterior vitreous detachment must be diagnosed on the basis of topography (Figure 5-6). Hemorrhage in the vitreous body usually settles inferiorly and comes in contact with the retina in highly reflective layers.

In making the distinction between vitreous membranes and retinal detachment, it is sometimes difficult to delineate the structures. In certain cases, subretinal limiting blood may be trapped and may mimic a fibrovascular membrane or a localized retinal detachment. Furthermore, the distinc-

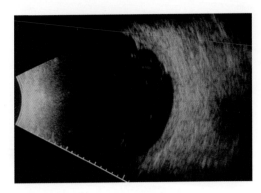

Figure 5-7 *Posterior vitreous detachment with focal areas of traction noted on B-scan.*

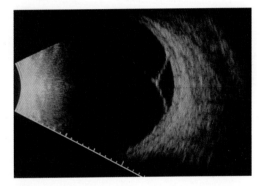

Figure 5-8 *Tractional retinal detachment, with fibrous tissue at apex of detachment.*

tion between a partly detached posterior hyaloid and the retina is difficult to ascertain (Figure 5-7). With a kinetic B-scan examination, it is sometimes possible to discern which of the echoes originate from the retina and which from aggregated blood and vitreous.[39]

Besides differentiating between the retina and the posterior hyaloid, ultrasonography may sometimes be useful for the detection of fibrovascular membranes on the retinal surface.[40] Three important consequences of diabetic epiretinal vasoproliferation are as follows[41]:

1. Fibrous contraction within epiretinal membrane formation, with accompanying tangential traction

2. An exaggerated adhesion between the vitreous gel and the retina in the vascularized epiretinal membrane

3. A separation of the cortical gel from the retinal surface except at the sites of exaggerated adhesion

Fibrovascular tissue, including membranes and cells, can grow on or within the surface of the posterior hyaloid and can be detected with ultrasound Fibrovascular tissue may also lead to splits in the cortical vitreous, which may be confused with posterior vitreous detachment.[42] Contraction of fibrous tissue on the retinal surface (tangential traction) and along the detached posterior hyaloid (anteroposterior traction) may ultimately lead to a tractional retinal detachment. Diabetic tractional retinal detachment has a characteristic concave configuration (Figure 5-8). The elevation of the retina is angular and immobile on kinetic testing; fibrovascular proliferation is usually present at the summit of the traction; and the retinal surface has an anterior concavity between the limit of the detachment and the vitreoretinal adhesion.[43]

In many cases, extensive tractional retinal detachments may have an associated rhegmatogenous component, which results in some mobility on dynamic testing and anterior convexity.[44] In many cases, fibrovascular proliferation on the surface of the retina is extensive, and crucial clinical decisions regarding timing and technique of vitreous surgery are often based on the ultrasonic diagnosis of retinal detachment, especially if the macula is involved.

5-5

CONCLUSION

Fluorescein angiography is particularly helpful in managing diabetic retinopathy associated with CSME. It facilitates the recognition of MAs and other leaking abnormalities that require photocoagulation per ETDRS criteria. Fluorescein angiography is typically obtained prior to the treatment of CSME and at subsequent visits, when additional treatment is considered. In some cases, it may be helpful in identifying neovascularization of the retina and/or disc, as well as areas of retinal capillary nonperfusion.

Contact B-scan ultrasonography is typically indicated in PDR when vitreous hemorrhage, cataract, or other media opacities preclude a view of the fundus. If tractional retinal detachment of the posterior pole or rhegmatogenous retinal detachment is present in an eye with vitreous hemorrhage and no fundus view, ultrasonography enables the clinician to recognize the detachment. This may lead to a decision to intervene with vitrectomy earlier, rather than waiting for the hemorrhage to clear.

REFERENCES

1. Klein R, Klein BE, Neider MW, et al: Diabetic retinopathy as detected using ophthalmoscopy, a nonmydriatic camera and a standard fundus camera. *Ophthalmology* 1985;92:485–491.

2. Moss SE, Klein R, Kessler SD, Richie KA: Comparison between ophthalmoscopy and fundus photography in determining severity of diabetic retinopathy. *Ophthalmology* 1985;92:62–67.

3. Gonzalez ME, Gonzalez C, Stern MP, et al: Concordance in diagnosis of diabetic retinopathy by fundus photography between retina specialists and standardized reading center. Mexico City Diabetes Study Retinopathy Group. *Arch Med Res* 1995;26:127–130.

4. Gonzalez ME, Gonzalez C, Stern MP, et al: Concordance between retina specialists and a preferred practice pattern in treatment and follow-up criteria for diabetic retinopathy. *Arch Med Res* 1996;27:205–211.

5. O'Hare JP, Hopper A, Madhaven C, et al: Adding retinal photography to screening for diabetic retinopathy: a prospective study in primary care. *Br Med J* 1996;312:679–682.

6. Kinyoun JL, Martin DC, Fujimoto WY, Leonetti DL: Ophthalmoscopy versus fundus photographs for detecting and grading diabetic retinopathy. *Invest Ophthalmol Vis Sci* 1992;33:1888–1893.

7. Harding SP, Broadbent DM, Neoh C, et al: Sensitivity and specificity of photography and direct ophthalmoscopy in screening for sight threatening eye disease: the Liverpool Diabetic Eye Study. *Br Med J* 1995;311:1131–1135.

8. Hellstedt T, Palsi VP, Immonen I: A computerized system for localization of diabetic lesions from fundus images. *Acta Ophthalmol* 1994;72: 352–356.

9. Taylor R: Practical community screening for diabetic retinopathy using the mobile retinal camera: report of a 12 centre study. British Diabetic Association Mobile Retinal Screening Group. *Diabetic Med* 1996;13:946–952.

10. Young S, George LD, Lusty J, Owens DR: A new screening tool for diabetic retinopathy: the Canon CR5 45NM retinal camera with Frost Medical Software RIS-lite digital imaging system. *J Audiov Media Med* 1997;20:11–14.

11. George LD, Halliwell M, Hill R, et al: A comparison of digital retinal images and 35 mm colour transparencies in detecting and grading diabetic retinopathy. *Diabetic Med* 1998;15: 250–253.

12. Ryder RE, Kong N, Bates AS, et al: Instant electronic imaging systems are superior to Polaroid at detecting sight-threatening diabetic retinopathy. *Diabetic Med* 1998;15:254–258.

13. MacClean AL, Maumenee AE: Hemangioma of the choroid. *Am J Ophthalmol* 1959;57: 171–176.

14. Novotny HR, Alvis DL: A method of photographing fluorescein in the human retina. *Circulation* 1961;24:72–77.

15. Yannuzzi LA, Rohrer KT, Tindel LJ, et al: Fluorescein angiography complication survey. *Ophthalmology* 1986;93:611–617.

16. Stein MR, Parker CW: Reactions following intravenous fluorescein. *Am J Ophthalmol* 1971; 72:861–868.

17. Diabetes Control and Complications Trial Research Group: Color photography versus fluorescein angiography in the detection of diabetic retinopathy in the Diabetes Control and Complications Trial. *Arch Ophthalmol* 1987;105: 1344–1351.

18. Nielsen NV: Fluorescein angiography in persons with slightly abnormal glucose tolerances. *Acta Endocrinol* 1980;238(suppl):77–84.

19. Nielsen NV: The normal fundus fluorescein angiogram, IV: a classification of the normal fundus fluorescein angiogram based on angiographic findings in clinically healthy subjects and in diabetics without ophthalmoscopically abnormalities. *Acta Ophthalmol* 1985;63:459–462.

20. Bresnick GH, Davis MD, Myers FL, de Venecia G: Clinicopathologic correlations in diabetic retinopathy, II: clinical and histologic appearances of retinal capillary microaneurysms. *Arch Ophthalmol* 1977;95:1215–1220.

21. Hellstedt T, Vesti E, Immonen I: Identification of individual microaneurysms: a comparison between fluorescein angiograms and red-free and colour photographs. *Graefes Arch Klin Exp Ophthalmol* 1996;234(suppl 1):S13–S17.

22. Diabetes Control and Complications Trial Research Group: Progression of retinopathy with intensive versus conventional treatment in the Diabetes Control and Complications Trial. *Ophthalmology* 1995;102:647–661.

23. Diabetes Control and Complications Trial Research Group: The effect of intensive diabetes treatment on the progression of diabetic retinopathy in insulin-dependent diabetes mellitus: the Diabetes Control and Complications Trial. *Arch Ophthalmol* 1995;113:36–51.

24. Friberg TR, Lace J, Rosenstock J, Raskin P: Retinal microaneurysm counts in diabetic retinopathy: colour photography versus fluorescein angiography. *Can J Ophthalmol* 1987;22:226–229.

25. Kohner EM, Henkind P: Correlation of fluorescein angiogram and retinal digest in diabetic retinopathy. *Am J Ophthalmol* 1970;69:403–414.

26. Jalli PY, Hellstedt TJ, Immonen IJ: Early versus late staining of microaneurysms in fluorescein angiography. *Retina* 1997;17:211–215.

27. Early Treatment Diabetic Retinopathy Study Research Group: Photocoagulation for diabetic macular edema. ETDRS Report Number 1. *Arch Ophthalmol* 1985;103:1796–1806.

28. Early Treatment Diabetic Retinopathy Study Research Group: Photocoagulation for diabetic macular edema. ETDRS Report Number 4. *Int Ophthalmol Clin* 1987;27:265–272.

29. Bresnick GH, Condit R, Syrjala S, et al: Abnormalities of the foveal avascular zone in diabetic retinopathy. *Arch Ophthalmol* 1984;102:1286–1293.

30. Tamura T, Tamura M: Perifoveal capillary network and visual prognosis in diabetic retinopathy. *Ophthalmologica* 1982;185:141–146.

31. Bresnick GH: Diabetic maculopathy: a critical review highlighting diffuse macular edema. *Ophthalmology* 1983;90:1301–1317.

32. Early Treatment Diabetic Retinopathy Study Research Group: Focal photocoagulation treatment of diabetic macular edema: relationship of treatment effect to fluorescein angiographic and other retinal characteristics at baseline. ETDRS Report Number 19. *Arch Ophthalmol* 1995;113:1144–1155.

33. Early Treatment Diabetic Retinopathy Study Research Group: Early photocoagulation for diabetic retinopathy. ETDRS Report Number 9. *Ophthalmology* 1991;98:766–785.

34. Shimizu K, Kobayashi Y, Muraoka K: Mid-peripheral fundus involvement in diabetic retinopathy. *Ophthalmology* 1981;88:601–612.

35. Early Treatment Diabetic Retinopathy Study Research Group: Fundus photographic risk factors for progression of diabetic retinopathy. ETDRS Report Number 12. *Ophthalmology* 1991;98:823–833.

36. Hodes BL: Eye disorders: using ultrasound in ophthalmologic diagnosis. *Postgrad Med* 1976;59:197–203.

37. Hermsen V: The use of ultrasound in the evaluation of diabetic vitreoretinopathy. *Int Ophthalmol Clin* 1984;24:125–141.

38. DiBernardo CW, Schachat AP, Fekrat S: *Ophthalmic Ultrasound: A Diagnostic Atlas.* New York: Thieme; 1998:1:3–45.

39. Byrne SF, Green RL: *Ultrasound of the Eye and Orbit.* St Louis: CV Mosby Co; 1992:53–88.

40. Restori M, McLeod D: Ultrasound in previtrectomy assessment. *Trans Ophthalmol Soc UK* 1977;97:232–234.

41. Arzabe CW, Akiba J, Jalkh AE, et al: Comparative study of vitreoretinal relationships using biomicroscopy and ultrasound. *Graefes Arch Klin Exp Ophthalmol* 1991;229:66–68.

42. Chu TG, Lopez PF, Cano MR, et al: Posterior vitreoschisis: an echographic finding in proliferative diabetic retinopathy. *Ophthalmology* 1996;103:315–322.

43. McLeod D, Restori M: Ultrasonic examination in severe diabetic eye disease. *Br J Ophthalmol* 1979;63:533–538.

44. Yoshida A, Cheng HM, Lashkari K, et al: Comparison between B-scan ultrasound and MRI in the detection of diabetic vitreous hemorrhage. *Ophthalmic Surg* 1992;23:693–696.

CHAPTER 6

Photocoagulation for Diabetic Macular Edema and Diabetic Retinopathy

James C. Folk, MD
Kean T. Oh, MD

Laser photocoagulation treatment is effective for both diabetic macular edema (DME) and proliferative diabetic retinopathy (PDR). This chapter reviews clinical evaluation, indications, treatment strategies, and complications of laser photocoagulation.

DME is the most common cause of moderate visual loss in diabetic patients. DME usually occurs before PDR, but may coexist with both PDR and nonproliferative diabetic retinopathy (NPDR). DME may develop at any time and may even be present at the initial diagnosis of type 2 (non–insulin-dependent) diabetes, probably because the real time of onset of the systemic disease is usually unknown in these patients. PDR initially involves the growth of new retinal blood vessels on the surface of the retina and/or optic nerve head. PDR typically occurs 15 years or more after the onset of the disease in type 1 (insulin-dependent) diabetic patients, but can occur as early as 5 years after diagnosis in 2% of patients.

6-1

SYMPTOMS AND MEDICAL HISTORY

The Diabetes Control and Complications Trial (DCCT)[1,2] and the United Kingdom Prospective Diabetes Study (UKPDS)[3] have shown that tight glucose control delays the onset and progression of diabetic retinopathy (DCCT for type 1 patients and UKPDS for type 2 diabetes). Managing diabetic retinopathy with medical therapy is reviewed in Chapter 8, "Medical Management of Diabetic Retinopathy."

6-1-1 Macular Edema

Most patients with DME experience blurred vision, but patients without involvement of the center of the macula may have excellent visual acuity and no visual complaints. Once DME occurs, treatment is more likely to stabilize vision than to improve it. For these reasons, it is important to examine asymptomatic diabetic patients regularly for DME, rather than waiting for symptoms of visual loss to occur, at which time the DME may be more advanced and less responsive to treatment.

6-1-2 Proliferative Retinopathy

Patients with PDR are often asymptomatic until the new vessels bleed or cause traction on the retina. By the time symptoms occur, the PDR may be advanced and difficult to control. This is another reason that periodic dilated fundus examinations are so important in diabetic patients, even when the patients are asymptomatic. Vitreous hemorrhage causes symptoms of floaters and blurred vision. Blurred vision may also be due to traction on the macula, tractional retinal detachment, combined rhegmatogenous and tractional retinal detachment, extensive capillary dropout or ischemia, or accompanying DME.

6-2

CLINICAL EVALUATION

6-2-1 Macular Edema

The best method to diagnose DME is stereoscopic examination of the macula at the slit lamp (and stereoscopic 30° color fundus photography of the macula).[4] A Hruby lens works well if the pupil is well dilated, the media are clear, the patient is cooperative, and the examiner is experienced. A thin, planoconcave contact lens gives the best view of the macula.

If no DME is seen on detailed examination of the macula and no neovascularization is present, the patient is observed at intervals depending on the severity of the retinopathy. Patients with mild or no retinopathy are observed yearly; patients with moderate retinopathy without DME are examined in 6 months; patients with severe NPDR, DME that is not clinically significant, or neovascularization that is not high-risk are seen every 3 months.

6-2-2 Proliferative Retinopathy

The clinical evaluation of patients with diabetic retinopathy is outlined in Table 6-1. Indirect ophthalmoscopy determines the presence of hemorrhage, vitreoretinal traction, retinal detachment, the extent of previous laser treatment, and large areas of neovascularization. A 78- or 90-diopter lens or fundus contact lens at the slit lamp allows detection of neovascularization on the retina or optic disc.

Fluorescein angiographic features of diabetic retinopathy are described in Chapter 5, "Photography, Angiography, and Ultrasonography in Diabetic Retinopathy."

THEORETICAL CONSIDERATIONS AND RESULTS IN PHOTOCOAGULATION

6-3-1 Macular Edema

The Early Treatment Diabetic Retinopathy Study (ETDRS) proved that laser treatment reduces moderate visual loss in patients with clinically significant macular edema (CSME) and less severe retinopathy (see Chapter 4, "Clinical Studies on Treatment for Diabetic Retinopathy").[5] The mechanism of action for laser treatment is uncertain. On fluorescein angiography, most of the leakage in eyes with focal DME appears to be caused by microaneurysms (MAs) or retinal vessels in the inner and middle retina. Focal burns appear to coagulate these MAs, which then stop leaking, and may result in improvement in the DME (Figure 6-1).

In eyes with diffuse DME, fluorescein angiography demonstrates diffuse leakage from retinal vessels, suggesting that leakage from MAs may not be the only cause of DME formation. Similarly, direct coagulation of MAs may not be the only mechanism of decreasing DME. Argon green, krypton red, and diode infrared laser, whether used as a grid pattern or as direct treatment to the MAs, all appear to be effective in reducing DME. Krypton red and diode infrared are poorly absorbed by the red blood vessels in the inner retina, suggesting that treatment of the retinal pigment epithelium (RPE) may play a role in reducing DME.

Both krypton and argon laser treatments to the outer retina have been shown to cause endothelial cell proliferation in retinal capillaries and veins in the inner retina.[6,7]

TABLE 6-1

Checklist for Evaluation of Patient With Diabetic Retinopathy

1. Medical history: duration of diabetes, method and dosage of glucose control, blood pressure, kidney function, heart disease, smoking, other medications (especially anticoagulants), allergies

2. Ocular history, including symptoms of floaters or blurred vision, glaucoma, previous laser treatment or ocular surgery

3. Predilation examination, especially in new patients, with check for neovascularization of iris; gonioscopy if iris neovascularization is present

4. Indirect ophthalmoscopy after dilation to look for vitreous hemorrhage, area of retinal traction or detachment, extent and location of previous laser treatment, and large areas of neovascularization

5. Slit-lamp examination using 78- or 90-diopter lens (or direct ophthalmoscope or contact lenses) mainly to look for neovascularization of disc (NVD) and neovascularization elsewhere (NVE)

6. Examination with contact lens mainly to detect DME but also to examine optic disk to detect subtle NVD

Figure 6-1 *(A) 67-year-old with CSME emanating from cluster of MAs superotemporally. Visual acuity is 20/25. (B) Fluorescein angiogram shows MAs scattered around posterior pole. (C) Leakage late is mainly from clusters of MAs superotemporally. (D) Posttreatment photograph of focal laser treatment applied to MAs: treatment within circle of exudate is somewhat light. (E) Patient returned 3.5 months later with residual DME superotemporally involving fovea. Photograph shows appropriate re-treatment intensity of MAs superotemporally. (F) Followup 6 months after second treatment shows resolving DME and hard exudates. (G) Early- and (H) late-phase fluorescein angiogram 9 months after second treatment: laser scars are seen superotemporally. There are some residual MAs in both treated and untreated areas superonasally and inferonasally. These MAs do not appear to be leaking much late in angiogram. More importantly, CSME was not seen on contact lens biomicroscopy. (I) Followup 2 years after second focal laser treatment. Visual acuity is 20/20, and fovea is flat. Few exudates remain temporally, but are well outside fovea and need not be treated. Initial light focal laser treatment did not close MAs or eliminate DME. Second treatment, of adequate intensity, ultimately resolved DME with good visual result.*

Note *With the exception of Figure 6-7, the figures in this chapter are reprinted from Folk JC, Pulido JS:* Laser Photocoagulation of the Retina and Choroid. *Ophthalmology Monograph 11. San Francisco: American Academy of Ophthalmology; 1997.*

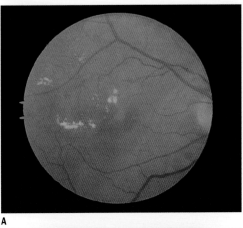

A

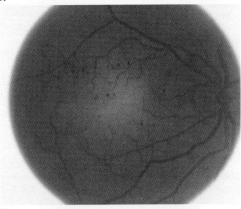

B

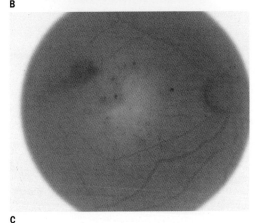

C

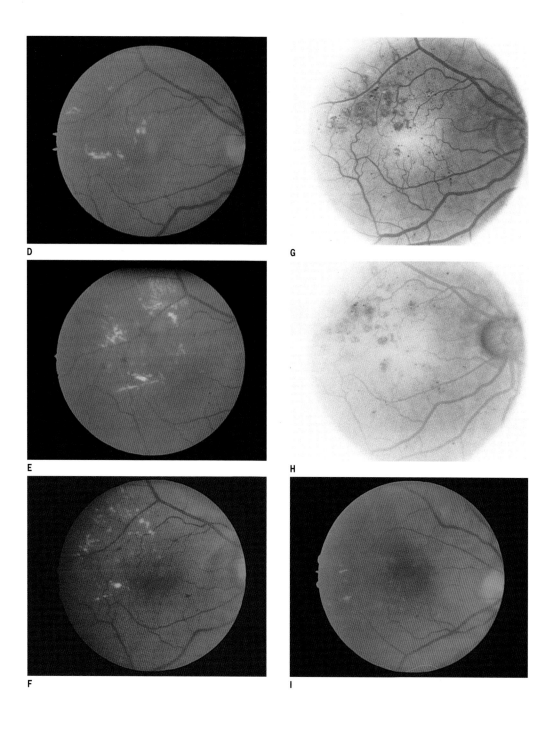

D

G

E

H

F

I

TABLE 6-2

Definition of Clinically Significant Macular Edema

Any one of the following in decreasing order of severity:

1. Retinal thickening, or hard exudates associated with retinal thickening involving center of fovea

2. Any retinal thickening, or hard exudates adjacent to retinal thickening extending within 500 µm of center of fovea

3. Retinal thickening involving 1 disc area or more of retina, part of which is within 1 disc diameter (DD) of center of macula

The proliferative effect on endothelial cells is greatest overlying the lesions and with the krypton laser. However, even areas distant from the site of the laser treatment (but within the same vessel distribution) may show some mitotic activity of endothelial cells.

One theory of the mechanism by which laser treatment reduces DME is that damage to the outer blood–retina barrier causes the elaboration of a chemical or substance that, in turn, causes mitosis of endothelial cells. After treatment, these vessels leak less or absorb more, effecting a reduction of the DME and accompanying hard exudate.

Another theory is that laser treatment destroys some of the photoreceptors and RPE, which are the layers that consume most (perhaps 75%) of the oxygen used by the retina. Posttreatment scarring also causes retinal thinning, which allows for better diffusion of oxygen from the choroid. After laser treatment, oxygen consumption in the retina is reduced and the supply to the thinned retina from the choroid is increased.

Retinal capillaries, especially in patients with severe DME, are often dilated before treatment and become narrower or less dilated after laser treatment.[8] This constriction of retinal vessels reduces the intravascular hydrostatic pressure.

Regardless of the mechanism of laser effect, the patient may experience stabilized or improved visual acuity as the DME resolves, when the leakage is reduced after laser treatment.

Patients with CSME, as defined by the ETDRS, are candidates for photocoagulation treatment (Table 6-2). Although the

ETDRS did not evaluate patients with visual acuity less than 20/200, treatment may still be considered to stabilize visual acuity. Patients with hard exudates in the fovea have a poor prognosis, but are still considered for treatment when the exudates are associated with DME. Likewise, patients with marked capillary nonperfusion involving the macula may have reduced visual acuity and may not respond as well to laser treatment compared to patients with good perfusion.[9]

6-3-2 Proliferative Retinopathy

The Diabetic Retinopathy Study (DRS) showed that scatter laser treatment or xenon light photocoagulation treatment reduced severe visual loss by 50% or more in patients with PDR who had high-risk characteristics (Table 6-3 and Figure 6-2).[10] The ETDRS results suggest that, because 50% of patients with early PDR or very severe NPDR developed high-risk characteristics during 1 year of followup, clinicians may consider scatter laser treatment before the onset of high-risk PDR (Figure 6-3).

The mechanism of scatter laser treatment is considered to be destruction of large portions of ischemic retina, thereby reducing the retina's oxygen demand and allowing more oxygen from the choroid to diffuse into retinal tissue by inducing retinal thinning. In contrast to patients with high-risk PDR, both the DRS and the ETDRS show that lesser degrees of retinopathy have a lower risk of severe visual loss and that some patients may not develop high-risk PDR even after 5 years of followup. However, if treatment is not applied to patients with severe NPDR or early PDR, they should be observed frequently.

TABLE 6-3

Indications for Scatter Laser Treatment of PDR

Definite Indications*

1. NVD equal to or greater than that shown in DRS standard photograph 10A, which is about ¼ to ⅓ disc area in extent with or without vitreous or preretinal hemorrhage

2. Vitreous or preretinal hemorrhage with any NVD (even less than that shown in DRS standard photograph 10A) or hemorrhage with NVE greater than ½ disc area in extent

Fairly Definite Indications

1. Neovascularization of angle with or without PDR

2. Neovascularization of iris with retinal neovascularization with or without vitreous or preretinal hemorrhage

Possible Indications†

Moderate PDR

1. NVD less than that shown in DRS standard photograph 10A

2. NVE at least ½ disc area without vitreous or preretinal hemorrhage

3. NVE less than ½ disc area with vitreous or preretinal hemorrhage

---

Very Severe NPDR

Two or three of the following (**4-2-1** rule):

1. MAs and hemorrhages equal to or greater than that shown in DRS standard photograph 2A in **4** or more standard photographic fields

2. Venous beading equal to or greater than that shown in DRS standard photograph 6A in **2** or more fields

3. Intraretinal microvascular abnormalities (IRMAs) equal to or greater than that shown in DRS standard photograph 8A in at least **1** field

DRS high-risk characteristics.
†*ETDRS showed that high-risk characteristics developed during 1 year of followup in 50% of these eyes.*

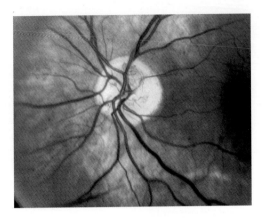

Figure 6-2 *DRS standard photograph 10A. New vessels equaling or exceeding those in this photograph are sufficient to place eye in high-risk category.*

Published with permission from Diabetic Retinopathy Study Research Group: Photocoagulation treatment of proliferative diabetic retinopathy: the second report of Diabetic Retinopathy Study findings. Ophthalmology 1978;85:82–106.

TABLE 6-4

Factors Influencing Decision for Photocoagulation

1. Degree of retinopathy

2. Poor compliance

3. Course of fellow eye

4. Systemic diseases (renal, hypertensive, etc)

5. Pregnancy

6. Pending cataract surgery

Many factors influence the decision for photocoagulation treatment (Table 6-4). Although the results of the DRS are well defined, clinical judgment must still be used when deciding whether to treat.[11] In spite of the physician's evaluation and recommendations, some patients do not want treatment, whereas others want to be treated immediately. In patients with poor vision in one eye because of severe retinopathy or treatment delay, earlier treatment should be considered in the second eye.

Patients with neovascularization of the anterior chamber angle are especially considered for early scatter treatment, even if neovascularization of the retina is not present. The differential diagnosis may include central retinal vein occlusion and the ocular ischemic syndrome. A fluorescein angiogram may demonstrate delayed arteriolar filling and dilated retinal veins. When the carotid artery has major occlusive disease, a carotid Doppler study may demonstrate an obstruction.

6-4

PRETREATMENT DISCUSSION

For patients undergoing photocoagulation treatment, informed consent is required prior to the procedure. These patients usually need numerous followup visits and often require supplementary laser treatments. Despite standard photocoagulation treatment, retinopathy may progress and be accompanied by vision loss. Patients should be educated through discussions with clinicians and office staff, as well as through educational handouts (Tables 6-5 and 6-6), which may be reviewed at home.

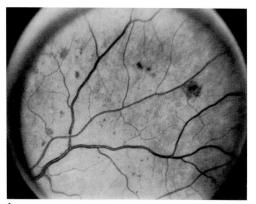

A

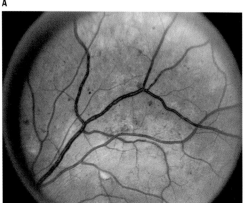

B

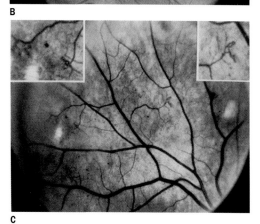

C

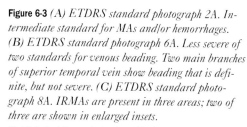

Figure 6-3 *(A) ETDRS standard photograph 2A. Intermediate standard for MAs and/or hemorrhages. (B) ETDRS standard photograph 6A. Less severe of two standards for venous beading. Two main branches of superior temporal vein show beading that is definite, but not severe. (C) ETDRS standard photograph 8A. IRMAs are present in three areas; two of three are shown in enlarged insets.*

Published with permission from Early Treatment Diabetic Retinopathy Study Research Group: Grading diabetic retinopathy from stereoscopic color fundus photographs: an extension of the modified Airlie House classification. ETDRS Report Number 10. Ophthalmology *1991;98:786–806.*

TABLE 6-5

Points to Include in Discussion Before Laser Treatment of DME

1. Diabetes is causing leakage of fluid and results in swelling, or edema, of retina.

2. Laser treatment helps reduce this leakage and edema.

3. Laser has been proven to be effective at preserving vision, compared to no treatment.

4. Usually, the best to hope for is stabilization of vision, rather than improvement, even with successful treatment.

5. Many patients require more than one and even three or four laser treatments to resolve the edema.

6. DME does not disappear in every patient despite good laser treatment.

7. Vision may also decrease for a few days to weeks after treatment because of temporary worsening of DME. Vision may continue to worsen over the long term despite laser treatment.

8. Laser treatment sometimes causes dark or hazy spots just off center that usually but not always disappear.

9. Patients should contact their internist or primary care physician to make sure that blood pressure, glucose, fluid balance, and any infections are under control.

10. Patients must return for scheduled followup visits.

Many patients forget information communicated orally, especially when they are confronted with the possibility of visual loss or blindness.

Information concerning the sound, flash, and discomfort of the laser treatment is usually given once patients are seated at the laser. Patients should be informed that some pain is to be expected when the retina is being treated adequately, but that they should let the clinician know if the pain becomes severe. Possible strategies to lessen the pain include avoiding a particularly sensitive area, decreasing the power, decreasing the burn duration, increasing the spot size, or resorting to peribulbar anesthesia.

6-5

LENSES AND FOCUSING

The planoconcave contact lens is the most commonly used lens for DME treatment. Some clinicians use indirect-type lenses for macular treatment, such as the Volk Area Centralis, Mainster High Magnification, or Mainster Standard, which are described in Table 6-7. These lenses have the advantage of a wider field of view, but the image is inverted and often magnified or minified, necessitating a change in spot size setting.[12] Also, their stereoscopic effect may be less than that of planoconcave lenses.

A variety of contact lenses are available for administering scatter laser photocoagulation treatment. The Goldmann lenses, which have been used for many years, produce an upright image with good magnification and resolution. The small ("pan-

TABLE 6-6

Points to Include in Discussion Before Laser Treatment of PDR

1. Diabetes has caused new and abnormal blood vessels to grow on surface of retina in back of eye. These blood vessels attach themselves to back of vitreous, or jelly-like part of eye. Vitreous then starts to pull forward toward front of eye, dragging abnormal blood vessels along because they are stuck to it. [Show piece of paper being dragged forward.] These vessels can then rupture and cause bleeding inside eye. Vessels grow from retina so that retina can also be dragged forward, causing detached retina with loss of vision.

2. Laser treatment to peripheral retina may halt this process. Areas of retina are not getting enough blood and produce substance that causes abnormal vessels to grow. If treated, these areas no longer produce this substance and blood vessels shrink. This reduces risk of hemorrhage or retinal detachment.

3. This laser treatment has been proven to be effective in national study of more than 1700 patients. Half of these patients had treatment to peripheral retina, and half did not. Half who received treatment did much better than half who did not.

4. Laser treatment often reduces peripheral vision and night vision. It occasionally reduces central, or reading, vision, although usually not by much and not for long. Sometimes, the treatment leads to patients needing reading glasses sooner than they would have otherwise or stronger lenses if they already have reading glasses. These side effects are small prices to pay to reduce risk of severe loss of vision.

5. Although laser treatment is effective, patients still could have bleeding in eye or retinal detachment in future. Such hemorrhage or detachment is caused by diabetes not by laser. In fact, it usually means patients need more laser treatment.

6. If patients lose vision, they should let clinician know right away.

7. Patients must return for scheduled followup visits, so that clinician can check on retinopathy and its response to treatment.

cake" or planoconcave) Goldmann lens has a single central opening for treating the posterior pole and near periphery. The three-mirror Goldmann lens has a central opening for treating the posterior pole and side mirrors for treating the midperipheral and peripheral retina. A significant disadvantage of the Goldmann lenses is their small field of view, which requires continual manipulation of the lens and slit lamp to complete the scatter treatment.

The Rodenstock Panfunduscope image is inverted, like that of the indirect ophthalmoscope, but the field of view is 3.3 times greater than that of a Goldmann lens. Scatter treatment can be applied to a large area of retina in a single image, and it is easy to visualize the disc and macula. The tubular design of the Panfunduscope is convenient for treating patients with prominent eyebrows. The magnification and resolution of this lens are lower than with a Goldmann lens. In addition, the Panfunduscope's spherical aberration may cause large, oblong burns at the periphery of a field of view, but this is not clinically important.

TABLE 6-7

Contact Lenses for Fundus Photocoagulation

Contact Lens	Uses	Image	Lateral Magnification	Axial Magnification	Relative Magnification*	Spot Magnification†	Field of View
Goldmann	Macula Equator Periphery	Virtual Erect	0.93	0.86	1.00	1.08	36°
Mainster High Magnification	Macula	Real Inverted	1.25	1.56	1.34	0.81	75°
Volk Area Centralis	Macula Equator	Real Inverted	1.05	1.10	1.13	0.95	82°
Mainster Standard	Macula Equator	Real Inverted	0.96	0.92	1.03	1.05	90°
Panfunduscope	Equator Periphery	Real Inverted	0.71	0.51	0.76	1.41	120°
Volk TransEquator	Equator Periphery	Real Inverted	0.70	0.49	0.75	1.43	122°
Mainster Wide-Field	Equator Periphery	Real Inverted	0.68	0.46	0.73	1.47	125°
Volk QuadPediatric	Equator Periphery	Real Inverted	0.55	0.30	0.59	1.82	100°
Mainster Ultra Field PRP	Equator Periphery	Real Inverted	0.53	0.28	0.57	1.89	140°
Volk QuadrAspheric	Equator Periphery	Real Inverted	0.52	0.27	0.56	1.92	130°
Volk SuperQuad 160	Equator Periphery	Real Real	0.52	0.27	0.56	1.92	160°
Mainster PRP 165 Laser	Equator Periphery	Real Real	0.51	0.26	0.54	1.96	165°
Volk Equator Plus	Equator Periphery	Real Real	0.45	0.20	0.48	2.22	114°

*Lateral magnification in relation to Goldmann lens.
†Laser spot diameter at retina versus photocoagulator spot size setting; for example, if laser spot size was set at 100 µm and Panfunduscope lens was used with spot-magnification factor of 1.41, spot size on retina would be 141 µm.

Source: *Reprinted with permission from Bloom SM, Brucker AJ:* Laser Surgery of the Posterior Segment. *2nd ed. Philadelphia: Lippincott-Raven; 1997. Updated by Dr Bloom and slightly altered by Dr Folk.*

Ocular Instruments has developed a series of high-resolution indirect-ophthalmoscopy lenses for laser treatment. The Mainster Standard has slightly greater magnification than does a Goldmann lens and a field of view 2.5 times that of a Goldmann lens. The Standard was designed for focal and grid treatment in the posterior pole and near periphery. The Mainster Wide-Field has a slightly wider field of view and lower magnification than does the Panfunduscope. Its higher resolution results in a clearer view of the peripheral retina than that seen with the Panfunduscope. The Mainster Ultra Field PRP and Mainster PRP 165 Laser have even greater fields of view, although less magnification.

Volk Instruments has developed the Volk Equator Plus, Volk TransEquator, Volk QuadrAspheric, and Volk SuperQuad 160, which give progressively larger fields of view and are excellent for administering scatter laser treatment.

6-6

LASER WAVELENGTHS

Argon green is the most commonly used wavelength for the treatment of DME, but krypton red, diode green, and diode infrared lasers also are effective.[5,13–16] Dye yellow laser may be better than green for treating specific MAs because of its better absorption by hemoglobin.

Green, yellow, red, and infrared wavelengths all appear to be effective at causing involution of neovascularization.[17] The green or yellow wavelengths are more commonly used because they do not penetrate the choroid as much as the red or diode infrared wavelengths. Therefore, these wavelengths are less painful and less likely to perforate Bruch's membrane or lead to later choroidal swelling if the scatter treatment is extensive.

The red and diode infrared wavelengths penetrate vitreous hemorrhage and yellow lens nuclei better than the green wavelengths and are less absorbed by any inner retinal hemorrhage. The red and diode infrared wavelengths may also be better for treating patients with significant vitreoretinal traction because their deeper burns may reduce the risk of worsening traction after the scatter treatment. However, the same result probably can be accomplished by using lighter burns with green or yellow wavelengths or by dividing the scatter treatment into multiple sessions.

Despite theoretical advantages of particular wavelengths for the treatment of DME or PDR, several studies have demonstrated no differences in the efficacy of different wavelengths in treating diabetic retinopathy. The choice of laser, then, is dictated more by availability, media opacity, and physician preference.

TABLE 6-8

Checklist for Laser Treatment of DME

1. After informed consent, patient is seated comfortably at slit lamp. Two or more topical anesthetic drops are placed in eye. A frame (usually early midphase) of fluorescein angiogram is projected beside or behind patient in easy view of clinician.

2. Contact lens is placed on eye, and center of macula is identified by comparing vessels or prominent landmarks of fundus to angiogram. Lesions requiring treatment are also identified. Patient is asked to look at fixation device with fellow eye and not to stare into center of laser beam.

3. Usually, green or yellow wavelengths are used. Yellow wavelengths are preferable for treatment of MAs.

4. Laser is set for 50- to 100-µm spot size, 0.05- to 0.1-sec duration, and power of 80 mW. MA or area of diffuse DME is treated. Power is increased in 10-mW increments until desired end point, off-white burn, is reached.

5. Usually, lesions closest to center of macula are treated first and then lesions farther away are treated. MAs are treated with one or two moderate 100-µm burns. Areas of diffuse DME are treated with light-to-moderate burns (more than barely visible).

6. Care is taken when moving from more edematous areas to areas less so, because latter require less power for effective burns. Areas of intraretinal hemorrhage are not treated directly but may be surrounded. Areas of nonedematous retina are not treated unless (rarely) they contain MAs or focal lesions that are thought to be contributing to DME. Burns are not placed confluently except perhaps in areas of extreme leakage.

7. After treatment, lens is removed and patient is asked to return in 3 or 4 months. No drops or patches are needed for focal/grid treatments.

6-7

LASER TREATMENT TECHNIQUE

6-7-1 Macular Edema

Topical anesthesia is usually sufficient for focal/grid laser treatment (Table 6-8). The patient is seated comfortably at the laser slit lamp and asked to focus with the opposite eye on a fixation light or target. The clinician carefully studies the retinal vascular landmarks (on the fluorescein angiogram when available) to locate the fovea precisely. If the anatomy of the macula is distorted by diffuse DME, the clinician may locate the fovea by asking the patient to fixate on the center of a reduced slit beam or by looking at the laser-aiming beam. The patient should then be reminded not to follow the aiming beam during photocoagulation treatment. In eyes with cystic edema, the center of the fovea usually corresponds to the center of the largest central cyst.

Small laser spots (50- to 100-µm burns) are used for essentially the entire DME treatment (Table 6-9). Larger burns carry an increased risk of creating scotomas or visually significant progressive atrophy of the RPE. The burn duration is usually set at 0.05 to 0.1 sec, but 0.2 sec may also be used if the patient is steady or if the DME is se-

TABLE 6-9

Recommended Techniques for Laser Treatment

Argon Green Wavelength	Spot Size (µm)	Duration (sec)	Power (mW)	Intensity	Number	Placement
Diabetic Macular Edema						
Focal/direct	50–100	0.05–0.1	50–	Whiten or darken MAs	Sufficient to target all leaking MAs	500–3000 µm from center of macula, 300–500 µm if <20/40 and re-treatment
Focal/grid	50–200	0.05–0.1	10–	Mild, light burns	Cover areas of diffuse DME and capillary nonperfusion	Spaced >1 burn width apart, 500–3000 µm from center of macula, 500 µm from disc
Proliferative Diabetic Retinopathy						
Scatter (panretinal photocoagulation)	500	0.1	200–	Moderately intense burns	1200–1600	½ burn width apart, >2 DD from center of macula to equator, 500 µm from disc
Local (direct) to NVE	500 200 (center of patch)	0.1 0.2–0.5	200–	Moderately intense burns	Overlapping, confluent treatment, 500 µm around margins	>2 DD from center of macula, scar <2 DD in diameter

Source: *Reprinted with permission from Regillo CD, Brown GC, Flynn HW Jr:* Vitreoretinal Disease: The Essentials. *New York: Thieme; 1999.*

vere. The initial power setting varies with the media clarity, fundus pigmentation, and individual laser unit.

Usually, an MA or area of diffuse DME that is slightly distant from the fovea is treated first. The power is increased in controlled increments until the desired end point is reached: a burn of mild or light intensity that is off-white but definitely visible. The clinician then locates the fovea and decides how close to it the treatment should be applied. In general, the first session of laser treatment for DME should not be at or near the foveal avascular zone.

A focal leak is usually due to an MA, and one medium-intensity burn is placed over it. If the MA does not darken or whiten or if the burn was off-center, another burn is placed. After the second burn, as long as the RPE beneath the MA is moderately white, even if the MA has not changed color, the clinician moves on to the next lesion. White burns are usually applied to particularly prominent and leaky MAs that appear to be a major source of the DME (Figure 6-4).

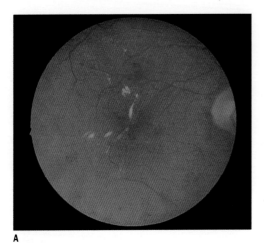

A

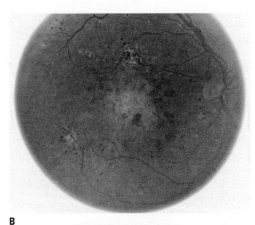

B

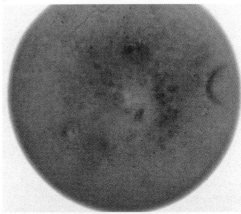

C

Figure 6-4 *(A) Non–insulin-dependent 60-year-old who had received combination focal and grid laser treatment 12 months previously. Grid was placed superiorly and nasally without attention to leaking MAs superiorly and inferotemporally. Patient returned with residual DME inferotemporally and superiorly. Visual acuity is 20/50. (B) Early fluorescein angiogram shows previous laser scars, mainly superiorly and nasally, and open MAs, mainly superiorly and inferotemporally. (C) Late fluorescein angiogram shows leakage mainly superiorly and inferotemporally. (D) Immediate posttreatment photograph shows focal laser treatment directed to MAs superiorly and inferotemporally; laser treatment resolved DME.*

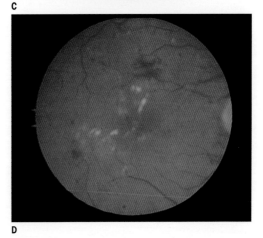

D

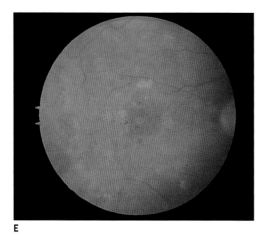

E

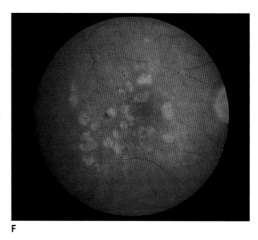

F

Initial treatment is applied up to 500 μm from the foveal center. If DME persists after the initial treatment, leaks closer to the fovea are treated and this treatment may extend up to 300 μm from the fovea. If possible, two or more burns are not placed confluently, especially close to the fovea because they may cause RPE atrophy and create scotomas. MAs located in areas of diffuse DME are treated directly; when numerous, this focal treatment may end up like a grid treatment localized on the MAs, and additional grid spots are unnecessary.

A grid pattern is placed using 100-μm burns in areas of diffuse DME without focal leaks (Figure 6-5). Large areas of diffuse DME (1500 μm or more from the fovea) may be treated with 200-μm burns. Burns are placed one and a half or two burn widths apart or closer if the leakage and DME are severe. Burns for grid treatment are usually slightly less prominent than burns for focal leaks but should be easily visible.

Figure 6-4 *(E) Almost 3 years after second treatment: dry macula and atrophic laser scars. Visual acuity is 20/40. (F) About 7 years after second treatment: dry macula and atrophic laser scars, which have expanded slightly. Visual acuity is 20/60. In this patient, light grid laser treatment not directed to MAs failed to resolve focal DME. Additional treatment to MAs did cause successful resolution.*

Figure 6-5 *(A) Insulin-dependent 59-year-old after one focal laser treatment. Patient continued to have diffuse DME with exudation throughout posterior pole of left eye. Visual acuity is 20/70. (B) Fluorescein angiogram shows dilated retinal capillaries and MAs throughout macula (C) with diffuse leakage into cystic spaces late in angiogram.*

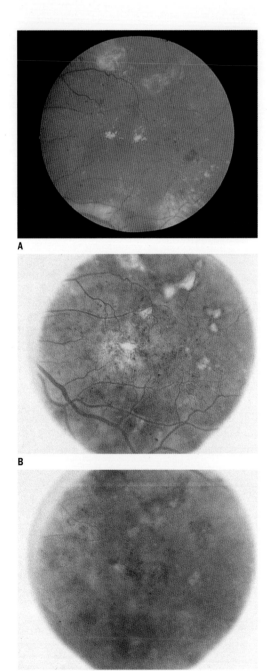

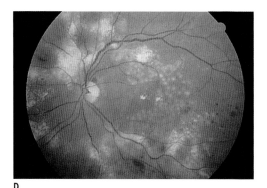

D

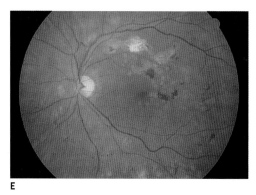

E

More power is needed to achieve a burn in more edematous areas than in less edematous ones. Burns may become too intense as the clinician moves from a swollen area to an area with minimal or no DME. Therefore, if possible, the clinician should treat the less edematous retina first and then increase the power as needed when moving to the more edematous retina. It is important to avoid placing intense burns close to the fovea because they often cause paracentral scotomas and occasionally choroidal neovascularization (Figure 6-6).

Treatment of areas of intraretinal hemorrhage are usually avoided, especially when using green or yellow wavelengths because energy absorption in the inner retina layers may cause substantial damage to the nerve fiber layer. Inner retinal burns appear as superficial, creamy-white burns in the area of the hemorrhage. The laser treatment can be placed at the border of the hemorrhage, rather than overlying it.

Patients with severe, diffuse DME and retinal ischemia may require extensive focal/grid laser treatment (Figure 6-7). The DME in these ischemic eyes may worsen, and the visual outcomes are frequently poor.

Figure 6-5 *(D) Photograph taken immediately after focal/grid treatment superiorly, nasally, and inferiorly to fovea. Treatment was also applied temporally and inferiorly just outside macula in areas of severe DME. MAs within area of treatment were treated focally. About 2 months later, patient received light scatter laser treatment to midperipheral retina in areas of severe retinal swelling and exudation because it was thought that these areas might be contributing to DME. (E) Followup 3 years after focal/grid treatment shows dry macula. Visual acuity is 20/50. This patient had MAs as well as diffuse DME with exudation secondary to dilated capillaries throughout posterior pole. Combination focal treatment to MAs and grid treatment was successful in resolving DME.*

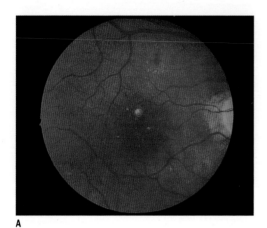

A

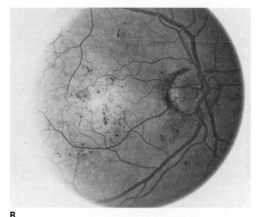

B

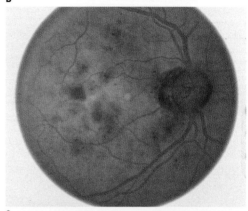

C

Figure 6-6 *(A) 63-year-old with focal and CSME in right eye. Visual acuity is 20/25. (B) Fluorescein angiogram reveals scattered MAs throughout macula that leak late (C). (D) Focal laser treatment to MAs. Laser spots appear to be small and intense. (E) About 9 months after treatment, patient presented with choroidal neovascularization and subretinal hemorrhage. Visual acuity is 20/100. Interestingly, no choroidal neovascularization was noted on either fundus examination or fluorescein angiography 4 months earlier. (F) Classic neovascularization now seen in superior fovea extending just into center of foveal avascular zone. (G) Neovascularization fills quickly and leaks profusely late (H). No treatment was given. (I,J) About 2 months after neovascularization was first noted, it has grown into large area of subfoveal neovascularization. Visual acuity is 20/500 and subsequently deteriorated to count fingers. Choroidal neovascularization developed after focal laser treatment with poor visual result. In retrospect, laser scars were rather small, intense, and fairly close to center of fovea.*

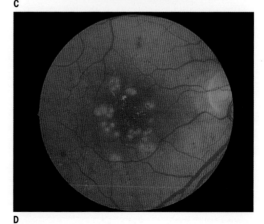

D

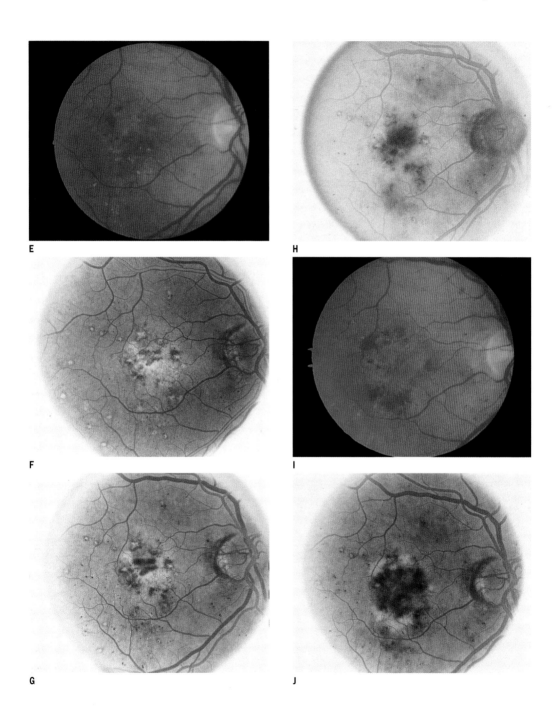

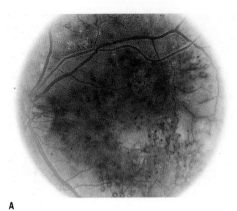

A

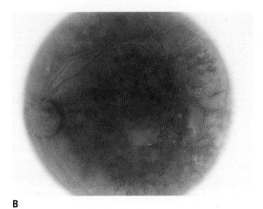

B

Figure 6-7 *Non–insulin-dependent 67-year-old with diffuse DME despite previous laser treatment in left eye. Visual acuity is 20/60. (A) Mid- and (B) late-phase fluorescein angiogram shows diffuse leakage throughout macula and capillary dropout temporally. (C) Photograph taken immediately after grid treatment. Treatment burns are closer to fovea temporally, where leakage was more severe. Treatment also extends temporally into area of capillary dropout. (D) Followup photograph 2 months later shows laser burns. DME is resolving but hard exudates are still present. All DME resolved and 3 years later visual acuity remains 20/60.*

In these severely ischemic eyes, segments of the macula may be treated in separate sessions at 2-week intervals. For instance, the segment between the 9- and 12-o'clock positions may be treated first, followed by the segment between the 12- and 3-o'clock positions. This divided-treatment strategy may reduce the posttreatment DME and improve the visual prognosis.

6-7-1-1 Complications of Treatment

The zone of cellular disruption caused by laser treatment is larger than the incident spot size.[18] Deep effects include disruption of Bruch's membrane, which may induce subretinal fibrosis[19] and may be visible clinically.[20,21] Fibrosis may be associated with severe subretinal lipid deposition, especially as the DME resolves.[22]

Choroidal neovascularization can also occur after laser treatment to the posterior pole and appears to be more common in patients who have received intense burns (see Figure 6-6).[23,24] The visual prognosis in patients with secondary choroidal neovascularization near the fovea is usually poor. Laser scars tend to enlarge over time and

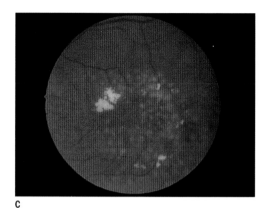

C

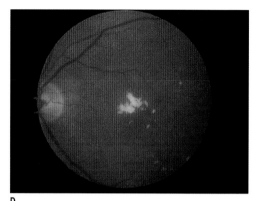

D

can cause visual loss from atrophy of the RPE and the photoreceptors.[25] Patients may also have bothersome paracentral scotomas, which are usually caused by confluent laser burns; single laser burns away from the macula usually do not cause scotomas. Table 6-10 lists complications of laser treatment for DME.

6-7-2 Proliferative Retinopathy

6-7-2-1 Use of Anesthetic While topical anesthesia is often sufficient for panretinal photocoagulation, retrobulbar or peribulbar anesthesia may be necessary for some patients. Pain tends to increase as the treatment session proceeds. If severe pain occurs during the application of the first few spots, retrobulbar anesthesia should be considered at that point. The pain may be diminished somewhat by increasing the spot size, decreasing the duration, switching from the red or diode infrared wavelengths to the green wavelengths, or dividing the treatment into more sessions of fewer spots. Treatment over the long posterior ciliary nerves at the 3- and 9-o'clock positions is

TABLE 6-10

Side Effects and Complications of Laser Treatment of DME

1. Paracentral scotomas
2. Transient increased edema/decreased vision
3. Choroidal neovascularization
4. Subretinal fibrosis
5. Photocoagulation scar expansion
6. Inadvertent foveolar burns

Source: *Reprinted with permission from Regillo CD, Brown GC, Flynn HW Jr:* Vitreoretinal Disease: The Essentials. *New York: Thieme; 1999.*

TABLE 6-11

Checklist for Scatter Laser Treatment of PDR

1. Spot size is set at 500 μm for Goldmann lenses, 350 μm for Mainster Wide-Field, Panfunduscope, or Volk TransEquator, and 250 to 300 μm for Volk QuadrAspheric, Volk SuperQuad 160, or Mainster Ultra Field PRP. Usually, magnification is set at 10× on slit lamp.

2. Generally, green or yellow wavelengths are used. Krypton red laser is also effective, as is diode infrared. Krypton red and diode infrared are more uncomfortable than green or yellow wavelengths. Longer wavelengths are useful when media opacities, such as cataract or vitreous hemorrhage, are present.

3. Burn duration is set at 0.1 sec; 0.2 sec may be used if anesthetic has been injected or for red wavelengths to reduce risk of perforating Bruch's membrane.

4. Power is set at 200 mW and increased in 50-mW increments until gray-white burn is achieved.

5. During one to three treatment sessions, total of 1200 laser burns are placed in midperiphery of retina out to vortex veins. Burns should go no closer than 1 DD from nasal edge of disc, 2 to 3 DD superiorly and inferiorly to macula, and 3 to 4 DD temporally.*

6. Inferior retina is treated first. When section of fundus is being treated, posterior is treated first and treatment is fanned out peripherally from there.

7. Small or medium-size areas of flat NVE are treated confluently with same spot size as used for scatter treatment, but with slightly increased power to achieve white burn (recommended but optional).

8. Treatment goes up to, but not over, areas of vitreoretinal traction or tractional retinal detachment.

9. NVD is not treated directly.

10. If patient has pain, reassurance is given. Scatter treatment can also be spread over more sessions, and size, power, or duration of burns can be reduced. If pain compromises needed scatter treatment, retrobulbar or peribulbar anesthetic can be used.

*More untreated space is left posteriorly if retinopathy is mild.

also more painful, so avoiding these areas or treating them at the end of a session may be helpful in completing treatment.

Retrobulbar or peribulbar anesthesia allows clinicians to use stronger and longer burns, possibly resulting in more effective treatment. Although the anesthetic eliminates eye movement, this does not limit treatment because many different lenses are now available to visualize different areas of the fundus.

6-7-2-2 Treatment Parameters   The DRS treatment protocol, which is generally followed by most practitioners, consists of placing 1200 burns, spaced one half burn width apart from posterior pole to the equator. Scatter burns should be of medium intensity or gray-white (Table 6-11). The laser spot size usually used is 500 μm with the Goldmann lenses and smaller with wide-angle lenses that magnify the spot (see Tables 6-7 and 6-11). Treatment borders are 1 DD nasal to the disc, just outside the temporal arcades, and 4 DD temporal to the fovea. If the retinopathy is severe, especially if there is marked capillary nonperfusion in the posterior pole, the treatment can be extended inside the temporal arcades and closer to the macula temporally.

The duration of scatter burns is usually set at 0.1 sec. A burn of shorter duration (0.05 sec) is less painful, but more power may be needed to cause an effect, and the risk of Bruch's membrane disruption is higher with shorter-duration burns. The power is carefully titrated upward from a lower initial setting.

The magnification of the slit lamp is chosen to result in a suitable field of view and to allow resolution of neovascularization and other details. Treatment extends through small areas (perhaps up to 3 DD) of NVE that are flat on the retina contiguously with the panretinal photocoagulation. Small spot sizes directed at the individual vessels in NVE should be avoided.

Many clinicians avoid treating areas covered by NVD and NVE. Evenly placed scatter treatment in a uniform pattern throughout the retina usually induces involution of the NVD and NVE. Large areas of NVE with traction or retinal detachment are not usually treated directly. Treatment is placed right up to, but not over, areas of vitreous traction or retinal detachment. NVD is not treated directly because of the risk of damage to the optic disc.

Scatter treatment of 1200 to 1500 burns is usually divided into two or three treatment sessions of 600 to 800 burns each. Most patients can better tolerate shorter sessions without retrobulbar anesthesia.

One treatment strategy is to treat the inferior retina before the superior retina. In this way, if vitreous hemorrhage occurs at any time between treatment sessions, sedimentation allows completion of the superior areas. Alternatively, the posterior retina may be treated first, and more peripheral areas in subsequent sessions.

Using the recommended spot sizes with the various lenses, about 1200 burns will satisfactorily cover the area between the posterior pole and the vortex veins. Additional burns may be placed between previous burns at subsequent or supplemental treatment sessions. Clinicians should avoid putting the burns too close together, especially posteriorly, because of the risk of visual field loss and delayed confluence of the laser scars after years of followup.

6-7-2-3 Single Versus Multiple Sessions Most clinicians apply scatter treatment in multiple sessions to reduce posttreatment pain, iritis, choroidal detachments with anterior rotation of the ciliary body and angle-closure glaucoma, worsening of the retinal edema, or serous retinal detachment. These complications usually resolve with time, and the ultimate visual acuity and outcomes appear to be the same when comparing single- and multiple-session treatment outcomes.[26]

Patients who have a history of iritis or glaucoma or who have narrow anterior chamber angles should have treatment in multiple sessions. Divided, shorter sessions of scatter treatment are also probably better for patients with CSME, as scatter treatment may exacerbate the edema.

TABLE 6-12

Tailoring Extent of Scatter Laser Treatment

**Characteristics Indicating Need
for More Extensive Treatment**

1. Extensive NVD especially; extensive NVE also but less so

2. Prominent background changes: hemorrhages (especially), venous beading, and IRMAs

3. Type 1 diabetes

4. Rapid progression of disease in fellow eye

5. Vitreous hemorrhage

6. Vitreoretinal traction

7. Anterior segment neovascularization

**Characteristics Indicating Need
for Less Extensive Treatment**

1. Neovascularization just meeting high-risk characteristics

2. Normal surrounding retina with few hemorrhages

3. Type 2 diabetes

4. Previous examinations documenting slow onset of retinopathy

5. Good result with laser treatment in fellow eye

Single-session, full-scatter treatment may be indicated in patients with severe PDR or with vitreous or preretinal hemorrhage. The full-scatter, single-session treatment avoids the delay of multiple sessions and may be considered for patients unable to comply with followup examinations. If patients require a retrobulbar or peribulbar anesthetic for any treatment, fewer sessions are usually advisable.

6-7-2-4 Intensity of Treatment The intensity and spacing of scatter treatment may be titrated to some degree in proportion to the degree of retinopathy (Table 6-12).[27] Patients with minimal disease may be treated with a somewhat lighter intensity. Patients with more severe disease, however, are treated more aggressively. Patients with two or more of the characteristics listed in the top half of Table 6-12 need prompt, aggressive treatment and often require far more than 1200 burns for involution of PDR.[28–30] With this aggressive treatment, it is often possible to achieve regression of neovascularization and retain good vision. A delay in delivering adequate laser treatment in more advanced cases may allow more severe PDR to progress to tractional retinal detachment or vitreous hemorrhage (Figure 6-8).

Patients with the characteristics in the lower half of Table 6-12 deteriorate more slowly, and less laser treatment may prevent progression. DME is usually treated first, followed by scatter treatment. A wider untreated margin around the optic disc and macula may be left and filled in later if the neovascularization does not regress. The burns may also be placed more than one half burn width apart, maximizing the remaining visual field (Figure 6-9).

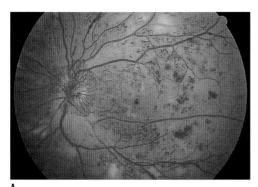

A

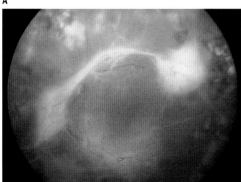

B

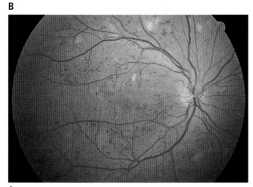

C

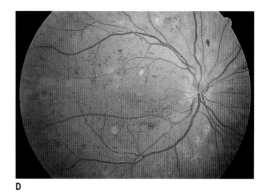

D

Figure 6-8 *(A) Type 1 (insulin-dependent) diabetic patient with severe neovascularization and background changes. This type of patient and eye needs aggressive scatter treatment. Initial scatter treatment of 1000 spots was placed, but patient did not return for 3 months. (B) Despite additional treatment, after patient returned, traction and ischemia resulted in light-perception vision. It is unknown whether more treatment earlier would have salvaged sight in this severely involved eye. (C) Fellow eye had severe background changes and minimal NVE. Because of fulminant course in patient's left eye, scatter treatment was started. (D) Despite initial scatter treatment of 1400 burns, NVE was still present 6 weeks later and early NVD was developing.*

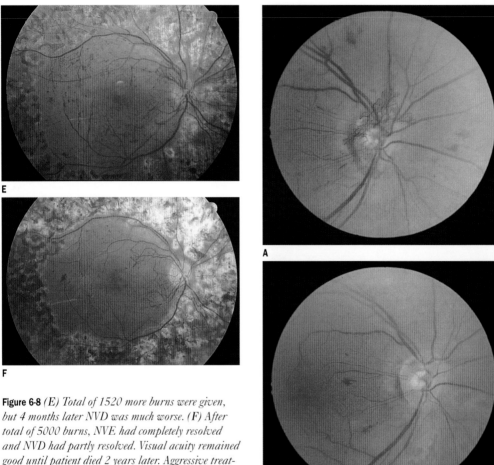

E

F

A

B

Figure 6-8 *(E) Total of 1520 more burns were given, but 4 months later NVD was much worse. (F) After total of 5000 burns, NVE had completely resolved and NVD had partly resolved. Visual acuity remained good until patient died 2 years later. Aggressive treatment probably saved vision in this severely involved fellow eye.*

Figure 6-9 *(A) Type 2 (non–insulin-dependent) diabetic patient with moderate NVD but few background changes. (B) Two scatter treatments of about 600 spots each caused prompt resolution of NVD. Burns were placed one burn width apart, and wide berth was given around posterior pole. This type of treatment maximized peripheral and night vision in this patient, whose PDR was relatively easy to control.*

6-8

POSTOPERATIVE FOLLOWUP

6-8-1 Macular Edema

The side effects after focal or grid laser treatment are usually mild. Some patients have increased blurred vision early after treatment, but very few notice laser-induced scotomas, especially if the foveal avascular zone is avoided (Table 6-13). Patients are asked to return in 2 to 4 months unless they have severe NPDR or PDR, which necessitates closer followup. The patient's internist or primary care physician is informed of the DME and asked to maximize control of the patient's blood pressure, fluid balance, serum lipids, renal status, and blood glucose levels as indicated. Of note, hard exudates may actually increase as the DME resolves. An increase in hard exudate alone is not an indication for additional laser treatment as long as the DME is resolving.

At the followup visit, the macula is examined to detect residual DME.[31,32] At about 3 months after the initial treatment, most clinicians add further treatment if CSME persists; DME that is not clinically significant is usually observed. If the fovea is dry but CSME persists, judgment is necessary in adding more laser treatment.

In borderline cases of DME, the amount of leakage or ischemia on fluorescein angiography influences the decision to re-treat. In the area of swelling, the clinician re-treats open MAs and diffuse areas of DME in a grid pattern. Re-treatment is applied up to 300 µm from the foveal center if proximal leaks are felt to be the cause of visual loss.

Patients are asked to return 2 to 4 months after the second focal/grid treatment. If the fovea is still edematous, the same process is repeated, depending on the clinician's judgment of the clinical situation.

A substantial minority (about 20%) of patients have persistent DME even after three or four treatments. The clinician may eventually do more harm than good in these patients by re-treating confluently large areas of perifoveal retina.

6-8-2 Proliferative Retinopathy

Usually, no topical medication is necessary after scatter laser treatment or 600 or fewer burns. Patients who have received more than 600 burns or who have substantial pain in the days after treatment may benefit from a short-acting cycloplegic. Patients with a history or evidence of intraocular inflammation may also be given a topical corticosteroid drop.

Immediately after laser treatment, most patients have mild pain and a minimal reduction in visual acuity. Therefore, they should be told to report promptly if they have severe pain or marked vision loss.

TABLE 6-13

Levels of Diabetic Retinopathy and Recommended Management

Age at Onset	First Fundus Exam	Followup (minimum)	Treatment
0–30 years	Within 5 years of diagnosis	Yearly	—
31 and older	On diagnosis	Yearly	—
Before pregnancy	Before conception or first trimester	3 months	—

Retinopathy Level	Fundus Findings		
A. Mild NPDR	At least one MA, mild hard exudates, cotton-wool spots, retinal hemorrhages (criteria not met for **B**)	9–12 months	—
B. Moderate NPDR	Retinal hemorrhages (>ETDRS standard photograph 2A), cotton-wool spots, venous beading, IRMAs present (criteria not met for **C**)	6 months	—
C. Severe NPDR	Any one or more of following criteria: **1.** Retinal hemorrhages/MAs (>ETDRS standard photograph 2A) in all four quadrants **2.** Venous beading in two or more quadrants **3.** IRMAs (>ETDRS standard photograph 8A) in one or more quadrants	4 months	Consider panretinal photocoagulation
D. Early PDR	New vessels present (criteria not met for **E**)	2–3 months	Consider panretinal photocoagulation
E. PDR with high-risk characteristics	Any one or more of following criteria: **1.** Neovascularization within 1 DD of disc with vitreous (or preretinal) hemorrhage **2.** Neovascularization within 1 DD of disc >¼–⅓ DD (>DRS standard photograph 10A) without vitreous (or preretinal) hemorrhage **3.** NVE (on retina) >½ DD with vitreous (or preretinal) hemorrhage	2–3 months	Immediate panretinal photocoagulation

Source: *Reprinted with permission from Regillo CD, Brown GC, Flynn HW Jr:* Vitreoretinal Disease: The Essentials. *New York: Thieme; 1999.*

These symptoms may indicate angle-closure glaucoma or severe iritis, both of which are uncommon complications that need to be treated promptly with cycloplegics, topical corticosteroids, topical glaucoma medications, or oral acetazolamide. Mild pain or decreased vision usually resolves spontaneously in a few days.

Several studies report followup after scatter treatment for PDR.[10,15,26] After at least 1200 laser burns, one study reported a reduction to two or fewer from three or more retinopathy risk factors within 3 weeks in 72% of patients.[33] Another study showed that 60% of patients responded to scatter laser treatment with regression of neovascularization within 3 months.[34] The responsive patients had much better long-term visual acuity outcomes compared to those who did not respond to initial treatment. Other studies have established the association between involution of neovascularization and good final outcome.[35]

The followup recommendations depend on the severity of the retinopathy and the response to initial treatment. After completion of the panretinal photocoagulation, patients are typically seen in 4 to 6 weeks. If the neovascularization has completely involuted, patients are scheduled for another examination in about 3 to 4 months. Most of the patients who initially respond will not require further laser treatment. Furthermore, patients who redevelop neovascularization later tend to respond well after additional treatment.

In patients with partial response by 4 to 6 weeks after laser treatment, additional treatment should be considered (Table 6-14 and Figure 6-10). Generally, small, active fronds or buds of neovascularization in-

TABLE 6-14

Tailoring Additional Scatter Laser Treatment on Followup

Characteristics Indicating Need for Additional Treatment

1. Amount of neovascularization increasing

2. New areas of neovascularization

3. Neovascularization still appears active: fine vessels, dilated buds, or tips covered with hemorrhage

4. Overall pattern of treatment looks light,* including: large area between burns, treatment does not extend to equator, too large an area of untreated retina posteriorly, or quadrant of retina left untreated

5. New vitreous hemorrhage

6. Area of NVE in area of retina treated minimally

7. Neovascularization of iris or angle

Characteristics Indicating No Need for Additional Treatment

1. Neovascularization has resolved

2. Neovascularization has lessened and coverage of retina by laser scars is good

3. Remaining neovascularization has only large trunk-like vessels

4. Good overall coverage of retina with no large untreated areas

5. Remaining untreated retina has minimal background changes

Not important if neovascularization has resolved.

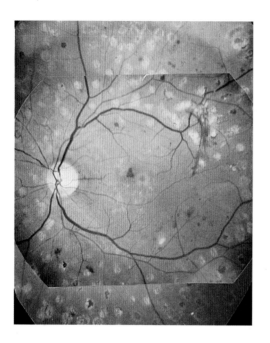

Figure 6-10 *Patient with residual NVE, some of which is fine in caliber after scatter treatment. Notice loose pattern of treatment, with large spaces between burns and areas of untreated retina, especially in quadrant of NVE. Additional treatment was applied, appropriately, and the neovascularization almost completely resolved.*

dicate persistent neovascular disease, and more treatment is usually recommended (Figure 6-11). Active new vessels often tend to leak more profusely on fluorescein angiography compared to older, involutional vessels.[36] Large-caliber vessels, which often remain after involution of small fronds, do not indicate active disease and are usually not re-treated (Figure 6-12).

Traction on elevated neovascularization may cause vitreous hemorrhage in spite of full scatter laser treatment. Patients should be warned that persistent vitreous hemorrhage may occur, but that the long-term prognosis is improved by the previous full scatter treatment. Most of the time, the recurrent hemorrhage is minimal and clears within a few weeks.

6-9

SPECIAL CASES

6-9-1 Macular Edema and Severe Retinopathy

When DME coexists with severe NPDR or early PDR, especially in type 1 (insulin-dependent) diabetic patients, scatter laser treatment may exacerbate DME and cause vision loss.[37,38] In these cases, the DME should ideally be treated first, followed by a period of close observation for progressive proliferative changes or by initiating light scatter treatment in the nasal and inferior quadrants.

When DME coexists with high-risk PDR, focal or grid laser treatment for DME and light scatter treatment to the nasal retina are delivered at the initial session. If high-risk PDR is very advanced, an addi-

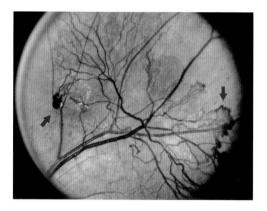

Figure 6-11 *Fine vessels with dilated tips (arrows), both of which indicate active neovascularization.*

Published with permission from Early Treatment Diabetic Retinopathy Study Research Group: Grading diabetic retinopathy from stereoscopic color fundus photographs: an extension of the modified Airlie House classification. ETDRS Report Number 10. Ophthalmology *1991;98:786–806.*

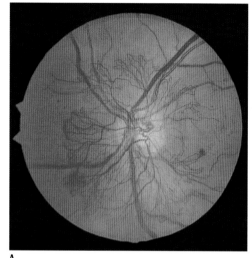

A

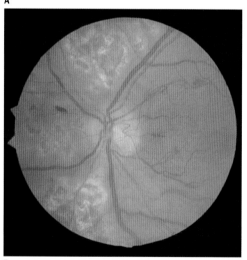

B

Figure 6-12 *(A) Extensive NVD before laser treatment. (B) After scatter treatment, most of NVD has resolved; only large trunks remain. This patient did well without additional scatter treatment.*

Published with permission from Folk JC: Diabetic retinopathy. In: Folk JC, Rakel RE, eds: Primary Care: Ophthalmology. *Vol 9, No 4. Philadelphia: WB Saunders Co; 1982:765.*

tional 1600 to 2000 scatter burns should be placed to effect regression of neovascularization. The macula should be re-evaluated for additional treatment 3 to 4 months after the initial focal/grid treatment.

6-9-2 Macular Edema and Cataract Surgery

DME may worsen following cataract surgery.[39] The DME sometimes progresses rapidly and responds poorly to laser treatment in this setting. Therefore, it is essential to treat leakage sites, if possible, before cataract surgery in order to resolve any DME. After treatment, it is advisable to wait 3 months or more before undertaking cataract surgery. Similarly, YAG capsulotomy should be delayed longer in eyes with DME. Pseudophakic cystoid macular edema (Irvine-Gass syndrome) may also occur after cataract surgery in diabetic patients. Fluorescein angiography in these post–cataract-surgery patients usually depicts the typical petaloid leakage pattern, while the retinopathy is mild or minimal. The optic disc hyperfluoresces late, indicating inflammation, in contrast to exacerbated DME. Pseudophakic cystoid macular edema should be treated with topical nonsteroidal agents, topical corticosteroids, or sub-Tenon's depot corticosteroids.

6-9-3 Macular Edema and Traction

A relatively small number of eyes with DME have a prominent posterior hyaloid attachment at the macula.[40,41] The fovea may be pulled forward by the hyaloid, losing its normal concavity, and is often cystic in appearance. DME may diminish after vitrectomy surgery when the macular traction is surgically removed.[42,43] Eyes with a taut, thickened posterior hyaloid face that appears to be firmly attached to the macula are considered candidates for surgery. On fluorescein angiography, the leakage is diffuse, with cystoid macular edema (seen late in the angiogram). The retinal vascular leakage is probably due to traction on inner retinal vessels surrounding the macula.

Macular pucker, distortion, or displacement (usually nasal) is caused by a partial vitreous detachment or by fibrovascular membranes from PDR. These patients often have blurred vision with metamorphopsia and even diplopia. Usually, the anatomic configuration is readily apparent on examination. A vitrectomy should be considered if visual acuity has decreased to 20/50 or less.

6-9-4 Proliferative Retinopathy and Traction

Early new vessels respond best to laser treatment before cicatricial changes occur. With additional maturation, fibrosis induces traction anteriorly and tangentially along the retina. This traction may range from retinal striae and macular pucker to traction or combined rhegmatogenous retinal detachment. Obviously, laser treatment is of less benefit when this process is well established.

The DRS demonstrated that scatter photocoagulation did not show higher rates of severe visual loss from treatment of eyes with increased traction (Figure 6-13).[44] However, many clinicians believe that scatter laser treatment can worsen the traction,

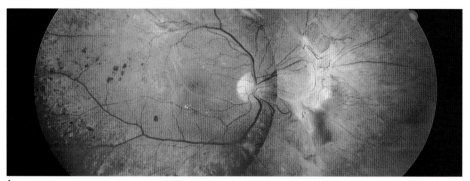

A

increase the macular distortion, or cause retinal detachment. Rather, DRS eyes with advanced fibrovascular traction had better visual outcomes with scatter treatment compared to untreated control eyes. Therefore, patients with high-risk PDR and tractional changes generally should receive standard full scatter laser treatment.

The burns should be placed up to the edge of, but not into, preretinal fibrosis or tractional retinal detachment. Fibrotic areas of NVE should usually not be treated directly, to avoid the risk of causing shrinkage of the fibrous tissue or weakening the adjacent retina. Patients presenting with extensive tractional or rhegmatogenous detachments should be considered for pars plana vitrectomy and scatter endolaser treatment.

6-9-5 Proliferative Retinopathy and Hemorrhage

Large subhyaloidal hemorrhages usually break into the vitreous cavity and disperse within a few weeks, prohibiting scatter treatment. For this reason, laser treatment should be performed promptly around the area of subhyaloidal hemorrhage before it disperses. Some eyes with subhyaloidal

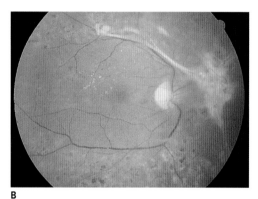

B

Figure 6-13 *(A) PDR with traction nasal to optic disc and along superior arcade extending into macula. Scatter treatment was applied surrounding, but not directly on, areas of traction. (B) On followup, traction had increased only minimally, neovascularization had resolved, and visual acuity was 20/25.*

Part A published with permission from Folk JC, Russell SR: *Appropriate wavelengths for posterior segment photocoagulation.* Focal Points: Clinical Modules for Ophthalmologists. *Vol VI, Module 7. San Francisco: American Academy of Ophthalmology; 1988.*

hemorrhages develop tractional changes around the area of blood; when this is apparent or if the hemorrhage does not clear from the macula, surgery should be considered. Young diabetic patients with active PDR are the most likely to develop these tractional changes.

If vitreous hemorrhage is already present, scatter laser treatment should be attempted in open areas. The krypton red or diode infrared wavelengths penetrate blood better than the green or yellow wavelengths, and may be useful in these patients.

6-10

PATIENT SUPPORT

Diabetic patients often develop a variety of complications of their disease at about the same time that their eyes deteriorate. They may also develop hypertension and kidney disease. Diabetic patients may become depressed because their bodies seem to be falling apart. They may be having difficulty at work because of their vision and health, yet not be eligible for disability because they are not legally blind.

It is important for physicians to be supportive of these patients by providing appropriate information (as requested) to the patients' employers to modify their jobs. Referrals to low vision clinics and support groups are also important.

6-11

CONCLUSION

Diabetes mellitus is the leading cause of blindness in Americans between the ages of 20 and 64 years. The DRS and the ETDRS have given clinicians excellent guidelines for the management of DME and PDR. Not all diabetic patients are alike, however, and clinicians must balance the guidelines with their own clinical judgment. This chapter has described the clinical signs of DME and PDR, paying careful attention to which eyes need treatment and which do not. The attempt has been to give clinicians practical information, such as points to include in the pretreatment discussion with the patient, the types of lenses to use, the goals and parameters of treatment, the do's and don'ts in treatment, and which findings on followup indicate a need for additional treatment. The chapter discussed briefly how laser treatment might control these diseases. Finally, the chapter described groups of patients who have a high risk of visual loss and need special care and treatment.

Diabetic retinopathy can be a challenging disease. It is a disease, however, in which close followup, careful examination, timely treatment matched to the patient's needs, and prompt referral when indicated can make a world of difference in the visual outcome.

ACKNOWLEDGMENT

This work was supported in part by Research to Prevent Blindness, Inc, New York, NY.

REFERENCES

1. Diabetes Control and Complications Trial Research Group: The relationship of glycemic exposure (HbA1c) to the risk of development and progression of retinopathy in the Diabetes Control and Complications Trial. *Diabetes* 1995;44: 968–983.

2. Diabetes Control and Complications Trial Research Group: The absence of a glycemic threshold for the development of long-term complications: the perspective of the Diabetes Control and Complications Trial. *Diabetes* 1996;45:1289–1298.

3. United Kingdom Prospective Diabetes Study Group: Intensive blood-glucose control with sulphonylureas or insulin compared with conventional treatment and risk of complications in patients with type 2 diabetes. UKPDS 33. *Lancet* 1998;352:837–853.

4. Kinyoun J, Barton F, Fisher M, et al: Detection of diabetic macular edema: ophthalmoscopy versus photography. ETDRS Report Number 5. *Ophthalmology* 1989;96:746–750; discussion 750–751.

5. Early Treatment Diabetic Retinopathy Study Research Group: Photocoagulation for diabetic macular edema. ETDRS Report Number 1. *Arch Ophthalmol* 1985;103:1796–1806.

6. Marshall J, Clover G, Rothery S: Some new findings on retinal irradiation by krypton and argon lasers. *Doc Ophthalmol Proc Ser* 1984;36: 21–37.

7. Clover GM: The effects of argon and krypton photocoagulation on the retina: implications for the inner and outer blood retinal barriers. In: Gitter KA, Schatz H, Yannuzzi LA, McDonald HR, eds: *Laser Photocoagulation of Retinal Disease.* (From International Laser Symposium of the Macula) San Francisco: Pacific Medical Press; 1988:11–17.

8. Gottfredsdottir MS, Stefansson E, Jonasson F, Gislason I: Retinal vasoconstriction after laser treatment for diabetic macular edema. *Am J Ophthalmol* 1993;115:64–67.

9. Early Treatment Diabetic Retinopathy Study Group: Focal photocoagulation treatment of diabetic macular edema: relationship of treatment effect to fluorescein angiographic and other retinal characteristics at baseline. ETDRS Report Number 19. *Arch Ophthalmol* 1995;113: 1144–1145.

10. Diabetic Retinopathy Study Research Group: Photocoagulation treatment of proliferative diabetic retinopathy: the second report of Diabetic Retinopathy Study (DRS) findings. *Ophthalmology* 1978;85:82–106.

11. Diabetic Retinopathy Study Research Group: Photocoagulation treatment of proliferative diabetic retinopathy: clinical application of Diabetic Retinopathy Study (DRS) findings. DRS Report Number 8. *Ophthalmology* 1981;88:583–600.

12. Mainster MA, Crossman JL, Erickson PJ, Heacock GL: Retinal laser lenses: magnification, spot size, and field of view. *Br J Ophthalmol* 1990; 74:177–179.

13. Akduman L, Olk RJ: Diode laser (810 nm) versus argon green (514 nm) modified grid photocoagulation for diffuse diabetic macular edema. *Ophthalmology* 1997;104:1433–1441.

14. Olk RJ: Modified grid argon (blue-green) laser photocoagulation for diffuse diabetic macular edema. *Ophthalmology* 1986;93:938–950.

15. Olk RJ: Argon green (514 nm) versus krypton red (647 nm) modified grid laser photocoagulation for diffuse diabetic macular edema. *Ophthalmology* 1990;97:1101–1112; discussion 1112–1113.

16. Khairallah M, Brahim R, Allagui M, Chachia N: Comparative effects of argon green and krypton red laser photocoagulation for patients with diabetic exudative maculopathy. *Br J Ophthalmol* 1996;80:319–322.

17. Krypton Argon Regression Neovascularization Study Research Group: Randomized comparison of krypton versus argon scatter photocoagulation for diabetic disc neovascularization. KARNS Report Number 1. *Ophthalmology* 1993; 100:1655–1664.

18. Wallow IH, Bindley CD: Focal photocoagulation of diabetic macular edema: a clinicopathologic case report. *Retina* 1988;8:261–269.

19. Rutledge BK, Wallow IH, Poulsen GL: Subpigment epithelial membranes after photocoagulation for diabetic macular edema. *Arch Ophthalmol* 1993;111:608–613.

20. Guyer DR, D'Amico DJ, Smith CW: Subretinal fibrosis after laser photocoagulation for diabetic macular edema. *Am J Ophthalmol* 1992; 113:652–656.

21. Han DP, Mieler WF, Burton TC: Submacular fibrosis after photocoagulation for diabetic macular edema. *Am J Ophthalmol* 1992;113:513–521.

22. Fong DS, Segal PP, Myers F, et al: Subretinal fibrosis in diabetic macular edema. ETDRS Report Number 23. *Arch Ophthalmol* 1997;115: 873–877.

23. Lewis H, Schachat AP, Haimann MH, et al: Choroidal neovascularization after laser photocoagulation for diabetic macular edema. *Ophthalmology* 1990;97:503–510; discussion 510–511.

24. Varley MP, Frank E, Purnell EW: Subretinal neovascularization after focal argon laser for diabetic macular edema. *Ophthalmology* 1988;95: 567–573.

25. Schatz H, Madeira D, McDonald HR, Johnson RN: Progressive enlargement of laser scars following grid laser photocoagulation for diffuse diabetic macular edema. *Arch Ophthalmol* 1991; 109:1549–1551.

26. Doft BH, Blankenship GW: Single versus multiple treatment sessions of argon laser panretinal photocoagulation for proliferative diabetic retinopathy. *Ophthalmology* 1982;89:772–779.

27. Rogell GD: Incremental panretinal photocoagulation: results in treating proliferative diabetic retinopathy. *Retina* 1983;3:308–311.

28. Vine AK: The efficacy of additional argon laser photocoagulation for persistent, severe proliferative diabetic retinopathy. *Ophthalmology* 1985;92:1532–1537.

29. Aylward GW, Pearson RV, Jagger JD, Hamilton AM: Extensive argon laser photocoagulation in the treatment of proliferative diabetic retinopathy. *Br J Ophthalmol* 1989;73:197–201.

30. Reddy VM, Zamora RL, Olk RJ: Quantitation of retinal ablation in proliferative diabetic retinopathy. *Am J Ophthalmol* 1995;119:760–766.

31. Early Treatment Diabetic Retinopathy Study Research Group: Treatment techniques and clinical guidelines for photocoagulation of diabetic macular edema. ETDRS Report Number 2. *Ophthalmology* 1987;94:761–774.

32. Early Treatment Diabetic Retinopathy Study Research Group: Photocoagulation for diabetic macular edema. ETDRS Report Number 4. *Int Ophthalmol Clin* 1987;27:265–272.

33. Doft BH, Blankenship G: Retinopathy risk factor regression after laser panretinal photocoagulation for proliferative diabetic retinopathy. *Ophthalmology* 1984;91:1453–1457.

34. Vander JF, Duker JS, Benson WE, et al: Long-term stability and visual outcome after favorable initial response of proliferative diabetic retinopathy to panretinal photocoagulation. *Ophthalmology* 1991;98:1575–1579.

35. Blankenship GW: Fifteen-year argon laser and xenon photocoagulation results of Bascom Palmer Eye Institute's patients participating in the Diabetic Retinopathy Study. *Ophthalmology* 1991;98:125–128.

36. Miller H, Miller B, Zonis S, Nir I: Diabetic neovascularization: permeability and ultrastructure. *Invest Ophthalmol Vis Sci* 1984;25:1338–1342.

37. Ferris FL III, Podgor MJ, Davis MD: Macular edema in Diabetic Retinopathy Study patients. DRS Report Number 12. *Ophthalmology* 1987;94:754–760.

38. Early Treatment Diabetic Retinopathy Study Research Group: Early photocoagulation for diabetic retinopathy. ETDRS Report Number 9. *Ophthalmology* 1991;98(suppl):766–785.

39. Jaffe GJ, Burton TC: Progression of nonproliferative diabetic retinopathy following cataract extraction. *Arch Ophthalmol* 1988;106:745–749.

40. Nasrallah FP, Jalkh AE, Van Coppenolle F, et al: The role of the vitreous in diabetic macular edema. *Ophthalmology* 1988;95:1335–1339.

41. Hikichi T, Fujio N, Akiba J, et al: Association between the short-term natural history of diabetic macular edema and the vitreomacular relationship in type II diabetes mellitus. *Ophthalmology* 1997;104:473–478.

42. Harbour JW, Smiddy WE, Flynn HW Jr, Rubsamen PE: Vitrectomy for diabetic macular edema associated with a thickened and taut posterior hyaloid membrane. *Am J Ophthalmol* 1996;121:405–413.

43. Tachi N, Ogino N: Vitrectomy for diffuse macular edema in cases of diabetic retinopathy. *Am J Ophthalmol* 1996;122:258–260.

44. Diabetic Retinopathy Study Research Group: Photocoagulation treatment of proliferative diabetic retinopathy: relationship of adverse treatment effects to retinopathy severity. DRS Report Number 5. *Dev Ophthalmol* 1981;2:248–261.

CHAPTER 7

Vitrectomy for Diabetic Retinopathy

William E. Smiddy, MD
Harry W. Flynn, Jr, MD

Prevention of retinopathy or reduction in rates of retinopathy progression via optimal glucose control[1-5] and laser treatment at earlier stages[3] has been advocated and implemented. Timely application of laser photocoagulation, with reapplication as needed, is the mainstay of treatment to reduce visual loss and to avoid the need for vitrectomy in patients with more advanced diabetic retinopathy complications.[6-13] However, despite timely treatment and preventive regimens, a substantial number of patients will develop complications of progressive retinopathy and may become candidates for vitrectomy.[14,15]

7-1

SURGICAL INDICATIONS

By the mid-1980s, the initial indications and surgical rationale for pars plana vitrectomy in diabetic patients were largely established.[16-27] As newer instrumentation, improved surgical technique, and further clinical experience have taken place over the past decade,[28] these indications have been refined. General categories of surgically approachable complications from diabetic retinopathy include eyes with induced media opacities and vitreoretinal

traction (Table 7-1). Even though these categories of indications for diabetic vitrectomy have changed little over the past 25 years, the timing of vitrectomy has been generally accelerated as improvements in surgical instrumentation have achieved better visual acuity outcomes.

7-1-1 Media Opacities

Historically, the first indication for pars plana vitrectomy was severe, nonclearing diabetic vitreous hemorrhage (Figure 7-1).[29-31] Vitreous hemorrhage is probably a result of vitreous traction on the vascular component of fibrovascular complexes from incomplete posterior vitreous detachment (PVD).[32-34] As timely application of panretinal photocoagulation (PRP) has become more widespread, the incidence of profound visual loss from dense vitreous hemorrhage has lessened. At the same time, development of new vitrectomy techniques and instruments allows successful outcomes even in complex cases. As a result, the distribution of cases undergoing vitrectomy for nonclearing vitreous hemorrhage decreased from 70% in 1977 to 20% in 1987 in one medical center.[30]

TABLE 7-1

Indications for Vitrectomy due to Severe Complications of Diabetic Retinopathy

Media Opacities

Nonclearing Hemorrhage

Vitreous

Subhyaloidal premacular hemorrhage

Anterior segment neovascularization with posterior segment opacity

Cataract Preventing Treatment

Tractional Defects

Progressive fibrovascular proliferation

Tractional retinal detachment involving macula

Combined tractional and rhegmatogenous retinal detachment

Macular edema associated with taut, persistently attached posterior hyaloid

Other Indications
(typically following previous vitrectomy)

Vitreous hemorrhage/ghost-cell glaucoma

Retinal detachment (tractional or rhegmatogenous)

Anterior hyaloidal fibrovascular proliferation

Fibrinoid syndrome

Epiretinal membrane (nonvascularized)

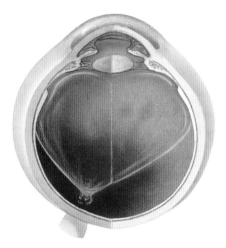

Figure 7-1 *Diabetic vitreous hemorrhage commonly presents as sudden decrease in vision. Depending on degree of hemorrhage, posterior pole may not be visible. Hemorrhage is usually due to traction on stump of neovascularization. Stump can be isolated or more broadly distributed. Drawing illustrates hemorrhage associated everywhere except at nerve head, where stump of neovascularization is present.*

Redrawn with permission of Johns Hopkins University from Michels RG: Proliferative diabetic retinopathy: pathophysiology of extraretinal complications and principles of vitreous surgery. Retina *1981;1:1–17.*

Several clinical features may influence the decision on timing of vitrectomy for diabetic vitreous hemorrhage. Earlier surgical intervention is generally recommended when no previous laser treatment has been performed, when the fibrovascular proliferation (FVP) complexes are more extensive, when the fellow eye has rapidly progressive visual loss, or when the fellow eye is blind. Surgical intervention may be more appropriately deferred, at least temporarily, when

there is a PVD, when extensive prior PRP
has been delivered, and when other labile
medical conditions coexist. Patients with
sustained hypertension or elevated levels of
glycosylated hemoglobin should receive
prompt and appropriate medical evaluation
of these systemic conditions. If a decision is
made to continue to defer surgery, echographic monitoring should be performed
to rule out retinal detachment.

Surgical intervention in the 1990s for
nonclearing diabetic vitreous hemorrhage
is usually considered earlier and may occur
within weeks or months for many patients.
However, some cases will have spontaneous
clearing and surgical intervention may be
deferred for a longer time in patients with
type 2 diabetes compared to patients with
type 1 diabetes. This delay allows time for
spontaneous clearing, possible delivery of
PRP, and subsequent regression of neovascularization. In contrast, vitrectomy is often
considered earlier (within months) for type
1 diabetic patients, especially if severe vitreous hemorrhage has shown no sign of
spontaneous clearing.[28]

Other coexisting clinical features define
subsets of vitrectomy indications for vitreous hemorrhage. Rubeosis iridis in an eye
with a recent vitreous hemorrhage, especially when no PRP has been applied, constitutes a relatively urgent indication for
intervention (Figure 7-2). An extensive
subhyaloidal hemorrhage over the macula
constitutes another surgical indication (Figure 7-3). The confinement of blood in the
subhyaloidal space indicates that the posterior hyaloid has not fully separated and remains as a scaffold for progressive FVP.[32,33]
Even though the hemorrhage may clear
over several months, this subhyaloidal hem-

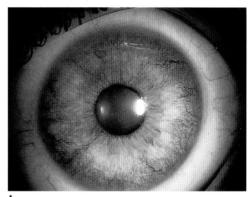

A

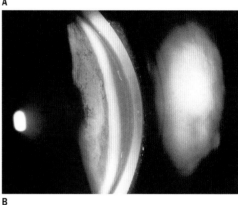

B

Figure 7-2 *(A) Rubeosis iridis characteristically appears first at pupillary border and then extends onto
iris surface. (B) However, in progressive cases, it is
rapidly seen in anterior chamber angle. Subsequent
neovascular glaucoma and precipitous loss of vision
may result, especially without prompt and extensive
PRP treatment.*

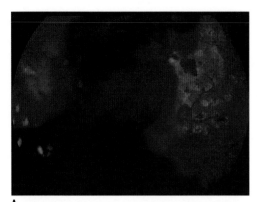

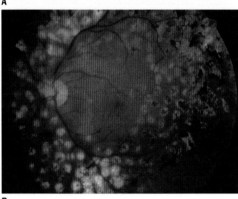

Figure 7-3 *(A) Patient presented with extensive sub-hyaloidal hemorrhage and visual acuity of 2/200. (B) Postoperative appearance following vitrectomy with supplementation of PRP. Visual acuity is 20/40.*

orrhage is usually associated with progressive FVP along the temporal vascular arcades, resulting in broad-based areas of vitreoretinal traction. Because of the relatively poor visual prognosis in these patients, even with spontaneous clearing, surgical intervention should be considered relatively early in the course (within a few months of onset). While waiting for the premacular hemorrhage to clear, however, the clinician should apply PRP in more peripheral areas.

In patients with vitreous hemorrhage, the assessment of the degree of cataract may be difficult. The vitreous hemorrhage may dim the red reflex and cause the nucleus to appear more opaque than in eyes without vitreous hemorrhage. Lens opacities may be sufficient to impair not only the patient's vision, but also the physician's ability to diagnose, monitor, and apply laser treatment to the retina. In such cases, cataract removal should be considered, either as a separate procedure or in combination with vitrectomy. Reports before the availability of endolaser photocoagulation documented a substantial rate of postoperative rubeosis iridis and generally poor visual outcomes in aphakic eyes or in those undergoing lensectomy at the time of vitrectomy.[35-38] However, more recent experience with extracapsular and phacoemulsification techniques for lens removal and with the ability to deliver intraoperative photocoagulation, improved outcomes have been reported with combined lensectomy and intraocular lens (IOL) implantation during vitrectomy in selected cases.[39-41]

Two general approaches have been reported. In the first approach, pars plana lensectomy is combined with vitrectomy maneuvers, and the anterior capsule (with central capsulotomy) is preserved for posterior chamber IOL support. With this approach, visual acuity has been reported to improve in more than 75% of patients, including about 25% who achieve 20/40 or better visual acuity.[39,40,42] In the second approach, cataract extraction using a standard limbal approach is performed, with the IOL insertion into the capsular bag, followed by the vitrectomy. With the latter approach, visualization of the posterior segment was reported to be excellent for the vitrectomy, but visual acuity outcomes were not as good in one report.[41] In this report, the discrepancy in visual results is most probably due to case selection. Indeed, modern surgical techniques for cataract extraction allow successful outcomes even in the presence of rubeosis iridis.[43]

7-1-2 Vitreoretinal Traction

The second general class of indications for pars plana vitrectomy in diabetic patients includes those with epiretinal and preretinal tractional components. This class of indications now constitutes the majority of patients undergoing vitrectomy for complications of diabetic retinopathy. There is a spectrum of tractional involvement, including macular heterotopia,[44] progressive FVP without retinal detachment, tractional retinal detachment, and rhegmatogenous retinal detachment where the retinal break is caused by progressive traction. Frequently, FVP with traction coexists with media opacities, and a dual set of indications for vitrectomy is present (Figure 7-4).

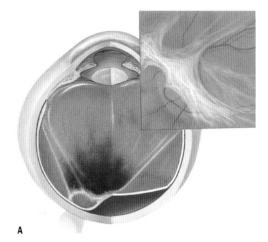

A

Figure 7-4 *(A) Frequently, media opacities and tractional components coexist. In this drawing, there is vitreous hemorrhage admixed with FVP, which is causing tractional retinal detachment. However, this may not be clinically evident due to obscuration of posterior pole by media opacities.*

Part A redrawn with permission of Johns Hopkins University from Michels RG: Proliferative diabetic retinopathy: pathophysiology of extraretinal complications and principles of vitreous surgery. Retina *1981;1:1–17.*

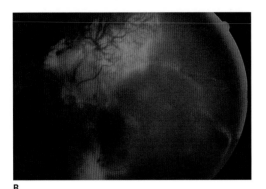

B

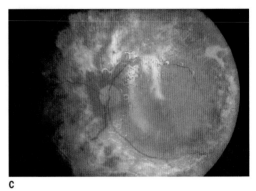

C

Figure 7-4 *(B) Patient presented with vision of hand motions. Clearly, there is vitreous hemorrhage, but view is clear enough to depict FVP along superotemporal arcade. (C) Appearance following vitrectomy with extensive membrane peeling and silicone oil infusion. Visual acuity is 20/400.*

Progressive FVP may occur despite appropriate PRP, especially in type 1 diabetic patients (Figure 7-5). In some patients, FVP may be very extensive and yet cause only slight visual loss. In more advanced stages, progressive FVP may be associated with marked loss of vision and a more guarded prognosis for visual improvement after vitrectomy. The lack of a PVD is an important factor associated with the visual prognosis in these patients. If the posterior hyaloid is still attached and has broad-based vitreoretinal connections, extensive scissors dissection of FVP may be required. Surgical relief of traction is accomplished with fewer complications when the zone of vitreoretinal attachment is less extensive, extends less anteriorly, and is more acute.

Tractional retinal detachment is today probably the single most common specific indication for vitrectomy in patients with progressive FVP (Figure 7-6). The pathogenesis of retinal detachment involves vitreous traction on fibrovascular tissues. Because peripheral or midperipheral tractional retinal detachments progress to involve the macula in only about 15% of cases per year,[45] caution is advised in recommending vitrec-

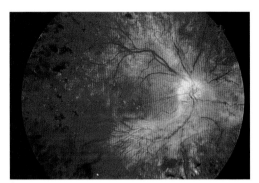

A

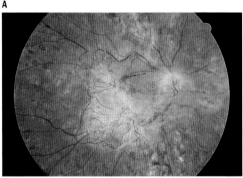

B

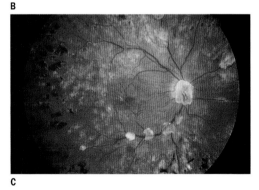

C

Figure 7-5 *(A) FVP typically progresses from neovascularization from nerve head and along arcade with, initially, relatively good visual acuity. This 29-year-old woman presented with 20/30 visual acuity. (B) With further progression over ensuing 3 months, visual acuity dropped to 20/200 as FVP enveloped posterior pole. (C) After vitrectomy, visual acuity returned to 20/30.*

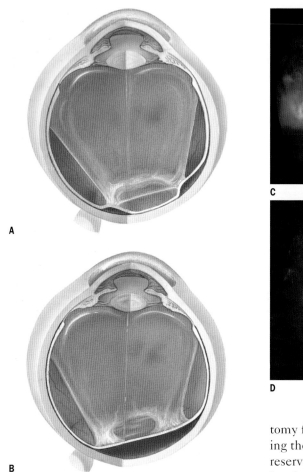

A

B

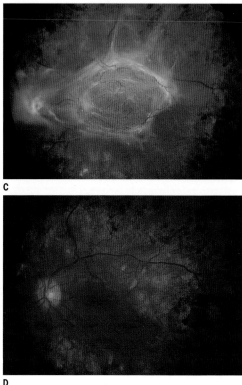

C

D

Figure 7-6 *(A) Tractional retinal detachment beginning outside of fovea due to traction from FVP along arcade and disc. (B) With further progression, "tabletop" configuration, in which macula is additionally affected, ensues. (C) Configuration is illustrated by this 39-year-old man, who presented with 2/200 vision. (D) Postoperatively, vision improved to 20/60.*

Parts A and B redrawn with permission of Johns Hopkins University from Michels RG: Proliferative diabetic retinopathy: pathophysiology of extraretinal complications and principles of vitreous surgery. Retina 1981;1:1–17.

tomy for localized detachments not involving the macula. Vitrectomy is generally reserved for cases in which the macula is involved or is clearly threatened by progressive retinal detachment.

As with cases of nonclearing diabetic vitreous hemorrhage, other factors influence the timing of surgical intervention. Patients with type 1 diabetes in whom coexisting media opacities have prevented delivery of adequate PRP and patients in whom a rapidly progressive course ensued in the fellow eye should be considered for earlier vitrectomy. Chronic macular detachment leads to a thinner, more atrophic retina, with more extensive and more tightly adherent fibro-vascular membranes. Consequently, the anatomic and visual prognoses are poorer in such patients. Therefore, when macular detachment has been present for 6 months or more, surgery is usually not recommended.

A third traction-related indication for diabetic vitrectomy is combined tractional and rhegmatogenous retinal detachment (Figure 7-7). The rhegmatogenous component results from progressive contraction of FVP. Pathognomonic of a rhegmatogenous cause is the appearance of hydration lines, with a more mobile, elevated retina. A more sudden and profound visual loss usually occurs as the rhegmatogenous component progresses. While in some eyes a rhegmatogenous component may be slowly progressive and could be closely monitored without surgery, prompt surgery is usually indicated. The retinal break typically occurs posterior to the equator, but is sometimes not detected during the preoperative examination. Common sites for retinal breaks include areas adjacent to previous chorioretinal scars or at the base of vitreoretinal adhesions.

A rare, more subtle traction-induced complication is macular edema induced by the traction of a taut, persistently attached posterior hyaloid. This subtype of diabetic macular edema characteristically does not respond to focal or grid laser photocoagulation. The vast majority of cases of diabetic macular edema do not appear to be induced by traction and should be considered for photocoagulation, in accordance with the results of the Early Treatment Diabetic Retinopathy Study.[46] Selected cases with this configuration respond to surgical release of the traction.[47] A subsequent study

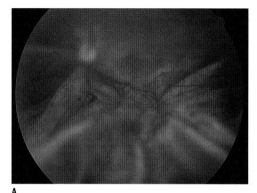

A

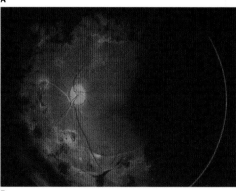

B

Figure 7-7 *(A) With continued traction, especially with more broad-based fibrovascular entities, rhegmatogenous component may develop in retina. This leads to more generalized retinal detachment, which may be apparent as rapid onset of decreased vision, extensive retinal detachment, and hydration lines. (B) Postoperative appearance of this patient.*

corroborated those results, but also emphasized both the rarity of the condition and the difficulty in accurately assessing such cases during the preoperative examination.[48]

7-1-3 Complications of Previous Vitrectomy

Another class of conditions that may constitute an indication for vitrectomy is the presence of one or more complications from a previous vitrectomy. Severe, recurrent vitreous hemorrhage (either before or after vitrectomy) not only is a media opacity, but also may induce a secondary glaucoma through a ghost-cell mechanism.[49–52] Most cases with vitreous hemorrhage and increased intraocular pressure are self-limited or respond to medical therapy. However, selected cases with poorly controlled intraocular pressure despite maximal medical treatment may respond to vitrectomy by debulking the substrate for outflow blockage.[53] In some cases, office-based fluid–gas exchange may provide sufficient elimination of blood, avoiding a second vitrectomy in the operating room.[54,55] In most cases, however, severe, recurrent vitreous hemorrhage after vitrectomy is a manifestation of reproliferation, retinal break formation, or other more severe complications.

Retinal detachment—either tractional or rhegmatogenous—after previous vitrectomy constitutes another indication for a second vitrectomy. Because such cases usually have a guarded visual prognosis, subsequent surgery may not be justified if the fellow eye has stable and satisfactory visual function.

An especially difficult condition is progressive anterior hyaloidal FVP occurring in the weeks to months following vitrectomy. These cases are usually managed by lensectomy and extensive anterior vitreous dissection, similar to techniques used for proliferative vitreoretinopathy.[56]

A rare postvitrectomy complication is the fibrinoid syndrome, which involves extensive fibrinous membrane cross-linking of the vitreous.[57] The fibrinoid syndrome may represent the response of an ischemic retina and increased vascular permeability induced by vitrectomy. Minor degrees of postoperative fibrin formation usually resolve spontaneously. When severe degrees of fibrin formation occur, the use of tissue plasminogen activator[58] or streptokinase[59] has been described. A second vitrectomy is considered in the more severe cases, but the visual prognosis is poor in these eyes with marked postoperative fibrin formation.

7-2

SURGICAL OBJECTIVES AND TECHNIQUES

The surgical objectives of vitrectomy for complications of diabetic retinopathy are numerous and are usually interrelated (Table 7-2). Basically, the objectives are to neutralize and, when possible, eliminate the components that have led to the visual loss. Specifically, this involves the removal of axial media opacities and preretinal traction, and delivery of appropriate laser treatment. New instruments and techniques for use in diabetic vitrectomy have emerged in response to the need to achieve these objectives more safely and reliably.

7-2-1 Media Opacities

Removal of axial opacities involves the vitrectomy instrument and, in some cases, lensectomy instruments. Endoillumination, an operating microscope, and an optical system provide standard visualization of the vitreous strands and surfaces. Newer instruments now offer better control of cutting rates, suction pressure, and fragmentation power and mode. Vitreous removal is facilitated with more complete posterior vitreous separation.

7-2-2 Vitreoretinal Traction

The elimination of traction involves removal of anteroposterior and tangential vitreoretinal traction, as well as removal of membrane-induced surface traction. Several different surgical techniques have been developed to achieve these goals.[60–69] While on the surface each technique seems to represent a totally different approach, all of them achieve the same objectives.

The first two techniques described below, segmentation and delamination, are generally combined as one technique, in contrast to the third method, the en bloc technique.

1. In the segmentation technique, the traction is sequentially dissected by removal of anteroposterior traction (Figure 7-8A), vertical scissors-dissection of bridging epiretinal traction (Figure 7-8B), and, finally, removal of residual islands of traction-incuding epiretinal membranes (Figure 7-8C).[60,61]

2. In the delamination technique, the anteroposterior traction is commonly removed first, using the segmentation technique.

TABLE 7-2

Objectives of Vitrectomy for Severe Diabetic Retinopathy

1. Remove axial opacities

2. Relieve anteroposterior traction

3. Relieve tangential traction

4. Segment or peel epiretinal membranes

5. Effect hemostasis

6. Treat all retinal breaks

7. Deliver laser treatment: limited or full PRP; local treatment of flat neovascularization elsewhere

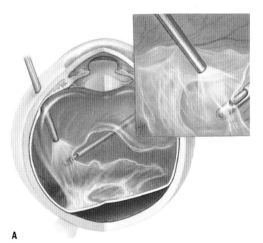

A

Figure 7-8 *Technique of vitreoretinal surgery, in which first media opacities and anteroposterior traction are relieved, followed by relief of bridging traction, (A) typically with vitreous cutter.*
Redrawn with permission of Johns Hopkins University from Michels RG: Proliferative diabetic retinopathy: pathophysiology of extraretinal complications and principles of vitreous surgery. Retina 1981;1:1–17.

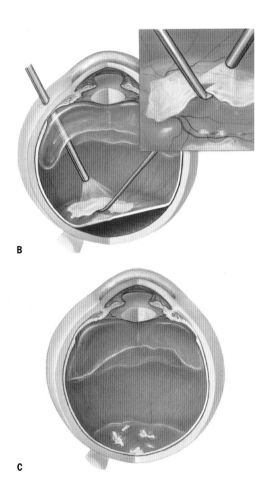

B

C

Figure 7-8 *(B) Vitreoretinal picks and scissors are used to segment preretinal membrane components. (C) Final result is removal of all posterior segment traction with remnant stumps of FVP. Sometimes, FVP is extensive and posterior hyaloid is well defined. In such cases, hyaloid may be peeled up in relatively confluent fashion and fewer fibrovascular stumps ensue. This is more similar to delamination technique (see Figure 7-9).*

With horizontal scissors, vertical scissors, and multifunction instruments (such as lighted picks, lighted forceps, and fiberoptic tissue manipulators), the preretinal tissue is removed at the retinal plane as one or more large pieces (Figure 7-9).[62,63] In this regard, it is similar to the en bloc technique, except that the anteroposterior traction of the vitreous has been previously removed, using the segmentation technique. Complete removal of the remaining fibrovascular stalks from the optic nerve head may include some axons, but does not adversely affect outcomes.[69]

3. In the en bloc technique, the surface traction is removed with horizontal scissors using the anteroposterior traction for countertraction on epiretinal proliferation (Figure 7-10).[64–68] The theoretical advantage of this technique is that the anteroposterior traction serves a "third-hand function" by retracting surface retinal tissue so that subsequent surface dissection is facilitated. The anteroposterior traction and vitreous are removed as the last step. Initially, there was some concern that this technique was associated with more intraoperative retinal breaks (35% in an early report),[67] but with further experience, the rate seems to be equivalent to other techniques (20% in more recent series).[68] Also, the consequences of a break when the traction has been more fully relieved are minimal compared to leaving traction unrelieved.

In many cases, the selected surgical technique is a hybrid of all three techniques. Scleral buckling is sometimes recommended to relieve peripheral retinal traction from unreachable or undissectable membranes.[70]

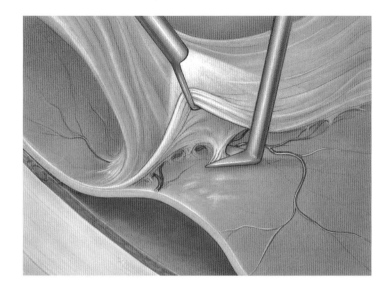

Figure 7-9 *Delamination technique. Although similar to en bloc technique, horizontal scissors are more commonly supplemented by use of lighted instruments, such as lighted picks and lighted forceps, to shave FVP from its retinal attachments. End result characteristically shows fewer fibrovascular stumps.*

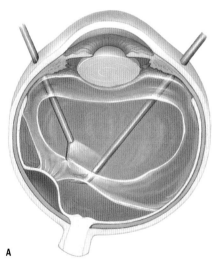

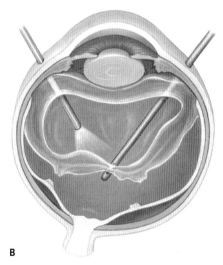

A

B

Figure 7-10 *En bloc technique. Initially, small-core vitrectomy is performed. (A) Posterior hyaloid space is entered and, typically, horizontal scissors are used to dissect vitreous from fibrovascular attachment. (B) Once this has been accomplished, vitreous cutter is used to remove remaining vitreous and FVP in one en bloc fashion.*

7-2-3 Control of Hemorrhage and Reproliferation

Intraoperative hemostasis facilitates completion of the other surgical objectives and optimizes the chance for surgical success by reducing postoperative fibrin and blood. While these are most apparent as media opacities, a potentially more deleterious factor is that they may contain promoters of cellular proliferation or serve as a substratum for reproliferation. Strategies include using intravitreal diathermy, increasing the infusion pressure, or using intraocular thrombin.[71,72] Optimal control of systemic blood pressure may lessen intraoperative and postoperative bleeding.

An important surgical objective is the delivery of endolaser PRP. Before 1983, intraoperative delivery techniques were not reliable. With the advent of laser endophotocoagulation[73–78] and indirect ophthalmoscopic laser delivery systems,[79,80] this objective can now be safely achieved in virtually all cases. The diode laser, which has been developed more recently, allows photocoagulation with certain logistical conveniences.[81,82] When media opacities or available instruments prohibit delivery of laser treatment or when more peripheral treatment is desired, panretinal cryopexy is an option.

7-2-4 Management of Severe Conditions

A necessary surgical objective is the treatment of retinal breaks. Retinal breaks may occur in up to 20% of diabetic vitrectomy cases and may lead to retinal detachment if untreated.[83] Most intraoperative breaks can be successfully managed by performing fluid–gas exchange and applying endolaser photocoagulation. Silicone oil may play a role in effecting long-term internal tamponade of multiple retinal breaks, usually in the setting of a reoperation for recurrent retinal detachment due to reproliferation of fibrovascular tissues causing proliferative vitreoretinopathy.[84–87] With anterior hyaloidal FVP, removal of the lens may allow more complete peripheral membrane dissection, but is usually reserved for reoperations.[88]

A final, but concurrent surgical objective is to treat and avoid future complications. Endolaser PRP, even if previous treatment has been applied, is usually delivered intraoperatively to reduce the likelihood of anterior segment neovascularization, to treat retinal breaks, and to maintain retinal reattachment. Intraoperative PRP has also been reported to reduce rates of postoperative vitreous hemorrhage. Preoperative anterior segment neovascularization often regresses in eyes with silicone oil, possibly by blocking diffusion of a vasoproliferative substance, and may constitute an indication for the use of silicone oil in selected cases.[89] Lensectomy may lead to an increased risk of postoperative rubeosis, but this rate is reduced after application of intraoperative PRP in more recent reports.

7-2-5 Instrumentation

A host of multifunction intraocular instruments have been developed to facilitate achieving the surgical objectives. The earliest vitreous-cutting probes combined the functions of infusion, suction, and cutting. Later generations of instruments separated these three tasks and allowed smaller sclerotomies, which lowered the risk of iatrogenic retinal dialysis. In recent years, the light probe has been modified to allow additional functions while remaining small enough to use a normal-sized sclerotomy. These instruments include the illuminated pick or forceps, the fiberoptic tissue manipulator for irrigation and aspiration, and the illuminated endolaser probe. A fourth sclerotomy has been advocated to allow insertion of a multiport illumination system, freeing up the second hand to use a pick or forceps.

Wide-angle viewing systems have been developed to facilitate the global view of the posterior pole, thereby lessening the risk of inducing unintended traction and retinal breaks in distant areas.[90,91] Another useful innovation has been the development of a variety of iris retractors.[92,93] While usually reserved for pseudophakic or aphakic patients, iris retractors facilitate achieving surgical objectives by maximizing the view of the posterior segment in patients with fixed, small pupils. Flexible iris retractors may be used in phakic patients.

7-3

OUTCOMES

Varying degrees of concomitant traction, capillary nonperfusion, retinal detachment, and macular edema may influence visual acuity outcomes in patients with diabetic retinopathy. Thus, very few cases present with vitreous hemorrhage as the sole cause of visual loss because concurrent diabetic maculopathy and extensive capillary nonperfusion also usually limit visual acuity.

7-3-1 Media Opacities

Over the past two decades, the results of vitrectomy for nonclearing diabetic hemorrhage have been reviewed extensively (Table 7-3).[18–20,29–32,94–100] A final visual acuity of ≥20/200 in 40% to 62% of patients has been reported and improved vision in 59% to 83% of patients. The Diabetic Retinopathy Vitrectomy Study (DRVS) demonstrated that early vitrectomy (1 to 4 months after the onset of severe vitreous hemorrhage) for type 1 diabetic patients yields visual acuity outcomes of 20/40 or better at 2 years in 36% of this subgroup, compared to only 12% with conventional management ($P = 0.001$).[31] The larger differential for type 1 versus type 2 patients is postulated to be due to the tendency for type 1 diabetic patients to have more extensive and aggressive neovascularization at an earlier stage. However, the rates of no light perception, visual acuity of ≥5/200, and visual acuity of ≥20/200 were similar for both groups.

Excellent surgical results have been reported for subhyaloidal hemorrhage removal.[101,102] Nearly all patients with visual acuity of 20/100 regained 20/40 or better after vitrectomy.

Combined cataract removal, vitrectomy, and endolaser treatment has been studied in relatively small series, with the finding that removal of the cataract does not increase the risk of rubeosis iridis or compromise the anatomic objectives.[39–42]

TABLE 7-3

Outcomes of Pars Plana Vitrectomy for Complications of Proliferative Diabetic Retinopathy

Complication	Improved Vision (%)	≥20/200 (%)	No Light Perception (%)
Vitreous hemorrhage	59–83	40–62	5–17
Fibrovascular proliferation	70	70	11
Tractional retinal detachment	59–80	21–58	11–19
Combined tractional and rhegmatogenous retinal detachment	32–53	25–36	9–23

Source: *Expanded from Blankenship GW: Proliferative diabetic retinopathy: principles and techniques of surgical treatment. In: Ryan SJ, ed:* Retina. *St Louis: CV Mosby Co; 1989;3:515–539.*

7-3-2 Vitreoretinal Traction

The first report of the DRVS showed that the nonsurgical management of patients with progressive FVP involved a very high rate of severe visual loss.[103] In a subsequent DRVS report, 370 patients with severe neovascularization were randomized to early vitrectomy or conventional management (deferral of vitrectomy to 1 year unless tractional detachment involved the macula). The rate of final vision ≥20/40 was 44% for the early-vitrectomy group compared to 28% in the conventional group with 4 years' followup (P = <0.05).[23]

Other investigators have found that preoperative factors indicating a more favorable postoperative result include age <40 years, preoperative vision ≥5/200, absence of iris neovascularization, and preoperative application of photocoagulation.[24] One series of 50 eyes, many with relatively good visual acuity, reported that 72% had improvement and only 10% lost vision after vitrectomy.[98] Thus, when patients have moderate visual loss (20/40 to 20/80) caused by progressive FVP, vitrectomy should be considered.[100]

The outcomes of vitrectomy for tractional retinal detachment involving the macula are somewhat worse than for vitreous hemorrhage alone.[14] Visual improvement of two lines or more has been reported in 59% to 80% of cases, but postoperative visual acuity reaches 20/200 or better in 21% to 58% (see Table 7-3).[16,25,64,99,102,104–109]

The outcomes of vitrectomy for combined tractional and rhegmatogenous retinal detachment are generally worse than for cases with purely tractional detachment. In this combined retinal detachment subgroup, visual improvement is reported in 32% to 53% and final visual acuity ≥20/200 in 25% to 36% (see Table 7-3).[22,110,111]

All too often, final visual acuity is limited despite successful achievement of the surgical and anatomic objectives. This outcome is usually attributable to generalized retinal ischemia, which may be evident as attenuated arterioles, capillary nonperfusion, and retinal thinning (featureless) (Figure 7-11).

7-3-3 Complications of Previous Vitrectomy

The outcomes of subsequent vitrectomy for complications after initial vitrectomy are poor, but visual acuity can be maintained or improved in some patients. In a series of 41 eyes undergoing reoperation, the authors reported that the indication for reoperation was associated with the visual prognosis; rhegmatogenous retinal detachment carried the worst visual prognosis.[112] Overall, 56% had final visual acuity of light perception or no light perception, including 32% with phthisis and 94% with preoperative rubeosis iridis. It is this group that most frequently requires silicone oil to achieve even modest degrees of success.[84-88]

7-4

COMPLICATIONS

The principal complications of vitrectomy in diabetic patients include recurrent vitreous hemorrhage, retinal detachment, and rubeosis iridis.[113-116] Some degree of postoperative vitreous hemorrhage occurs in virtually all cases, but is visually significant in about 30% of cases.[114] Management options include office-based fluid–gas exchange,[54,117] vitreous lavage, or a second vitrectomy. Before reoperation, a waiting period ranging from weeks to months is generally recommended to allow spontaneous clearing. The rates of postoperative retinal detachment and neovascular glaucoma vary with the preoperative diagnoses, and may occur in up to 20% of cases. In patients with poorly controlled neovascular glaucoma, procedures such as Molteno or Baerveldt seton placements may be considered, because standard glaucoma filtering surgery is usu-

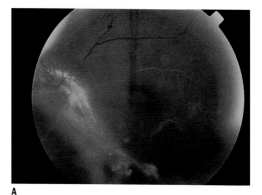

A

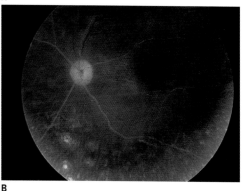

B

Figure 7-11 *(A) Patient presented with visual acuity of 20/400 and tractional elevation extending from disc and inferotemporal arcade into macula. Even preoperatively, marked vascular sclerosis extending into macula is evident. (B) Postoperative appearance shows visual acuity of 20/200 with total removal of preretinal components and supplementary PRP. However, narrowing of arterioles and capillary nonperfusion are now more evident and are probable cause of limited vision.*

ally unsuccessful in such cases.[118,119] Also, the risk of endophthalmitis after vitrectomy is higher in diabetic patients.[120] While there may be other potential postoperative complications, they are not unique to diabetic vitrectomy cases.

7-5

PUBLIC HEALTH CONSIDERATIONS

As the technical upper limits in treating certain conditions are asymptotically approached, much attention has been directed toward optimal application of preventive therapies.[2,3,121] Javitt and associates have shown the cost-effectiveness of proper application of subsequent collaborative laser studies sponsored by the National Eye Institute to the diabetic population at risk.[122] With appropriate and timely laser photocoagulation, disability and associated expenses can be minimized.

Currently, medical care expenditures are being increasingly examined. The high costs for complex surgical cases, such as pars plana vitrectomy, have come under particular scrutiny and, indeed, have been a target of significant reimbursement reductions. The field of evidence-based medicine has emerged to evaluate the effectiveness of various treatment resources. These studies have been mostly focused on the functional outcomes of patients undergoing cataract surgery.[123] Outcomes research relies heavily on "patient satisfaction" and patients' perceptions of their functional status, which are difficult to quantify because of their subjective nature.

Objective measures of functional status were developed and studied in a series of 213 diabetic patients who underwent vitrectomy for complications of proliferative diabetic retinopathy.[124] In this series, the operated eye became the better-seeing eye in 32% of patients and equal to the fellow eye in 16%. These patients had an average 61% disability of the visual system preoperatively (as determined by guidelines of the American Medical Association) due to the high frequency of disease in the fellow eye, but improved postoperatively to 50% disability. Improvements were greater in eyes without preoperative retinal detachment. Similar outcomes were found in analyses of nondiabetic vitreoretinal procedures,[125] and in the same study cohort outcomes were found to be worthwhile as measured by patient-satisfaction surveys.[126]

7-6

CONCLUSION

The indications and timing of pars plana vitrectomy for diabetic retinopathy continue to evolve, but have not changed conceptually. The thresholds for performing surgery in established indications have generally been lowered, and a few additional indications have been established. The lowered thresholds are attributable to improvements in both instrumentation and surgical techniques. Accordingly, more difficult cases are now being considered and postoperative recovery of vision is more consistent.

Although the postvitrectomy visual acuity outcomes are favorable compared to the natural history of diabetic retinopathy, they are still poor compared to the potential efficacy of preventive measures, such as improved control of glucose and timely application of laser treatment. Despite optimal medical and ophthalmologic management, substantial numbers of patients will have progressive retinopathy, leading to the need for laser treatment and pars plana vitrectomy.[14] Because long-term stability of initially successful treatment is good[127] and life expectancy following diabetic vitrectomy is relatively favorable,[128] pars plana vitrectomy remains an essential tool in the management of severe complications from diabetic retinopathy.

REFERENCES

1. Aiello LP, Gardner TW, King GL, et al: Diabetic retinopathy. *Diabetes Care* 1998;21:143–156.

2. American Diabetes Association: Diabetic retinopathy [position statement]. *Diabetes Care* 1998;21(suppl):547–549.

3. Patz A, Smith RE: The ETDRS and Diabetes 2000. *Ophthalmology* 1991;98:739–740.

4. Diabetes Control and Complications Trial Research Group: The effect of intensive treatment of diabetes on the development and progression of long-term complications in insulin-dependent diabetes mellitus. *New Engl J Med* 1993;329: 977–986.

5. Diabetes Control and Complications Trial Research Group: The effect of intensive diabetes treatment on the progression of diabetic retinopathy in insulin-dependent diabetes mellitus. *Arch Ophthalmol* 1995;113:36–51.

6. Aiello LM, Beetham WP, Balodimos MC, et al: Ruby laser photocoagulation in treatment of diabetic proliferating retinopathy: preliminary report. In: Goldberg MF, Fine SL, eds: *Symposium on the Treatment of Diabetic Retinopathy.* (Airlie House, 1968) Public Health Service Publ. No. 1890. Washington, DC: US Govt Printing Office; 1969:437–463.

7. Diabetic Retinopathy Study Research Group: Preliminary report on effects of photocoagulation therapy. *Am J Ophthalmol* 1976;81:383–396.

8. Diabetic Retinopathy Study Research Group: Photocoagulation treatment of proliferative diabetic retinopathy: the second report of the Diabetic Retinopathy Study findings. *Ophthalmology* 1978;85:82–106.

9. Diabetic Retinopathy Study Research Group: Four risk factors for severe visual loss in diabetic retinopathy: the third report from the Diabetic Retinopathy Study. *Arch Ophthalmol* 1979;97: 654–655.

10. Diabetic Retinopathy Study Research Group: Photocoagulation treatment of proliferative diabetic retinopathy: relationship of adverse treatment effects to retinopathy severity. DRS Report Number 5. *Dev Ophthalmol* 1981;2:248–261.

11. L'Esperance FA: The treatment of ophthalmic vascular disease by argon laser photocoagulation. *Ophthalmology* 1968;72:1077–1096.

12. Doft BH, Metz DJ, Kelsey SF: Augmentation laser for proliferative diabetic retinopathy that fails to respond to initial panretinal photocoagulation. *Ophthalmology* 1992;99:1728–1734; discussion 1734–1735.

13. Vine AK: The efficacy of additional argon laser photocoagulation for persistent, severe proliferative diabetic retinopathy. *Ophthalmology* 1985;92:1532–1537.

14. Flynn HW Jr, Chew EY, Simons BD, et al: Pars plana vitrectomy in the Early Treatment Diabetic Retinopathy Study. ETDRS Report Number 17. *Ophthalmology* 1992;99:1351–1357.

15. Aaberg TM: Results of 100 consecutive vitrectomy procedures. In: McPherson A, ed: New and *Controversial Aspects of Vitreoretinal Surgery.* St Louis: CV Mosby Co; 1977:245–249.

16. Aaberg TM: Pars plana vitrectomy for diabetic traction retinal detachment. *Ophthalmology* 1981;88:639–642.

17. Blankenship GW: Preoperative prognostic factors in diabetic pars plana vitrectomy. *Ophthalmology* 1982;89:1246–1249.

18. Michels RG, Rice TA, Rice EF: Vitrectomy for diabetic vitreous hemorrhage. *Am J Ophthalmol* 1983;95:12–21.

19. Oldendoerp J, Spitznas M: Factors influencing the results of vitreous surgery in diabetic retinopathy, I: iris rubeosis and/or active neovascularization at the fundus. *Graefes Arch Klin Exp Ophthalmol* 1989;227:1–8.

20. Sigurdsson H, Baines PS, Roxburgh ST: Vitrectomy for diabetic eye disease. *Eye* 1988;2: 418–423.

21. Diabetic Retinopathy Vitrectomy Study Research Group: Early vitrectomy for severe vitreous hemorrhage in diabetic retinopathy: two-year results of a randomized trial. DRVS Report Number 2. *Arch Ophthalmol* 1985;103:1644–1652.

22. Rice TA, Michels RG, Rice EF: Vitrectomy for diabetic rhegmatogenous retinal detachment. *Am J Ophthalmol* 1983;95:34–44.

23. Diabetic Retinopathy Vitrectomy Study Research Group: Early vitrectomy for severe proliferative diabetic retinopathy in eyes with useful vision: results of a randomized trial. DRVS Report Number 3. *Ophthalmology* 1988;95: 1307–1320.

24. de Bustros S, Thompson JT, Michels RG, Rice TA: Vitrectomy for progressive proliferative diabetic retinopathy. *Arch Ophthalmol* 1987;105: 196–199.

25. Hutton WL, Bernstein I, Fuller D: Diabetic traction retinal detachment: factors influencing final visual acuity. *Ophthalmology* 1980;87: 1071–1077.

26. Machemer R, Norton EW: A new concept for vitreous surgery, 3: indications and results. *Am J Ophthalmol* 1972;74:1034–1055.

27. Michels RG: Vitrectomy for complications of diabetic retinopathy. *Arch Ophthalmol* 1978;96: 237–246.

28. Smiddy WE, Flynn HW Jr: Vitrectomy in the management of diabetic retinopathy. *Surv Ophthalmol* 1999;43:491–507.

29. Machemer R, Blankenship G: Vitrectomy for proliferative diabetic retinopathy associated with vitreous hemorrhage. *Ophthalmology* 1981;88: 643–646.

30. Aaberg TM, Abrams GW: Changing indications and techniques for vitrectomy in management of complications of diabetic retinopathy. *Ophthalmology* 1987;94:775–779.

31. Diabetic Retinopathy Vitretomy Study Research Group: Early vitrectomy for severe vitreous hemorrhage in diabetic retinopathy: four-year results of a randomized trial. DRVS Report Number 5. *Arch Ophthalmol* 1990;108:958–964.

32. Machemer R: Pathogenesis of proliferative neovascular retinopathies and the role of vitrectomy: a hypothesis. *Int Ophthalmol* 1978;1:1–3.

33. Davis MD: Vitreous contraction in proliferative diabetic retinopathy. *Arch Ophthalmol* 1965; 74:741–751.

34. Faulborn J, Bowald S: Microproliferations in proliferative diabetic retinopathy and their relationship to the vitreous: corresponding light and electron microscopic studies. *Graefes Arch Klin Exp Ophthalmol* 1985;223:130–138.

35. Blankenship GW: The lens influence on diabetic vitrectomy results: report of a prospective randomized study. *Arch Ophthalmol* 1980;98: 2196–2198.

36. Aiello LM, Wand M, Liang G: Neovascular glaucoma and vitreous hemorrhage following cataract surgery in patients with diabetes mellitus. *Ophthalmology* 1983;90:814–820.

37. Blankenship GW, Cortez R, Machemer R: The lens and pars plana vitrectomy for diabetic retinopathy complications. *Arch Ophthalmol* 1979; 97:1263–1267.

38. Rice TA, Michels RG, Maguire MG, Rice EF: The effect of lensectomy on the incidence of iris neovascularization and neovascular glaucoma after vitrectomy for diabetic retinopathy. *Am J Ophthalmol* 1983;95:1–11.

39. Blankenship GW, Flynn HW Jr, Kokame GT: Posterior chamber intraocular lens insertion during pars plana lensectomy and vitrectomy for complications of proliferative diabetic retinopathy. *Am J Ophthalmol* 1989;108:1–5.

40. Kokame GT, Flynn HW Jr, Blankenship GW: Posterior chamber intraocular lens implantation during diabetic pars plana vitrectomy. *Ophthalmology* 1989;96:603–610.

41. Benson WE, Brown GC, Tasman W, McNamara JA: Extracapsular cataract extraction, posterior chamber lens insertion, and pars plana vitrectomy in one operation. *Ophthalmology* 1990; 97:918–921.

42. Chaudhry NA, Belforte A, Flynn HW Jr, et al: Combined cataract extraction and pars plana vitrectomy for proliferative diabetic retinopathy. *Invest Ophthalmol Vis Sci* 1998;39(S):3818.

43. Küchle M, Händel A, Naumann GO: Cataract extraction in eyes with diabetic iris neovascularization. *Ophthalmic Surg Lasers* 1998;29: 28–32.

44. Sato Y, Shimada H, Aso S, Matsui M: Vitrectomy for diabetic macular heterotopia. *Ophthalmology* 1994;101:63–67.

45. Charles S, Flinn CE: The natural history of diabetic extramacular traction retinal detachment. *Arch Ophthalmol* 1981;99:66–68.

46. Early Treatment Diabetic Retinopathy Study Research Group: Photocoagulation for diabetic macular edema. ETDRS Report Number 1. *Arch Ophthalmol* 1985;103:1796–1806.

47. Lewis H, Abrams GW, Blumenkranz MS, Campo RV: Resolution of diabetic macular edema associated with a thickened and taut premacular posterior hyaloid after vitrectomy. *Ophthalmology* 1991;98(S):146.

48. Harbour W, Smiddy WE, Flynn HW Jr, Rubsamen PE: Vitrectomy for diabetic macular edema associated with a thickened and taut posterior hyaloid membrane. *Am J Ophthalmol* 1996; 121:405–413.

49. Campbell DG, Simmons RJ, Tolentino FI, McMeel JW: Glaucoma occurring after closed vitrectomy. *Am J Ophthalmol* 1977;83:63–69.

50. Campbell DG, Simmons RJ, Grant WM: Ghost cells as a cause of glaucoma. *Am J Ophthalmol* 1976;81:441–450.

51. Han DP, Lewis H, Lambrou FH Jr, et al: Mechanisms of intraocular pressure elevation after pars plana vitrectomy. *Ophthalmology* 1989; 96:1357–1362.

52. Weinberg RS, Peyman GA, Huamonte FU: Elevation of intraocular pressure after pars plana vitrectomy. *Graefes Arch Klin Exp Ophthalmol* 1976;200:157–161.

53. Singh H, Grand MG: Treatment of blood-induced glaucoma by trans pars plana vitrectomy. *Retina* 1981;1:255–257.

54. Miller JA, Chandra SR, Stevens TS: A modified technique for performing outpatient fluid–air exchange following vitrectomy surgery. *Am J Ophthalmol* 1986;101:116–117.

55. Blankenship GW: Management of vitreous cavity hemorrhage following pars plana vitrectomy for diabetic retinopathy. *Ophthalmology* 1986;93:39–44.

56. Lewis H, Abrams GW, Williams GA: Anterior hyaloidal fibrovascular proliferation after diabetic vitrectomy. *Am J Ophthalmol* 1987;104:607–613.

57. Sebestyen JG: Fibrinoid syndrome: a severe complication of vitrectomy surgery in diabetics. *Ann Ophthalmol* 1982;14:853–856.

58. Williams GA, Lambrou FH, Jaffe GA, et al: Treatment of post-vitrectomy fibrin formation with intraocular tissue plasminogen activator. *Arch Ophthalmol* 1988;106:1055–1058.

59. Cherfan GM, el Maghraby A, Tabbara KF, et al: Dissolution of intraocular fibrinous exudate by streptokinase. *Ophthalmology* 1991;98:870–874.

60. Michels RG: Proliferative diabetic retinopathy: pathophysiology of extraretinal complications and principles of vitreous surgery. *Retina* 1981;1:1–17.

61. Meredith TA, Kaplan HJ, Aaberg TM: Pars plana vitrectomy techniques for relief of epiretinal traction by membrane segmentation. *Am J Ophthalmol* 1980;89:408–413.

62. Charles S: *Vitreous Microsurgery.* Baltimore: Williams & Wilkins; 1981:107–120.

63. Meredith TA: Epiretinal membrane delamination with a diamond knife. *Arch Ophthalmol* 1997;115:1598–1599.

64. Abrams GW, Williams GA: "En bloc" excision of diabetic membranes. *Am J Ophthalmol* 1987;103:302–308.

65. McCuen BW II, Hickingbotham D: A fiberoptic diathermy tissue manipulator for use in vitreous surgery. *Am J Ophthalmol* 1984;98:803–804.

66. Abrams GW: Dissection methods in vitrectomy for diabetic retinopathy. In: Franklin RM, ed: *Retina and Vitreous.* Proceedings of Symposium on Retina and Vitreous, New Orleans Academy of Ophthalmology. Amsterdam/New York: Kluger; 1993:101–113.

67. Williams DF, Williams GA, Hartz A, et al: Results of vitrectomy for diabetic traction retinal detachments using the en bloc excision technique. *Ophthalmology* 1989;96:752–758.

68. Han DP, Murphy ML, Mieler WF: A modified en bloc excision technique during vitrectomy for diabetic traction retinal detachment: results and complications. *Ophthalmology* 1994;101:803–808.

69. Pendergast SD, Martin DF, Proia AD, et al: Removal of optic disc stalks during diabetic vitrectomy. *Retina* 1995;15:25–28.

70. Han DP, Pulido JS, Mieler WF, Johnson MW: Vitrectomy for proliferative diabetic retinopathy with severe equatorial fibrovascular proliferation. *Am J Ophthalmol* 1995;119:563–570.

71. de Bustros S, Glaser BM, Johnson MA: Thrombin infusion for the control of intraocular bleeding during vitreous surgery. *Arch Ophthalmol* 1985;103:837–839.

72. Thompson JT, Glaser BM, Michels RG, de Bustros S: The use of intravitreal thrombin to control hemorrhage during vitrectomy. *Ophthalmology* 1986;93:279–282.

73. Charles S: Endophotocoagulation. *Retina* 1981;1:117–120.

74. Peyman GA, Grisolano JM, Palacio MN: Intraocular photocoagulation with the argon-krypton laser. *Arch Ophthalmol* 1980;98:2062–2064.

75. Fleischman JA, Swartz M, Dixon JA: Argon laser endophotocoagulation: an intraoperative trans–pars plana technique. *Arch Ophthalmol* 1981;99:1610–1612.

76. Liggett PE, Lean JS, Barlow WE, Ryan SJ: Intraoperative argon endophotocoagulation for recurrent vitreous hemorrhage after vitrectomy for diabetic retinopathy. *Am J Ophthalmol* 1987; 103:146–149.

77. Landers MB III, Trese MT, Stefansson E, Bessler M: Argon laser intraocular photocoagulation. *Ophthalmology* 1982;89:785–788.

78. Parke DW II, Aaberg TM: Intraocular argon laser photocoagulation in the management of severe proliferative vitreoretinopathy. *Am J Ophthalmol* 1984;97:434–443.

79. Friberg TR: Clinical experience with a binocular indirect ophthalmoscope laser delivery system. *Retina* 1987;7:28–31.

80. Whitacre MM, Manoukian N, Mainster MA: Argon indirect ophthalmoscopic photocoagulation: reduced potential phototoxicity with a fixed safety filter. *Br J Ophthalmol* 1990;74:233–234.

81. Smiddy WE: Diode endolaser photocoagulation. *Arch Ophthalmol* 1992;110:1172–1174.

82. Sasoh M, Smiddy WE: Diode laser endophotocoagulation. *Retina* 1995;15:388–393.

83. Oyakawa RT, Schachat AP, Michels RG, Rice TA: Complications of vitreous surgery for diabetic retinopathy, I: intraoperative complications. *Ophthalmology* 1983;90:517–521.

84. Rinkoff JS, de Juan E Jr, McCuen BW II: Silicone oil for retinal detachment with advanced proliferative vitreoretinopathy following failed vitrectomy for proliferative diabetic retinopathy. *Am J Ophthalmol* 1986;101:181–186.

85. Yeo JH, Glaser BM, Michels RG: Silicone oil in the treatment of complicated retinal detachments. *Ophthalmology* 1987;94:1109–1113.

86. Heimann K, Dahl B, Dimopoulos S, Lemmen KD: Pars plana vitrectomy and silicone oil injection in proliferative diabetic retinopathy. *Graefes Arch Klin Exp Ophthalmol* 1989;227: 152–156.

87. Brourman ND, Blumenkranz MS, Cox MS, Trese MT: Silicone oil for the treatment of severe proliferative diabetic retinopathy. *Ophthalmology* 1989;96:759–764.

88. Ehud A, Varda C, Joseph M, Giora T: Management of complicated retinal detachment by vitrectomy and silicone oil injection. *Metab Pediatr Syst Ophthalmol* 1988;11:63–66.

89. McCuen BW II, Rinkoff JS: Silicone oil for progressive anterior ocular neovascularization after failed diabetic vitrectomy. *Arch Ophthalmol* 1989;107:677–682.

90. Spitznas M: A binocular indirect ophthalmomicroscope (BIOM) for non-contact wide-angle vitreous surgery. *Graefes Arch Klin Exp Ophthalmol* 1987;225:13–15.

91. Spitznas M, Reiner J: A stereoscopic diagonal inverter (SDI) for wide-angle vitreous surgery. *Graefes Arch Klin Exp Ophthalmol* 1987;225: 9–12.

92. de Juan E Jr, Hickingbotham D: Flexible iris retractor. *Am J Ophthalmol* 1991;111:776–777.

93. Arpa P: A new device for pupillary dilation in vitreous surgery. *Retina* 1992;12(suppl): S87–S89.

94. Blankenship GW: Proliferative diabetic retinopathy: principles and techniques of surgical treatment. In: Ryan SJ, ed: *Retina*. St Louis: CV Mosby Co; 1989;3:515–539.

95. Peyman GA, Raichand M, Huamonte FU, et al: Vitrectomy in 125 eyes with diabetic vitreous haemorrhage. *Br J Ophthalmol* 1976;60:752–755.

96. Rice TA, Michels RG: Long-term anatomic and functional results of vitrectomy for diabetic retinopathy. *Am J Ophthalmol* 1980;90:297–303.

97. Thompson JT, Auer CL, de Bustros S, et al: Prognostic indicators of success and failure in vitrectomy for diabetic retinopathy. *Ophthalmology* 1986;93:290–295.

98. Grewing R, Mester U: Early vitrectomy for progressive diabetic proliferations covering the macula. *Br J Ophthalmol* 1994;78:433–436.

99. Thompson JT, de Bustros S, Michels RG, et al: Results of vitrectomy for proliferative diabetic retinopathy. *Ophthalmology* 1986;93:1571–1574.

100. Diabetic Retinopathy Vitrectomy Study Research Group: Early vitrectomy for severe proliferative diabetic retinopathy in eyes with useful vision: clinical application of results of a randomized trial. DRVS Report Number 4. *Ophthalmology* 1988;95:1321–1334.

101. Packer AJ: Vitrectomy for progressive macular traction associated with proliferative diabetic retinopathy. *Arch Ophthalmol* 1987;105:1679–1682.

102. O'Hanley GP, Canny CL: Diabetic dense premacular hemorrhage: a possible indication for prompt vitrectomy. *Ophthalmology* 1985;92:507–511.

103. Diabetic Retinopathy Vitrectomy Study Research Group: Two-year course of visual acuity in severe proliferative diabetic retinopathy with conventional management. DRVS Report Number 1. *Ophthalmology* 1985;92:492–502.

104. Miller SA, Butler JB, Myers FL, Bresnick GH: Pars plana vitrectomy: treatment for tractional macula detachment secondary to proliferative diabetic retinopathy. *Arch Ophthalmol* 1980;98:659–664.

105. Rice TA, Michels RG, Rice EF: Vitrectomy for diabetic traction retinal detachment involving the macula. *Am J Ophthalmol* 1983;95:22–33.

106. Thompson JT, de Bustros S, Michels RG, Rice TA: Results and prognostic factors in vitrectomy for diabetic traction retinal detachment of the macula. *Arch Ophthalmol* 1987;105:497–502.

107. Tolentino FI, Freeman HM, Tolentino FL: Closed vitrectomy in the management of diabetic traction retinal detachment. *Ophthalmology* 1980;87:1078–1089.

108. Nakae R, Saito Y, Nishikawa N, et al: Results of vitrectomy for diabetic traction retinal detachment involving the macula: a comparison of six-month and three-year postoperative findings. *Nippon Ganka Gakkai Zasshi* 1989;93:271–275.

109. Meier P, Weidemann P: Vitrectomy for traction macular detachment in diabetic retinopathy. *Graefes Arch Klin Exp Ophthalmol* 1997;235:569–574.

110. Rice TA, Michels RG, Rice EF: Vitrectomy for diabetic rhegmatogenous retinal detachment. *Am J Ophthalmol* 1983;95:34–44.

111. Thompson JT, de Bustros S, Michels RG, Rice TA: Results and prognostic factors in vitrectomy for diabetic traction-rhegmatogenous retinal detachment. *Arch Ophthalmol* 1987;105:503–507.

112. Brown GC, Tasman WS, Benson WE, et al: Reoperation following diabetic vitrectomy. *Arch Ophthalmol* 1992;110:506–510.

113. Aaberg TM, Van Horn DL: Late complications of pars plana vitreous surgery. *Ophthalmology* 1978;85:126–140.

114. Schachat AP, Oyakawa RT, Michels RG, Rice TA: Complications of vitreous surgery for diabetic retinopathy, II: postoperative complications. *Ophthalmology* 1983;90:522–530.

115. Novak MA, Rice TA, Michels RG, Auer C: Vitreous hemorrhage after vitrectomy for diabetic retinopathy. *Ophthalmology* 1984;91:1485–1489.

116. Wand M, Madigan JC, Gaudio AR, Sorokanich S: Neovascular glaucoma following pars plana vitrectomy for complications of diabetic retinopathy. *Ophthalmic Surg* 1990;21:113–118.

117. Martin DF, McCuen BW II: Efficacy of fluid–air exchange for postvitrectomy diabetic vitreous hemorrhage. *Am J Ophthalmol* 1992;114:457–463.

118. Lloyd MA, Heuer DK, Baerveldt G, et al: Combined Molteno implantation and pars plana vitrectomy for neovascular glaucomas. *Ophthalmology* 1991;98:1401–1405.

119. Varma R, Heuer DK, Lundy DC, et al: Pars plana Baerveldt tube insertion with vitrectomy in glaucomas associated with pseudophakia and aphakia. *Am J Ophthalmol* 1995;119:401–407.

120. Cohen SM, Flynn HW Jr, Murray TG, Smiddy WE: Endophthalmitis after pars plana vitrectomy. Postvitrectomy Endophthalmitis Study Group. *Ophthalmology* 1995;102:705–712.

121. *Diabetic Retinopathy.* Preferred Practice Pattern. San Francisco: American Academy of Ophthalmology; 1989.

122. Javitt JC, Aiello LP, Bassi LJ, et al: Detecting and treating retinopathy in patients with type I diabetes mellitus: savings associated with improved implementation of current guidelines. *Ophthalmology* 1991;98:1565–1574.

123. Steinberg EP, Tielsch JM, Schein OD, et al: National study of cataract surgery outcomes: variation in 4-month postoperative outcomes as reflected in multiple outcome measures. *Ophthalmology* 1994;101:1131–1141.

124. Smiddy WE, Feuer W, Irvine WD, et al: Vitrectomy for complications of proliferative diabetic retinopathy: functional outcomes. *Ophthalmology* 1995;102:1688–1695.

125. Scott IU, Smiddy WE, Merikansky A, Feuer W: Vitreoretinal surgery outcomes: impact on bilateral visual function. *Ophthalmology* 1997:104:1041–1048.

126. Scott IU, Smiddy WE, Feuer W, Merikansky A: Vitreoretinal surgery outcomes: results of a patient satisfaction/functional status survey. *Ophthalmology* 1998;105:795–803.

127. Blankenship GW, Machemer R: Long-term diabetic vitrectomy results: report of a 10 year follow-up. *Ophthalmology* 1985;92:503–506.

128. Gollamudi SR, Smiddy WE, Schachat AP, et al: Long-term survival rate after vitreous surgery for complications of diabetic retinopathy. *Ophthalmology* 1991;98:18–22.

Medical Management of Diabetic Retinopathy

Jay S. Skyler, MD

Medical management for diabetic retinopathy is largely that of prevention. Controlled clinical trials have demonstrated that aggressive glycemic control reduces the risk of retinopathy and slows the progression of retinopathy. As a consequence, current recommendations for glycemic control are to aim for fasting plasma glucose to be <110 mg/dL and HbA_{1c} to be <7% (normal range about 3.0% to 6.0%). Controlled clinical trials also have demonstrated that aggressive blood pressure control reduces the risk of retinopathy. As a consequence, current recommendations for blood pressure control are to aim for systolic blood pressure to be <130 mm Hg and diastolic blood pressure to be <85 mm Hg in adults with diabetes. No specific medical therapy has yet been shown to be effective, although a number of therapies are under evaluation in clinical trials.

8-1

GLYCEMIC CONTROL

Analyses from a number of epidemiologic studies and randomized, controlled clinical trials suggest a significant relationship between glycemia and retinopathy.[1–11] In

these studies, integrated glycemic control is measured by glycosylated hemoglobin—either HbA_{1c} or HbA_1 (which includes HbA_{1c}, as well as HbA_{1a} and HbA_{1b}) or total glycosylated hemoglobin (which measures slightly different components).

8-1-1 Epidemiologic Study

8-1-1-1 Wisconsin Epidemiologic Study of Diabetic Retinopathy
One of the longest, largest, and most carefully conducted epidemiologic studies is the Wisconsin Epidemiologic Study of Diabetic Retinopathy (WESDR).[2–5] (For a detailed discussion of the Wisconsin study, see Chapter 2, "Epidemiology of Eye Disease in Diabetes.")

In all three cohorts (younger-onset, older-onset treated with insulin, and older-onset not treated with insulin), there was, at both 4 and 10 years' followup, a statistically significant relationship between baseline HbA_1 and (1) incidence of retinopathy, (2) progression of retinopathy by two or more steps on a modified scale developed by the Early Treatment Diabetic Retinopa-

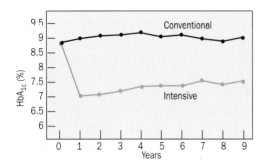

Figure 8-1 *Measurement of glycosylated hemoglobin (HbA$_{1c}$) in DCCT patients with type 1 diabetes, assigned to conventional or intensive treatment. Median values are shown. Differences are statistically significant at all time points after baseline (P <0.001).*

Adapted with permission from Diabetes Control and Complications Trial Research Group: The effect of intensive treatment of diabetes on the development and progression of long-term complications in insulin-dependent diabetes mellitus. N Engl J Med 1993;329:683–689. Copyright © 1993, Massachusetts Medical Society. All rights reserved.

thy Study (ETDRS), and (3) progression to proliferative diabetic retinopathy (PDR).[4,5] At the 10-year followup, there was also a statistically significant relationship between baseline HbA$_1$ and (1) macular edema in the younger-onset cohort and the older-onset cohort considered as a whole and (2) visual loss in the younger-onset cohort and the older-onset cohort treated with insulin, but not in the older-onset cohort not treated with insulin. In the older-onset cohort, however, nondiabetic causes of visual loss (for example, cataract, glaucoma, or macular degeneration) complicated data interpretation.

8-1-2 Intervention Studies

Observational epidemiologic studies, however, cannot demonstrate a treatment effect. A number of randomized, controlled clinical trials have demonstrated the beneficial effect on retinopathy of lowering glycemia to close to normal.

8-1-2-1 Diabetes Control and Complications Trial The Diabetes Control and Complications Trial (DCCT), a randomized, multicenter, controlled clinical trial, demonstrated that intensive treatment of type 1 diabetes, with the goal of meticulous glycemic control, decreased the frequency and severity of retinopathy, nephropathy, and neuropathy.[6] (For a detailed discussion of the DCCT, see Chapter 4, "Clinical Studies on Treatment for Diabetic Retinopathy.")

The intensive-therapy group achieved a median HbA$_{1c}$ of 7.2% versus 9.1% in the conventional group (*P* <0.001) (Figure 8-1). Mean blood glucose was 155 mg/dL in the intensive-therapy group and 230 mg/dL in

TABLE 8-1

Effects of Glycemic Control on Ophthalmologic End Points in DCCT:
Risk Reduction for Intensive Therapy Versus Conventional Therapy*

Outcome Measure	Combined Cohorts (%)	Primary Cohort (%)	Secondary Cohort (%)
Clinically important sustained progression	70.3	78.5	64.5
1 yr duration of diabetes prior to entry	92		
5 yr duration of diabetes prior to entry	77		
10 yr duration of diabetes prior to entry	64		
15 yr duration of diabetes prior to entry	53		
Adolescents		53	70
Progression to severe nonproliferative diabetic retinopathy or worse			60.8
Progression to neovascularization			46.3
Clinically significant macular edema			22.1 NS†
Laser photocoagulation	56		
Initial appearance of any retinopathy		27	

**Percentage risk reduction for various DCCT outcome measures in entire study group (combined cohorts), primary-prevention cohort, and secondary-intervention cohort.*

†*NS = not significant.*

the conventional-therapy group. This separation in median glycemic values between the two groups was maintained for 4 to 9 years, with mean duration of followup 6.5 years, for a total of approximately 9300 patient-years of observation. Of 1430 subjects alive at the end of the study, 1422 came for evaluation of outcomes.

Risk reductions for ophthalmologic end points in the DCCT are shown in Table 8-1. Cumulative 8.5-year rates of clinically important, sustained progression of diabetic retinopathy, that is, ≥3 steps change sustained at two consecutive 6-month visits, were: 54.1% with conventional treatment and 11.5% with intensive treatment in the

primary-prevention cohort, and 49.2% with conventional treatment and 17.1% with intensive treatment in the secondary-intervention cohort.[6-8]

Using multiple regression analyses employing generalized estimating equations, and a number of regression models to assess risks, it was found that total glycemic exposure was the dominant factor associated with risk of retinopathy progression.[9] Total glycemic exposure is defined as baseline HbA_{1c} related to duration of diabetes prior

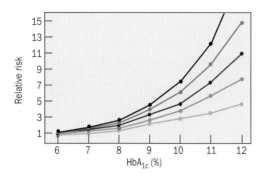

Figure 8-2 *Stylized relative risks for development of various complications as function of mean HbA$_{1c}$ during followup in DCCT. For purposes of illustration, relative risk of various complications is set to 1 at HbA$_{1c}$ of 6%. Lines depict stylized relationship for risk of: sustained progression of retinopathy (burgundy); progression to clinical nephropathy (urinary albumin excretion ≥300 mg/24 hr) (blue); progression to severe NPDR or to PDR (pink); progression to clinical neuropathy (green); and progression to microalbuminuria (urinary albumin excretion ≥40 mg/24 hr) (orange).*

Adapted from Skyler JS: Diabetic complications: the importance of glucose control. Endocrinol Metab Clin North Am *1996;25:243–254.*

to study entry, mean study HbA$_{1c}$ related to time in the study, and the interaction between these variables. Within each treatment group, mean HbA$_{1c}$ during the trial was the dominant predictor of retinopathy progression, with a continuous risk gradient without an apparent glycemic threshold (Figure 8-2).

Benefit was seen for those who were still in adolescence at entry, retinopathy progression being significantly reduced by 53% for those in the primary-prevention cohort and by 70% for those in the secondary-intervention cohort.[10]

Consistent with earlier studies, a transient worsening of retinopathy was observed at the 6-month and/or 12-month visit in 13.1% of patients assigned to intensive therapy and in 7.6% of patients assigned to conventional therapy (odds ratio [OR] 2.06), with subsequent recovery and no long-term impact.[11] The most important risk factors for early worsening were higher levels of HbA$_{1c}$ at screening and rapid reduction of HbA$_{1c}$ in the first 6 months. This finding has led to the recommendation that there be careful ophthalmologic monitoring before initiation of intensive therapy in those patients at or past the moderate nonproliferative stage and, in patients approaching high-risk characteristics, consideration of photocoagulation prior to initiation of intensive therapy, particularly if the HbA$_{1c}$ is high.[11]

8-1-2-2 Stockholm Diabetes Intervention Study and Meta-Analysis The beneficial effects and impact of effective glycemic control on retinopathy in type 1 diabetes were also seen in the much smaller (102 subjects) Stockholm Diabetes Intervention Study

(SDIS).[12] The SDIS was also combined with a number of other, smaller, prospective intervention studies subjected to meta-analysis.[13] The meta-analysis of 271 subjects in six studies showed that, compared to conventionally treated patients, after more than 2 years of intensive therapy, the risk of retinopathy progression was significantly lower (OR 0.49; 95% confidence interval [CI] 0.28 to 0.85; $P = 0.011$). In the 186 subjects in four studies in which progression to PDR or photocoagulation was assessed, the meta-analysis showed that intensive therapy reduced risk (OR 0.44; 95% CI 0.22 to 0.87; $P = 0.018$).

8-1-2-3 Kumamoto University Study A study reported from Kumamoto University in Japan involved 110 nonobese patients with type 2 diabetes.[14] Of these, 102 subjects completed the 6-year study, which was designed to be similar to the DCCT except for involving subjects with type 2 diabetes. Thus, the Kumamoto study contrasted intensive insulin therapy (multiple daily injections: preprandial regular and bedtime intermediate-acting insulin) and conventional insulin therapy (once- or twice-daily intermediate-acting insulin) in two cohorts: a primary-prevention cohort and a secondary-intervention cohort.

Over the 6 years of followup, glycemic outcomes and risk reductions were almost identical to those found in the DCCT. The intensive-therapy group achieved a mean HbA_{1c} over the 6 years of the study of 7.1% versus a value in the conventional-therapy group of 9.4% ($P <0.001$). Mean fasting blood glucose was 157 mg/dL in the intensive group and 221 mg/dL in the conventional group. Two-step progression of reti-

nopathy was significantly reduced by 69% overall: by 76% in the primary-prevention cohort and by 65% in the secondary-intervention cohort. In the secondary-intervention cohort, progression to severe nonproliferative diabetic retinopathy (NPDR) or to PDR was reduced by 40%, as was the need for laser photocoagulation.

8-1-2-4 United Kingdom Prospective Diabetes Study
The United Kingdom Prospective Diabetes Study (UKPDS), a randomized, multicenter, controlled clinical trial, demonstrated that an intensive-treatment policy in type 2 diabetes, with the goal of meticulous glycemic control, decreased diabetic complications, including retinopathy.[15,16] The UKPDS was conducted in twenty-three centers. Enrollment was between 1977 and 1991, and end-of-study evaluations were performed during 1997. A total of 5102 subjects with newly diagnosed type 2 diabetes were enrolled. They were 25 to 63 years of age at entry (median 53 years). The primary outcome measures in the UKPDS were three aggregate end points: any diabetes-related end point, diabetes-related death, and all-cause mortality. Retinopathy was assessed by four-field fundus photography performed at baseline and every 3 years, read at the Hammersmith Hospital (London) Reading Center, and graded according to a modified EDTRS protocol.

Subjects were randomly assigned to either intensive treatment or conventional treatment. Intensive treatment aimed at

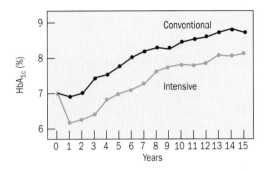

Figure 8-3 *Measurement of glycosylated hemoglobin (HbA$_{1c}$) in UKPDS patients with type 2 diabetes, assigned to conventional or intensive treatment. Median values are shown. Differences over course of study are statistically significant (P <0.0001).*

Adapted with permission from UK Prospective Diabetes Study Group: Intensive blood-glucose control with sulfonylureas or insulin compared with conventional treatment and risk of complications in patients with type 2 diabetes. UKPDS 33. Lancet *1998;352:837–853.*

achieving fasting plasma glucose of 110 mg/dL, using various pharmacologic agents. Conventional treatment attempted control with diet alone, adding pharmacologic therapy when symptoms developed or fasting plasma glucose exceeded 270 mg/dL. Although many analyses focused on various treatment modalities used, the primary analysis was based on the "intention-to-treat principle," comparing subjects assigned to intensive treatment with those assigned to conventional treatment.

The intensive-treatment group achieved a median HbA$_{1c}$ of 7.0% versus 7.9% in the conventional-treatment group (P <0.001). Although there was a progressive deterioration in glycemia over time, degree of glycemic separation was maintained for 6 to 20 years, with a median duration of followup of 10 years (Figure 8-3).

Risk reductions for ophthalmologic end points in the UKPDS are shown in Table 8-2. Patients assigned intensive treatment had a significant 25% risk reduction in microvascular end points (P <0.01) compared with conventional treatment, most of which was due to fewer cases of retinal photocoagulation, for which there was a 29% risk reduction (P <0.005). Reduction in risk was of borderline significance for cataract extraction (P <0.05). After 6 years' followup and thereafter, a smaller proportion of patients in the intensive-treatment group than in the conventional-treatment group had a two-step deterioration in retinopathy; this finding was significant even when retinal photocoagulation was excluded. At 6 and 9 years' followup, there was a 17% risk reduction, while at 12 years' followup, there was a 21% risk reduction (Figure 8-4).

TABLE 8-2

Effects of Glycemic Control on Ophthalmologic End Points in UKPDS

End Point	Absolute Risk: Events per 1000 Patient-Years		Log-Rank *P*	Risk Reduction for Intensive Glycemic Control
	Intensive Therapy	Conventional Therapy		
Microvascular*	8.6	11.4	0.0099	25%
Retinal photocoagulation	7.9	11.0	0.0031	29%
Vitreous hemorrhage	0.7	0.9	0.51	0%
Blind in one eye	2.9	3.5	0.39	0%
Cataract extraction	5.6	7.4	0.046	24%

*Any retinal or renal end point.

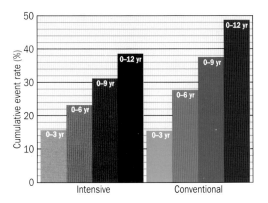

Figure 8-4 *Proportion of UKPDS patients assigned to conventional or intensive treatment with two-step progression of diabetic retinopathy at 3-year intervals. Differences are statistically significant for 0 to 6 years (P = 0.017), 0 to 9 years (P = 0.012), and 0 to 12 years (P = 0.015).*

Adapted from data contained in UK Prospective Diabetes Study Group: Intensive blood-glucose control with sulfonyl-ureas or insulin compared with conventional treatment and risk of complications in patients with type 2 diabetes. UKPDS 33. Lancet *1998;352:837–853.*

8-1-3 Current Recommendations

The current glycemic recommendations of the American Diabetes Association (ADA) appear in their "Standards of Medical Care for Patients With Diabetes Mellitus" (Table 8-3).[17] The goal is, ideally, fasting plasma glucose <110 mg/dL and HbA_{1c} <7% (normal range about 3.0% to 6.0%). The ADA uses the term "Action Suggested" to define another category, which might also be de-

TABLE 8-3

ADA Recommendations for Glycemic Control

Index	Normal	Goal	"Action Suggested" (Not Acceptable)
Fasting/preprandial plasma glucose	<110 mg/dL	80–120 mg/dL	<80 mg/dL >140 mg/dL
Bedtime plasma glucose	<120 mg/dL	100–140 mg/dL	<100 mg/dL >160 mg/dL
HbA$_{1c}$ (%)*	<6.0%	<7.0%	>8.0%

Referenced to nondiabetic range of 4% to 6%.

Source: *American Diabetes Association: Standards of medical care for patients with diabetes mellitus.* Diabetes Care *1998;21 (suppl 1):S23–S31.*

fined as "unacceptable glycemic control," that is, fasting plasma glucose >140 mg/dL and HbA$_{1c}$ >8%.

Contemporary diabetes management is based on the concept of "targeted glycemic control." Therapy, based on glycemic goals, utilizes progressive, step-wise additions of whatever treatment modality is necessary to achieve glycemic goals. Medical nutritional therapy and promotion of physical activity are fundamental and needed for all patients, as is basic diabetes education.

Intensive insulin therapy is mandatory in type 1 diabetes. This is accomplished, as in the DCCT, with insulin administered either by continuous subcutaneous insulin infusion (CSII) with a pump or by multiple daily injections (MDI); frequent self-monitoring of blood glucose (SMBG); and meticulous attention to balancing insulin dose, food intake, and energy expenditure.[18]

In type 2 diabetes, progressive pharmacologic therapy is required, the specific choice based on disease severity and glycemic targets.[19] There are a growing number of classes of pharmacologic agents available to control glycemia:

1. Insulin secretagogs (that is, sulfonylureas and repaglinide), which stimulate insulin production

2. Insulin sensitizers (that is, biguanides and thiazolidinediones), which enhance muscle glucose uptake and decrease hepatic glucose production

3. Alpha-glucosidase inhibitors, which retard carbohydrate absorption

4. Replacement of insulin deficiency with insulin or insulin analogs

The availability of agents with differing and complementary mechanisms of action allows them to be used in various combinations, thus increasing the likelihood that satisfactory glycemic control can be achieved in any given patient.

BLOOD PRESSURE CONTROL

Epidemiologic studies have long suggested a relationship between blood pressure elevation and retinopathy progression. For example, a prospective study of Swiss patients with diabetes mellitus revealed a lower incidence of diabetic retinopathy development among patients taking antihypertensive medications compared to patients with untreated systolic hypertension.[20] In a population-based epidemiologic study of Pima Indians with type 2 diabetes, NPDR was associated with mean blood pressure, and PDR was associated with diastolic blood pressure.[21,22]

8-2-1 Epidemiologic Studies

8-2-1-1 Wisconsin Epidemiologic Study of Diabetic Retinopathy
In the Wisconsin study mentioned above, there was found to be an important relationship between hypertension and the incidence and progression of diabetic retinopathy.[23] In the younger-onset cohort of diabetic patients, elevation of both systolic and diastolic blood pressure was associated with an increased risk of development of PDR. In the older-onset cohort, results differed between those taking insulin and those not taking insulin. In the older-onset cohort taking insulin, elevation of both systolic and diastolic blood pressure was associated with a significant increase in progression to PDR.

On the other hand, in the older-onset cohort not taking insulin, comparison of systolic blood pressure and diastolic blood pressure quartiles did not reveal any relationship between blood pressure and incidence of diabetic retinopathy or progression to PDR. However, among these same patients, if untreated hypertensive subjects were compared to normotensive subjects, there was a 2-fold increase in risk of progression to PDR. (For a detailed discussion of the Wisconsin study, see Chapter 2, "Epidemiology of Eye Disease in Diabetes.")

8-2-1-2 Hypertension in Diabetes Study
The Hypertension in Diabetes Study (HDS) was embedded in the UKPDS by using a factorial design.[24,25] The HDS was conducted in twenty centers with 1148 patients who had type 2 diabetes and coexisting hypertension. The design was a randomized, controlled trial comparing "tight" control of blood pressure aiming at a blood pressure of <150/85 mm Hg, with the use of an angiotensin-converting enzyme (ACE) inhibitor (captopril) or a beta blocker (atenolol) as main treatment, with "less tight" control aiming at a blood pressure of <180/105 mm Hg. Median followup was 8.4 years. The tight control group achieved a mean blood pressure of 144/82 mm Hg versus 154/87 mm Hg in the less-tight control group (P <0.0001) (Figure 8-5).

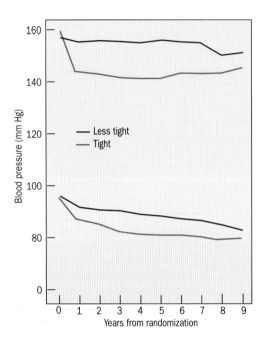

Figure 8-5 *Mean systolic and diastolic blood pressure over 9 years in HDS patients: 297 patients in group assigned to tight control of blood pressure and 156 in group assigned to less-tight control.*

Adapted from UK Prospective Diabetes Study Group: Tight blood pressure control and risk of macrovascular and microvascular complications in type 2 diabetes. UKPDS 38. Br Med J 1998;317:703–713, with permission from the BMJ Publishing Group.

Risk reductions for ophthalmologic end points in the HDS are shown in Table 8-4. Patients assigned tight control had a significant 37% risk reduction in microvascular end points (*P* <0.01) compared with less-tight control—predominantly due to a reduced risk of retinal photocoagulation, for which there was a 35% risk reduction (*P* <0.025).[24] After 7.5 years of followup, the group assigned to tight control also had a 34% reduction in risk (*P* <0.0005) in the proportion of patients with deterioration of retinopathy by two steps (Figure 8-6) and a 47% reduced risk (*P* <0.005) of deterioration in visual acuity by three lines of the ETDRS chart (Figure 8-7).

The HDS also sought to determine whether tight control of blood pressure with either a beta blocker or an ACE inhibitor has a specific advantage or disadvantage in preventing the macrovascular and microvascular complications of type 2 diabetes.[25] Blood pressure lowering with captopril or atenolol was similarly effective in reducing the incidence of diabetic complications. There was no evidence that either drug has any specific beneficial or deleterious effect, suggesting that blood pressure reduction in itself may be more important than the treatment used. However, it should be pointed out that the tight control group in this study did not achieve the degree of blood pressure control currently recommended. It is unknown whether a difference between therapeutic strategies would emerge if further reduction of blood pressure were achieved.

TABLE 8-4

Effects of Blood Pressure Control on Ophthalmologic End Points in HDS/UKPDS

End Point	Absolute Risk: Events per 1000 Patient-Years		Log-Rank *P*	Risk Reduction for Tight Blood Pressure Control
	Tight Control	Less-Tight Control		
Microvascular*	12.0	19.2	0.0092	37%
Retinal photocoagulation	10.2	16.6	0.023	35%
Vitreous hemorrhage	0.5	1.7	0.76	0%
Blind in one eye	3.1	4.4	0.34	0%
Cataract extraction	6.2	4.7	0.35	0%

Any retinal or renal end point.

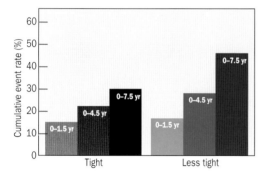

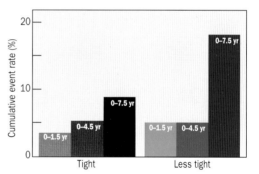

Figure 8-6 *Proportion of HDS patients assigned to tight control of blood pressure or to less-tight control with two-step progression of diabetic retinopathy at various intervals. Differences are statistically significant for 0 to 4.5 years (P = 0.019) and 0 to 7.5 years (P = 0.0038).*

Adapted from data contained in UK Prospective Diabetes Study Group: Tight blood pressure control and risk of macrovascular and microvascular complications in type 2 diabetes. UKPDS 38. Br Med J 1998;317:703–713.

Figure 8-7 *Proportion of HDS patients assigned to tight control of blood pressure or to less-tight control with deterioration of visual acuity by three lines of ETDRS chart at various intervals. Difference is statistically significant for 0 to 7.5 years (P = 0.0006).*

Adapted from data contained in UK Prospective Diabetes Study Group: Tight blood pressure control and risk of macrovascular and microvascular complications in type 2 diabetes. UKPDS 38. Br Med J 1998;317:703–713.

8-2-2 Current Recommendations

In patients with diabetes, current blood pressure recommendations of the ADA appear in their "Standards of Medical Care for Patients With Diabetes Mellitus"[17] and in a consensus statement on "Treatment of Hypertension in Diabetes."[26] Similar recommendations are contained in "The Sixth Report of the Joint National Committee on Prevention, Detection, Evaluation, and Treatment of High Blood Pressure"[27] and elsewhere.

The primary goal of therapy for (nonpregnant) adults (>18 years of age) with diabetes is to decrease blood pressure to, and maintain it at, <130 mm Hg systolic and <85 mm Hg diastolic. In children, blood pressure should be decreased to the corresponding age-adjusted 90th-percentile values. For patients with an isolated systolic hypertension of >180 mm Hg, the initial goal of treatment is to reduce the systolic blood pressure to <160 mm Hg. For those with systolic blood pressure of 160 to 179 mm Hg, the goal is a reduction of 20 mm Hg. If these goals are achieved and well tolerated, further lowering to <140 mm Hg may be appropriate.

Many experts are concerned about the selection of antihypertensive agents in individuals with diabetes.[28] The class of drugs that has been best demonstrated in clinical trials to benefit diabetic patients is the ACE inhibitors, particularly with respect to renal function and cardiovascular disease. Presumably, angiotensin-II receptor blockers (ARBs) also have the same beneficial effects. In addition, some ACE inhibitors

have beneficial effects on insulin sensitivity. On the other hand, thiazide diuretics may reduce insulin sensitivity, thus aggravating insulin resistance. Thiazide diuretics also may decrease insulin secretion. Beta blockers also have negative effects on glycemic control by reducing insulin sensitivity and insulin secretion in type 2 diabetes, by masking hypoglycemic symptoms in insulin-treated patients, and by inhibiting recovery from hypoglycemia in type 1 patients.

Both thiazide diuretics and beta blockers also may aggravate dyslipidemia, raising both triglycerides and low-density lipoproteins (LDLs). On the other hand, neutral-to-beneficial effects on insulin sensitivity and lipids are seen with calcium channel blockers (CCBs) and alpha-adrenergic blockers. Beta blockers have potential negative effects on exercise tolerance and sexual function. For all of these reasons, the classes of antihypertensive drugs favored in diabetic patients are ACE inhibitors, ARBs, alpha-adrenergic blockers, and perhaps CCBs. When needed, low-dose diuretics may be used, as may loop diuretics.

8-3

ANGIOTENSIN-CONVERTING ENZYME INHIBITORS

It has been demonstrated that even in normotensive individuals with diabetes, ACE inhibitors have beneficial effects on kidney function. Several small studies suggested specific beneficial effects of ACE inhibitors on reducing the progression of diabetic retinopathy as well. Although these studies were not statistically significant, they gave impetus to a larger study.

8-3-1 Intervention Study

8-3-1-1 EURODIAB Controlled Trial of Lisinopril in Insulin-Dependent Diabetes Mellitus

The EURO-DIAB Controlled Trial of Lisinopril in Insulin-Dependent Diabetes Mellitus (EUCLID), a randomized, multicenter, controlled clinical trial, was conducted in 354 patients with type 1 diabetes aged 20 to 59 in fifteen European centers.[29] Patients were not hypertensive and were either normoalbuminuric (85%) or microalbuminuric (15%). Patients were randomized to receive either the ACE inhibitor lisinopril or placebo. Retinal photographs were taken at baseline and followup (24 months). Retinopathy was classified from photographs on a five-level scale (none, minimal nonproliferative, moderate nonproliferative, severe nonproliferative, photocoagulated or proliferative).

Retinopathy progressed by at least one level in 13.2% of patients taking lisinopril and 23.4% of patients taking placebo (50% risk reduction, $P < 0.02$). This 50% reduction was the same when adjusted for clinical center and glycemic control. Lisinopril also decreased retinopathy progression by two or more grades (73% risk reduction, $P < 0.05$) and progression to PDR (82% risk reduction, $P < 0.03$) (Figure 8-8). In the EUCLID, however, patients with better glycemic control had the most benefit from ACE inhibitors, suggesting that the combination may be the best therapeutic approach.

The EUCLID findings lend support to the notion that ACE inhibitors may have an important role in limiting the progression of retinopathy in patients with type 1 diabe-

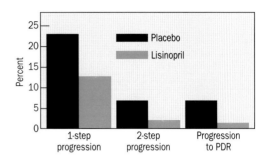

Figure 8-8 *Proportion of EUCLID patients assigned to ACE inhibitor lisinopril or to placebo with specified degree of progression of diabetic retinopathy over a 2-year interval. Differences are statistically significant for one-step progression (P <0.02), for two-step progression (P <0.05), and for progression to PDR (P <0.03).*

Adapted from data contained in Chaturvedi N, Sjolie AK, Stephenson JM, et al: Effect of lisinopril on progression of retinopathy in normotensive people with type 1 diabetes. Lancet *1998;351:28–31.*

tes. Nevertheless, the effects of ACE inhibitors on the development and regression of retinopathy must be studied further in large, randomized, controlled trials before changes in clinical practice are advocated.

8-4

DYSLIPIDEMIC CONTROL

Diabetic dyslipidemia, particularly in patients with poor glycemic control, is characterized by increased levels of total cholesterol, LDLs, and triglycerides and by decreased levels of high-density lipoproteins (HDLs).[30] Data from the WESDR showed that there was a significant trend for increasing severity of diabetic retinopathy and retinal hard exudate with increasing cholesterol in insulin-using persons.[31] Data from the ETDRS showed that elevated total serum cholesterol and LDL cholesterol is associated with a significant increase in the presence of retinal lipid exudate.[32]

In the ETDRS, patients with total cholesterol levels >240 mg/dL were twice as likely to have retinal lipid exudate as were those patients with serum cholesterol of <200 mg/dL. Moreover, among those patients with minimal or no retinal lipid exudate at baseline, elevated total cholesterol, LDL cholesterol, and triglycerides was associated with more rapid onset of retinal lipid exudate. Even after adjusting statistically for retinal thickening, retinal lipid exudate was associated with a 2-fold risk of decreased visual acuity at 5 years of followup.

Older studies[33–35] suggested that treatment of dyslipidemia is beneficial for retinal lipid exudates. In one small series (six patients), lipid exudate diminished after 1-year treatment of hyperlipidemia (total cholesterol decreased from 231 mg/dL to 165 mg/dL) with dietary instruction and pravastatin, an inhibitor of 3-hydroxy-3-methylglutaryl (HMG) coenzyme A reductase. Visual acuity did not change appreciably.[36]

Data from the ETDRS suggest that treatment of hyperlipidemia may help stabilize retinal status and possibly visual acuity.[37] However, there are no data to suggest that visual acuity can be improved with treatment of hyperlipidemia. Moreover, whether such treatment has a long-term beneficial effect on visual outcome is unknown.

8-5

PLATELET INHIBITORS

Diabetes is associated with increased platelet aggregability.[38] As a consequence, there have been a number of investigations of various platelet-aggregation inhibitors, including aspirin, dipyridamole, and ticlopidine.

8-5-1 Aspirin

Many older studies suggested an association between salicylate use (both aspirin and para-amino salicylic acid) and decreased risk of diabetic retinopathy.[39] Several small series tended to either support or refute this claim. The ETDRS set out to answer the question systematically, controlling for other potential confounding variables.

The ETDRS included a double-masked, placebo-controlled comparison of the effect of aspirin versus placebo on progression of diabetic retinopathy and incidence of vitreous hemorrhage.[40,41] There was no significant difference between aspirin and placebo. Aspirin did not slow the progression of diabetic retinopathy. The ETDRS also found that the relative risk for myocardial infarction in the first 5 years in those randomized to aspirin therapy was lowered significantly to 0.72 (95% CI 0.55 to 0.95).

This finding, together with abundant data of the beneficial effects of aspirin from a cardiovascular and neurologic standpoint,[42,43] has led the ADA to advocate the use of aspirin therapy as a secondary prevention strategy in diabetic men and women who have evidence of large-vessel disease, including a history of myocardial infarction, vascular bypass procedure, stroke or transient ischemic attack, peripheral vascular disease, claudication, and/or angina.[44] The ADA also recommends considering aspirin therapy as a primary prevention strategy in high-risk men and women with type 1 or type 2 diabetes. The potential benefit of these recommendations seems to outweigh any (unproven) increased risk of vitreous hemorrhage (which is a treatable condition).

8-5-2 Aspirin Plus Dipyridamole

Aspirin alone and aspirin plus dipyridamole were evaluated in a double-masked, placebo-controlled European clinical trial, the Dipyridamole and Aspirin Microangiopathy of Diabetes (DAMAD) Study.[45] The effect of these drugs was quantified by macular microaneurysm counts in 475 patients with NPDR assigned randomly to aspirin alone, aspirin plus dipyridamole, or placebo. The mean yearly increase in microaneurysm count was less for the two treatment groups (aspirin alone and aspirin plus dipyridamole) than for the placebo group. This was true for patients with type 1 or type 2 diabetes. The clinical significance of this finding remains uncertain. Neovascularization of the disc and retina occurred to the same degree in all three groups. At present, any potential benefit of dipyridamole needs to be confirmed in a larger, longer clinical trial before further recommendations can be made.

8-5-3 Ticlopidine

In France, the Ticlopidine Microangiopathy of Diabetes (TIMAD) Study Group evaluated another platelet-aggregation inhibitor, ticlopidine, on the progression of microaneurysm counts in patients with diabetes and NPDR.[46] Microaneurysm counts were obtained from fluorescein angiography and included the macula as well as four peripheral fundus fields. For insulin-treated patients, ticlopidine was associated with a 7-fold decrease in microaneurysm count during 3 years of followup compared to placebo. In non–insulin-treated patients, ticlopidine had no observable benefit over placebo. Deterioration of retinal status to PDR occurred in 9 of 215 patients in the placebo group and in 3 of 220 patients in the ticlopidine-treated group. There was no ocular bleeding in the ticlopidine group. Reversible neutropenia, gastrointestinal upset, rash, elevated liver-function tests, and bleeding at sites other than the eye occurred. As with dipyridamole, more clinical trials of ticlopidine are required before definitive recommendations can be made.

8-6

EXPERIMENTAL MEDICAL THERAPIES

8-6-1 Aldose-Reductase Inhibitors

Glucose is converted to its sugar alcohol, sorbitol, by the enzyme aldose reductase.[47] Treatment of experimental animals with inhibitors of aldose reductase can prevent the development of sugar cataracts. In diabetic retinopathy, an early histopathologic alteration is the loss of retinal capillary pericytes, followed later by thickening of the capillary basement membrane. Aldose reductase localizes to retinal capillary pericytes on immunohistochemical staining. Aldose-reductase inhibitors prevent diabetes-like retinal vascular changes in some animal models. Therefore, it is potentially possible to alter the progression of diabetic retinopathy with aldose-reductase inhibitors.

The Sorbinil Retinopathy Trial, a prospective, randomized clinical trial, tested this hypothesis by comparing the aldose-reductase inhibitor sorbinil (250 mg/day) to placebo.[48] The goal was to determine whether sorbinil could delay the onset or slow the progression of diabetic retinopathy. A total of 497 patients entered the study (248 assigned to sorbinil and 249 to placebo), and followup examinations ranged from 12 to 56 months (median 41 months). Retinopathy was assessed by standardized fundus photography graded at the University of Wisconsin Reading Center. There was no significant difference in retinopathy progression between the treatment and control groups. However, the duration of followup may have been too short to observe treatment effects.

There are no aldose-reductase inhibitors currently on the market. Several remain in clinical development. It remains to be determined whether interruption of this pathway will alter the course of diabetic retinopathy.

8-6-2 Rheologic Agents

Pentoxifylline, a hemorheologic agent that increases red blood cell (RBC) deformability and decreases whole-blood viscosity, is used to improve blood flow in patients with claudication secondary to peripheral vascular disease. Pentoxifylline increases retinal blood flow velocity.[49] In a clinical study reported by Ferrari and associates, urinary albumin excretion and total protein excretion decreased during 48 months of followup in patients treated with 1200 mg per day of oral pentoxifylline.[50] In this study, diabetic retinopathy, assessed by fluorescein angiography, decreased in 13 of 27 patients with NPDR at baseline over a 48-month period of treatment with pentoxifylline. The investigators did not describe how diabetic retinopathy was quantified and graded.

8-6-3 Agents to Improve Capillary Fragility

Calcium dobesilate was developed to improve capillary fragility and decrease capillary leakage.[51] A flurry of studies in the mid to late 1970s examined its effects on diabetic retinopathy. Although initial studies seemed promising, controlled studies failed to demonstrate significant benefit.[52]

8-6-4 Histamine-Receptor Antagonists

In animal models with experimental diabetes, there is increased retinal histamine production.[53] Histamine reduces the expression of tight-junction proteins in retinal endothelial cells, and histamine H_1- and H_2-receptor antagonists reduce retinal vascular permeability.[54] This is the basis of a potential role of histamine in diabetic macular edema. In a double-masked, placebo-controlled 6-month pilot study of fourteen patients with type 1 diabetes, combined astemizole and ranitidine therapy significantly reduced blood–retina barrier permeability, as measured by vitreous fluorometry.[55] This finding led to a double-masked, placebo-controlled study, the Astemizole Retinopathy Trial, which is being conducted to examine the effects of the histamine-receptor antagonist astemizole in patients with macular edema that is not clinically significant.

8-6-5 Inhibitors of Endothelial Cell Proliferation

Hypoxic retinal tissue produces vascular endothelial cell growth factor (VEGF), which stimulates endothelial cell mitosis.[56] VEGF interaction with endothelial cell membrane receptors initiates a cascade of events, including activation of intracellular protein kinase C, which eventuates in endothelial cell division. In a monkey model of retinal vascular ischemia, antibodies to VEGF successfully prevented iris neovascularization when injected into the vitreous cavity.[56] Experimentally, inhibitors of protein kinase C block endothelial tube formation in vitro[57] and intraocular neovascularization caused by retinal ischemia.[58] Two double-masked, placebo-controlled clinical trials are currently being conducted to test the effects of an orally effective beta-isoform-selective inhibitor of protein kinase C: one in patients with diabetic macular edema and the other in patients with diabetic retinopathy.

8-7

CONCLUSION

The medical management of diabetic retinopathy currently is primarily preventive. In the future, however, specific interventions might emerge that would allow interdiction of the pathophysiologic processes leading to the development and progression of diabetic retinopathy. The ADA has developed specific recommendations concerning diabetic retinopathy for the primary care physician and diabetologist.[59] The rationale for these recommendations is developed and presented in an ADA technical review.[60] An excellent review for nonophthalmologists has appeared as well.[61]

The challenge for the primary care physician and diabetologist is to attain excellent glycemic control, aggressive control of blood pressure, and normalization of lipids, while assuring that every patient has appropriate dilated fundus examinations at least annually. With such an approach, appropriate medical intervention can occur to reduce the risk of blindness and lessen the burden from diabetic retinopathy.

REFERENCES

1. Skyler JS: Diabetic complications: the importance of glucose control. *Endocrinol Metab Clin North Am* 1996;25:243–254.

2. Klein R: Hyperglycemia and microvascular and macrovascular disease in diabetes. *Diabetes Care* 1995;18:258–268.

3. Klein R, Klein BE, Moss SE: Relation of glycemic control to diabetic microvascular complications in diabetes mellitus. *Ann Intern Med* 1996;124:90–96.

4. Klein R, Klein BE, Moss SE, et al: Glycosylated hemoglobin predicts the incidence and progression of diabetic retinopathy. *J Am Med Assoc* 1988;260:2864–2871.

5. Klein R, Klein BE, Moss SE, Cruickshanks KJ: Relationship of hyperglycemia to the long-term incidence and progression of diabetic retinopathy. *Arch Intern Med* 1994;154:2169–2178.

6. Diabetes Control and Complications Trial Research Group: The effect of intensive treatment of diabetes on the development and progression of long-term complications in insulin-dependent diabetes mellitus. *N Engl J Med* 1993;329:977–986.

7. Diabetes Control and Complications Trial Research Group: The effect of intensive diabetes treatment on the progression of diabetic retinopathy in insulin-dependent diabetes mellitus: Diabetes Control and Complications Trial. *Arch Ophthalmol* 1995;113:36–51.

8. Diabetes Control and Complications Trial Research Group: Progression of retinopathy with intensive versus conventional treatment in the Diabetes Control and Complications Trial. *Ophthalmology* 1995;102:647–661.

9. Diabetes Control and Complications Trial Research Group: The relationship of glycemic exposure (HbA$_{1c}$) to the risk of development and progression of retinopathy in the Diabetes Control and Complications Trial. *Diabetes* 1995;44:968–983.

10. Diabetes Control and Complications Trial Research Group: Effect of intensive diabetes treatment on the development and progression of long-term complications in adolescents with insulin-dependent diabetes mellitus: Diabetes Control and Complications Trial. *J Pediatr* 1994;125:177–188.

11. Diabetes Control and Complications Trial Research Group: Early worsening of diabetic retinopathy in the Diabetes Control and Complications Trial. *Arch Ophthalmol* 1998;116:874–886.

12. Reichard P, Nilsson BY, Rosenqvist U: The effect of long-term intensified insulin treatment on the development of microvascular complications of diabetes mellitus. *N Engl J Med* 1993;329: 304–309.

13. Wang PH, Lau J, Chalmers TC: Meta-analysis of effects of intensive blood-glucose control on late complications of type I diabetes. *Lancet* 1993;341:1306–1309.

14. Ohkubo Y, Kishikawa H, Araki E, et al: Intensive insulin therapy prevents the progression of diabetic microvascular complications in Japanese patients with non–insulin-dependent diabetes mellitus: a randomized prospective 6-year study. *Diabetes Res Clin Pract* 1995;28:103–117.

15. UK Prospective Diabetes Study Group: Intensive blood-glucose control with sulfonylureas or insulin compared with conventional treatment and risk of complications in patients with type 2 diabetes (UKPDS 33). *Lancet* 1998;352:837–853.

16. UK Prospective Diabetes Study Group: Effect of intensive blood-glucose control with metformin on complications in overweight patients with type 2 diabetes (UKPDS 34). *Lancet* 1998; 352:854–865.

17. American Diabetes Association: Standards of medical care for patients with diabetes mellitus. *Diabetes Care* 1998;21(suppl 1):S23–S31.

18. Hirsch IB: Intensive treatment of type 1 diabetes. *Med Clin North Am* 1998;82:689–719.

19. Feinglos MN, Bethel MA: Treatment of type 2 diabetes mellitus. *Med Clin North Am* 1998;82: 757–790.

20. Teuscher A, Schnell H, Wilson PW: Incidence of diabetic retinopathy and relationship to baseline plasma glucose and blood pressure. *Diabetes Care* 1988;11:246–251.

21. Knowler WC, Bennett PH, Ballintine EJ: Increased incidence of retinopathy in diabetics with elevated blood pressure: a six-year follow-up study in Pima Indians. *N Engl J Med* 1980; 302:645–650.

22. Nagi DK, Pettitt DJ, Bennett PH, et al: Diabetic retinopathy assessed by fundus photography in Pima Indians with impaired glucose tolerance and NIDDM. *Diabetic Med* 1997;14: 449–456.

23. Klein BE, Klein R, Moss SE, Palta M: A cohort study of the relationship of diabetic retinopathy to blood pressure. *Arch Ophthalmol* 1995; 113:601–606.

24. UK Prospective Diabetes Study Group: Tight blood pressure control and risk of macrovascular and microvascular complications in type 2 diabetes: UKPDS 38. *Br Med J* 1998;317:703–713.

25. UK Prospective Diabetes Study Group: Efficacy of atenolol and captopril in reducing risk of macrovascular and microvascular complications in type 2 diabetes: UKPDS 39. *Br Med J* 1998; 317:713–720.

26. American Diabetes Association: Treatment of hypertension in diabetes [consensus statement]. *Diabetes Care* 1993;16:1394–1401.

27. The sixth report of the Joint National Committee on prevention, detection, evaluation, and treatment of high blood pressure. *Arch Intern Med* 1997;157:2413–2446.

28. Marks JB, Raskin P: Nephropathy and hypertension in diabetes. *Med Clin North Am* 1998; 82:877–907.

29. Chaturvedi N, Sjolie AK, Stephenson JM, et al: Effect of lisinopril on progression of retinopathy in normotensive people with type 1 diabetes: EUCLID Study Group. EURODIAB Controlled Trial of Lisinopril in Insulin-Dependent Diabetes Mellitus. *Lancet* 1998;351:28–31.

30. Garber AJ: Vascular disease and lipids in diabetes. *Med Clin North Am* 1998;82:931–948.

31. Klein BE, Moss SE, Klein R, Surawicz TS: The Wisconsin Epidemiologic Study of Diabetic Retinopathy, XIII: relationship of serum cholesterol to retinopathy and hard exudate. *Ophthalmology* 1991;98:1261–1265.

32. Chew EY, Klein ML, Ferris FL III, et al: Association of elevated serum lipid levels with retinal hard exudate in diabetic retinopathy. ETDRS Report Number 22. *Arch Ophthalmol* 1996;114:1079–1084.

33. Kempner W, Peschel RL, Schlayer C: Effect of rice diet on diabetes mellitus associated with vascular disease. *Postgrad Med* 1958;24:359–371.

34. Van Eck WF: The effect of a low fat diet on the serum lipids in diabetes and its significance in diabetic retinopathy. *Am J Med* 1959;27:196–211.

35. Harrold BP, Marmion VJ, Gough KR: A double-blind controlled trial of clofibrate in the treatment of diabetic retinopathy. *Diabetes* 1969;18:285–291.

36. Gordon B, Chang S, Kavanagh M, et al: The effects of lipid lowering on diabetic retinopathy. *Am J Ophthalmol* 1991;112:385–391.

37. Ferris FL III, Chew EY, Hoogwerf BJ: Serum lipids and diabetic retinopathy: Early Treatment Diabetic Retinopathy Study Research Group. *Diabetes Care* 1996;19:1291–1293.

38. Colwell JA, Winocour PD, Halushka PV: Do platelets have anything to do with diabetic microvascular disease? *Diabetes* 1983;32(suppl 2):14–19.

39. Powell ED, Field RA: Diabetic retinopathy and rheumatoid arthritis. *Lancet* 1964;2:17–18.

40. Early Treatment Diabetic Retinopathy Study Research Group: Effects of aspirin treatment on diabetic retinopathy. ETDRS Report Number 8. *Ophthalmology* 1991;98:757–765.

41. Chew EY, Klein ML, Murphy RP, et al: Effects of aspirin on vitreous/preretinal hemorrhage in patients with diabetes mellitus. ETDRS Report Number 20. *Arch Ophthalmol* 1995;113:52–55.

42. Antiplatelet Trialists' Collaboration: Collaborative overview of randomised trials of antiplatelet therapy, I: prevention of death, myocardial infarction, and stroke by prolonged antiplatelet therapy in various categories of patients. *Br Med J* 1994;308:81–106.

43. Colwell JA: Aspirin therapy in diabetes [review]. *Diabetes Care* 1997;20:1767–1771.

44. American Diabetes Association: Aspirin therapy in diabetes [position statement]. *Diabetes Care* 1998;21:(suppl 1):S45–S46.

45. DAMAD Study Group: Effect of aspirin alone and aspirin plus dipyridamole in early diabetic retinopathy: a multicenter randomized controlled clinical trial. *Diabetes* 1989;38:491–498.

46. TIMAD Study Group: Ticlopidine treatment reduces the progression of nonproliferative diabetic retinopathy. *Arch Ophthalmol* 1990;108:1577–1583.

47. Kinoshita JH: Aldose reductase in the diabetic eye: XLIII Edward Jackson memorial lecture. *Am J Ophthalmol* 1986;102:685–692.

48. Sorbinil Retinopathy Trial Research Group: A randomized trial of sorbinil, an aldose reductase inhibitor, in diabetic retinopathy. *Arch Ophthalmol* 1990;108:1234–1244.

49. Sonkin PL, Kelly LW, Sinclair SH, Hatchell DL: Pentoxifylline increases retinal capillary blood flow velocity in patients with diabetes. *Arch Ophthalmol* 1993;111:1647–1652.

50. Ferrari E, Fioravanti M, Patti AL, et al: Effects of long-term treatment (4 years) with pentoxifylline on haemorheological changes and vascular complications in diabetic patients. *Pharmatherapeutica* 1987;5:26–39.

51. Sévin R, Cuendet JF: The action of calcium dobesilate on capillary permeability in diabetics. *Ophthalmologica* 1971;162:33–40.

52. Stamper RL, Smith ME, Aronson SB, et al: The effect of calcium dobesilate on nonproliferative diabetic retinopathy: a controlled study. *Ophthalmology* 1978;85:594–606.

53. Carroll WJ, Hollis TM, Gardner TW: Retinal histamine synthesis is increased in experimental diabetes. *Invest Ophthalmol Vis Sci* 1988; 29:1201–1204.

54. Hollis TM, Gardner TW, Vergis GJ, et al: Antihistamines reverse blood–ocular barrier breakdown in experimental diabetes. *J Diabetic Complications* 1988;2:47–49.

55. Gardner TW, Eller AW, Friberg TR, et al: Antihistamines reduce blood–retinal barrier permeability in type I (insulin-dependent) diabetic patients with nonproliferative retinopathy: a pilot study. *Retina* 1995;15:134–140.

56. Aiello LP, Bursell SE, Clermont A, et al: Vascular endothelial growth factor–induced retinal permeability is mediated by protein kinase C in vivo and suppressed by an orally effective beta-isoform-selective inhibitor. *Diabetes* 1997;46: 1473–1480.

57. Ishii H, Jirousek MR, Koya D, et al: Amelioration of vascular dysfunctions in diabetic rats by an oral PKC beta inhibitor. *Science* 1996;272: 728–731.

58. Danis RP, Bingaman DP, Jirousek M, Yang Y: Inhibition of intraocular neovascularization caused by retinal ischemia in pigs by PKC beta inhibition with LY333531. *Invest Ophthalmol Vis Sci* 1998;39:171–179.

59. American Diabetes Association: Diabetic retinopathy [position statement]. *Diabetes Care* 1998;21:(suppl 1):S47–S49.

60. Aiello LP, Gardner TW, King GL, et al: Diabetic retinopathy. *Diabetes Care* 1998;21:143–156.

61. Neely KA, Quillen DA, Schachat AP, et al: Diabetic retinopathy. *Med Clin North Am* 1998; 82:847–876.

CHAPTER 9

Cataract Management in Diabetes

Mitchell S. Fineman, MD
William E. Benson, MD

Individuals who have diabetes mellitus not only develop cataracts more frequently than nondiabetic patients, but do so at a younger age.[1–3] They account for about 10% of people with visually significant cataracts and represent about 6% of the population of the United States.[4–7] Cataract is a frequent cause of visual loss in older-onset diabetic patients and is second only to proliferative diabetic retinopathy (PDR) in younger-onset diabetic patients.[8] Although the main indication for cataract extraction in diabetic patients is visual rehabilitation, it is occasionally required when the lens opacity prevents adequate diagnosis or treatment of retinopathy.[9]

Diabetic patients have a higher risk of both anterior and posterior segment complications following cataract surgery.[10] One of the most significant anterior segment complications is neovascularization of the iris (NVI), because it usually progresses to neovascular glaucoma.[11–15] Other anterior segment complications include pigment dispersion with precipitates on the surface of the intraocular lens (IOL), fibrinous exudate or membrane in the anterior chamber, and posterior synechiae (Figure 9-1).[16–18] The incidence of pseudophakic pupillary block with secondary angle-closure glaucoma[19] and postoperative posterior capsular

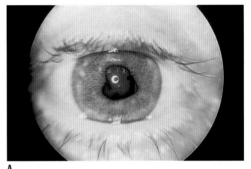

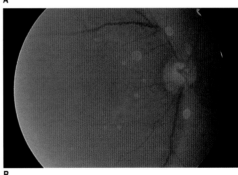

Figure 9-1 *(A) Posterior synechiae in diabetic eye following extracapsular cataract extraction (ECCE). (B) Resulting small size of pupil caused poor view of fundus and difficulties with peripheral laser photocoagulation.*

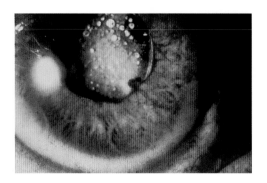

Figure 9-2 *Slit-lamp photograph of diabetic eye demonstrating severe posterior capsular opacification 2 months following cataract extraction. Posterior synechia is visible between 4- and 5-o'clock positions.*

opacification (Figure 9-2)[20,21] is also reported to be greater in diabetic patients. Following cataract surgery in diabetic patients, macular edema, macular ischemia,[22–29] PDR,[25,30] vitreous hemorrhage,[11,30] and tractional retinal detachment[30] may appear or worsen.

The best predictor of visual and anatomic outcomes after cataract surgery is the preoperative severity of retinopathy.[11,24,25] Other factors affecting the postoperative visual outcome are the age and sex of the patient,[31] insulin treatment,[29,32] glycemic control,[32,33] prior laser photocoagulation,[34] and previous vitrectomy.[35]

In this chapter, unless otherwise specified, the term *cataract surgery* means extracapsular cataract extraction (ECCE) or phacoemulsification with placement of a posterior chamber IOL, because these techniques currently are used in nearly all cataract operations performed in the United States.

9-1

PREOPERATIVE SEVERITY OF RETINOPATHY

9-1-1 No or Mild Retinopathy

The current results of cataract surgery in diabetic patients with no or minimal retinopathy are comparable to those in nondiabetic persons.[25,36–39] About 85% of eyes can be expected to achieve a postoperative visual acuity of 20/40 or better.[40] However, the risk of angiographic pseudophakic cystoid macular edema (CME) is considerably higher than in nondiabetic patients, and the progression of retinopathy occurs in 15% of eyes within 18 months postoperatively.[25]

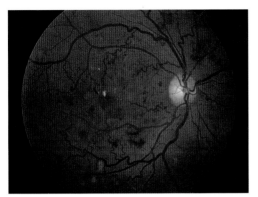

A Right eye

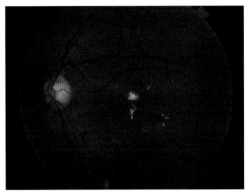

A Left eye

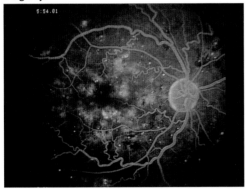

B Right eye

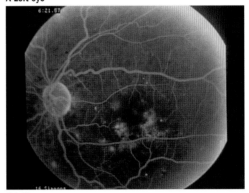

B Left eye

9-1-2 Nonproliferative Retinopathy Without Macular Edema

Cataract surgery is often followed by progression of established nonproliferative diabetic retinopathy (NPDR) or by NVI (Figure 9-3).[24–26,28,29,31,32,38] Sebestyen[36] and Wagner and associates[41] are the only investigators to find that cataract surgery did not lead to progression of pre-existing retinopathy. In one study, clinically significant macular edema (CSME) developed postoperatively in 50% of eyes that did not have it preoperatively.[31] In some cases, progression

Figure 9-3 *(A) Fundus photograph of right and left eyes of 57-year-old man with NPDR who underwent uncomplicated ECCE with implantation of posterior chamber IOL in right eye 5 months earlier. Retinopathy was symmetric before cataract surgery, but is asymmetric postoperatively. (B) Intravenous fluorescein angiography reveals asymmetry of NPDR, with significantly more microaneurysms and fluorescein leakage in right eye.*

of NPDR and CSME caused the postoperative visual acuity to be worse than the preoperative level (Figure 9-4).[22,24] Dowler and associates[40] performed a meta-analysis and calculated that 80% of eyes with preoperative NPDR and no macular edema achieve a visual acuity of 20/40 or better following ECCE.

In the Early Treatment Diabetic Retinopathy Study (ETDRS), evaluation of 1-year postoperative visual acuities for all eyes with mild-to-moderate NPDR at the annual visit prior to cataract surgery showed that 53% achieved better than 20/40, 90% better than 20/100, and only 10% 5/200 or worse.[42] Severity of retinopathy at the time of lens removal is the most important predictor of poor visual acuity outcome in the study by Dowler and associates[40] and in the ETDRS Report Number 25.[42]

Focal macular photocoagulation is applied preoperatively or postoperatively to limit the progression of CSME.[43] Prompt panretinal photocoagulation (PRP) frequently causes regression of NVI and PDR.

9-1-3 Nonproliferative Retinopathy With Macular Edema

Eyes with preoperative macular edema generally have a poor visual prognosis, even if they undergo focal macular photocoagulation preoperatively.[25,31] Retinopathy progresses in 30% of eyes, and 50% require supplemental postoperative focal macular photocoagulation for worsening macular edema. Only 50% have a postoperative improvement of visual acuity. A meta-analysis performed by Dowler and associates[40] found that 40% of eyes with preoperative NPDR and maculopathy achieve a visual acuity of 20/40 or better following ECCE. The presence of macular edema prior to cataract extraction worsened by 6-fold the odds of obtaining a final visual acuity better than 20/40.[40]

It is the clinical impression of many ophthalmologists that patients with macular edema who are treated with focal laser photocoagulation prior to cataract surgery have less progression than those who are not so treated. However, no controlled series has been published to support this opinion. Moreover, it is unlikely that such a study would ever be undertaken, because of concerns about withholding treatment. Even in eyes with previous focal macular photocoagulation, progression of the retinopathy occurs in 30% of eyes; 35% to 50% of eyes require supplemental focal macular photocoagulation for macular edema.

If CSME is present prior to cataract surgery but cannot be treated with macular laser photocoagulation because the cataract obscures the view, then focal macular photocoagulation in the early postoperative period is usually recommended.

9-1-4 Proliferative Retinopathy

There are three reasons why PDR is a risk factor for a poor visual acuity outcome:

1. The prevalence of macular edema is related to the overall severity of retinopathy. Macular edema is present in 3% of eyes with mild NPDR, in 38% of eyes with moderate-to-severe NPDR, and in 71% of eyes with PDR.[44]

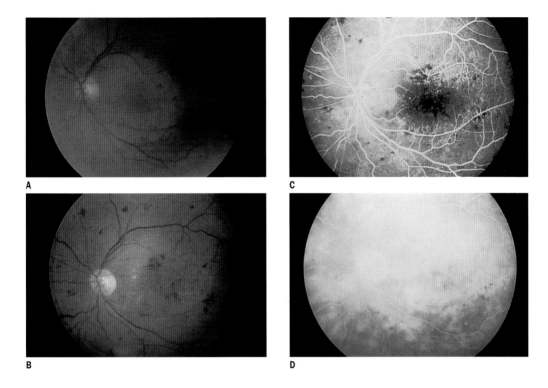

A

B

C

D

2. Patients with PDR have an increased risk of vitreous hemorrhage and retinal detachment.

3. Patients with PDR have a higher risk of NVI than do patients with NPDR.

When high-risk PDR is present, PRP should be performed prior to the cataract extraction, when possible. Yellow and red laser wavelengths may penetrate a nuclear sclerotic cataract better than green or blue-green wavelengths. If PRP is not possible and there is no vitreoretinal traction present, standard cataract surgery with IOL placement can be considered and laser treatment can be performed at the time of cataract surgery or shortly thereafter. Alter-

Figure 9-4 *(A) Fundus photograph of left eye of 65-year-old man with moderate cataract in setting of mild NPDR without CSME. Visual acuity of 20/70 was consistent with density of cataract. (B) About 8 weeks after ECCE, visual acuity had deteriorated to 20/200 and CSME was present. (C,D) Intravenous fluorescein angiography performed 8 weeks after cataract surgery reveals relatively few microaneurysms in full-venous phase (C) and diffuse leakage of fluorescein in macula in recirculation phase (D). Vision remained poor in this eye due to chronic macular edema despite medical and laser treatment.*

natively, a combined procedure, including cataract surgery, vitrectomy, and IOL insertion, can be considered (see Section 9-2-2).

Intracapsular cataract extraction in the presence of active retinal neovascularization was found to be associated with a significant risk of progression of PDR. In one study, 40% of eyes developed neovascular glaucoma within 6 weeks.[11] With current extracapsular and phacoemulsification surgical techniques, this risk is lower. However, neovascular glaucoma has been reported in eyes with an intact posterior capsule[13–15,25] and in eyes that had undergone preoperative PRP.[30] These findings are a reminder that PRP and preservation of the posterior capsule do not guarantee prevention of postoperative NVI.

Eyes that have active PDR have the worst visual prognosis. They have a higher rate of postoperative uveitis and associated fibrin membrane formation. Few can be expected to achieve a final visual acuity of 20/40 or better[45] unless simultaneous vitrectomy and endolaser PRP are performed.

Eyes that have quiescent PDR and undergo cataract extraction have a better visual prognosis compared to active PDR. Overall, about 50% of eyes that undergo cataract surgery after PRP achieve a visual acuity of 20/40 or better, but 25% have a final visual acuity of 20/200 or worse.[40] The final visual outcome is influenced most by the presence of preoperative macular edema. In the meta-analysis study by Dowler

and associates, a postoperative visual acuity of 20/40 or better was achieved in about 60% of eyes with quiescent PDR without macular edema and in about 10% of eyes with quiescent PDR with macular edema.[40] In one study, 33% of eyes required additional PRP in the postoperative period, 10% developed new or recurrent NVI, and 10% underwent a postoperative pars plana vitrectomy.[31]

9-2

METHOD OF CATARACT EXTRACTION AND VISUAL ACUITY OUTCOME

9-2-1 Extracapsular Cataract Extraction Versus Phacoemulsification

One study found no significant differences in the progression of the retinopathy, in the types of complications, or in the final visual acuity between eyes that underwent ECCE and those that had phacoemulsification.[46]

The ETDRS did not distinguish between the two types of cataract surgery on study patients.[42] At 1 year following lens surgery, visual acuity improvement of two lines from preoperative levels occurred in 64.3% of the operated eyes assigned to early photocoagulation and in 59.3% of eyes assigned to deferral of photocoagulation. In eyes assigned to early photocoagulation, 46% achieved visual acuity better than 20/40, 73% were better than 20/100, and 8% were 5/200 or worse at 1 year after surgery. Visual acuity results for eyes assigned to deferral of laser photocoagulation at 1 year were not as favorable: 36% achieved visual acuity better than 20/40, 55% were better than 20/100, and 17% were 5/200 or worse.

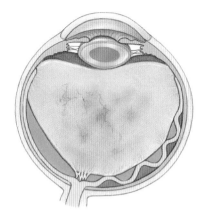

A

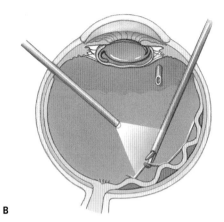

B

9-2-2 Combined Cataract Extraction and Vitrectomy

A common indication for combined cataract extraction and pars plana vitrectomy in eyes with severe retinopathy is a lens opacity that impairs the surgeon's ability to perform safe vitreoretinal surgery. Although it is possible to perform vitrectomy and cataract surgery as separate procedures, several studies have shown that they can be safely combined (Figure 9-5).[47,48] Some surgeons prefer pars plana lensectomy with placement of the IOL in front of the anterior capsule.[49,50] Others prefer ECCE or phacoemulsification with placement of the IOL in the bag or in the sulcus.[47,51–57] All three approaches are effective, and the method chosen usually depends on surgeon preference and the hardness of the lens.[58]

With all these techniques, approximately 80% of eyes have improved postoperative visual acuity. However, because many eyes have severe retinopathy preoperatively, final visual acuity is 20/40 or better in only about 30%. The most common cause for poor final visual acuity is pre-existing macular disease.[49]

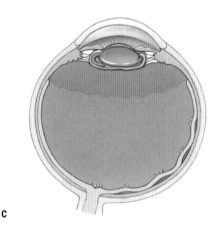

C

Figure 9-5 *(A) Significant lens opacity, which impairs surgical treatment of vitreoretinal disease. (B) After cataract surgery has been performed, standard 3-port pars plana vitrectomy is performed. (C) One operation results in pseudophakic eye with treated vitreoretinal disease.*

Although the combination of cataract surgery and pars plana vitrectomy has advantages for both the patient and the surgeon, it is not without risks. One study that predated the era of endophotocoagulation reported that the risk of postoperative NVI increased 3-fold and the risk of neovascular glaucoma increased 4-fold if the lens was removed during vitrectomy and the eye was left aphakic.[59] Severe preoperative retinal neovascularization and the absence of preoperative PRP were also associated with an increased incidence of postoperative NVI. However, Wand and associates did not find an association between postvitrectomy aphakia and the development of neovascular glaucoma in eyes with completed PRP.[60] This study found retinal reattachment and aggressive PRP to be the most important factors in reducing the incidence of postvitrectomy neovascular glaucoma. One minor concern is that the addition of vitrectomy to cataract surgery may result in a small, myopic, postoperative refractive error.[61]

FACTORS AFFECTING VISUAL OUTCOME

9-3-1 Age

The patient's age may be a predictor of final visual acuity following ECCE with placement of an IOL.[31] Patients aged 63 years or less were more likely to have a final visual acuity of 20/40 or better (58% versus 38%) and were less likely to have a final visual acuity of 20/200 or less (17% versus 38%) than older patients. The poor visual acuity outcomes in the older group were caused by progression and persistence of macular edema more often than by complications of PDR. Older patients were twice as likely to receive focal macular photocoagulation (41% versus 19%), but were less likely to receive scatter PRP (27% versus 38%) during the course of cataract management.

9-3-2 Sex

One study reported that diabetic women were more likely to have postoperative CSME than were diabetic men.[22] However, other studies failed to show an association between the sex of the patient and visual results following cataract surgery.[31]

9-3-3 Previous Vitrectomy

Eyes that required a vitrectomy prior to cataract surgery might be expected to have a poor visual prognosis, because nearly all have had severe retinopathy, the most significant predictor of poor final visual acuity. In addition, phacoemulsification is more difficult after vitrectomy because of reduced vitreous support of the lens and possibly weakened zonules.[62–65] On the other hand, there are reasons why vitrectomy prior to cataract surgery may actually improve the visual prognosis:

1. The development of endophotocoagulation allows intraoperative PRP before cataract extraction.[66–68]

2. Removal of vitreous traction may contribute to the regression of retinal and optic disc neovascularization.[69]

3. Separation of the vitreous from the macula may decrease the severity of the macular edema in some eyes.

Eyes with macular edema are much less likely to have posterior vitreous detachment than are eyes without macular edema.[70,71]

About 90% of eyes that have undergone vitrectomy before cataract extraction have an improvement in visual acuity following cataract surgery.[31,35,65] A final visual acuity of 20/40 or better is reported in only 50% of eyes and correlates with the presence of preoperative macular edema.[31] The majority of eyes do not have retinopathy progression, and very few of these eyes require a second pars plana vitrectomy. Therefore, cataract surgery has a high likelihood of visual acuity improvement in patients who have had a successful vitrectomy. However, structural changes in an eye that has undergone vitrectomy should alert the cataract surgeon to possible variations in the intraoperative dynamics of the cataract surgery.[62–65] Retinal ischemia may be an independent factor limiting visual recovery.

9-4

ROLE OF POSTERIOR CAPSULOTOMY

Preservation of the posterior lens capsule does not necessarily reduce neovascular complications or slow progression of retinopathy. In eyes with mild-to-moderate NPDR, progression of retinopathy and development of NVI within 1 year of cataract surgery may occur, even though the posterior capsule remains intact.[13–15]

The question of whether or not posterior capsulotomy increases the risk of neovascular glaucoma has no clear answer. In a 1985 study, eyes that underwent ECCE with a primary posterior capsulotomy and without placement of an IOL developed neovascular glaucoma more often than eyes with an intact posterior capsule.[12] Another study reported that neovascular glaucoma developed in pseudophakic eyes within 1 month after an Nd:YAG laser posterior capsulotomy.[72] However, other studies have failed to show evidence of an adverse effect from posterior capsulotomy following ECCE with placement of an IOL.[31] It is possible that the presence of a posterior chamber IOL may reduce the rate of NVI by restricting the access of vasoproliferative factors to the anterior chamber[73] and by decreasing the flow of oxygen from the anterior to the posterior segment.[74] In one large series, a posterior capsulotomy did not increase the risk of CSME.[31]

9-5

TREATMENT OF POSTOPERATIVE MACULAR EDEMA

The evaluation and treatment of macular edema following cataract extraction is difficult, because these eyes may have macular edema and pseudophakic CME (Irvine-Gass syndrome). Although the mechanism of CME following cataract extraction is incompletely understood, fluorophotometry readings suggest a role for breakdown of the blood–retina barrier.[75] In addition, it is known that diabetic eyes may have some breakdown of the blood–retina barrier, even in the absence of retinopathy or previous ocular surgery.[76–80] It is likely that the higher rate of CME seen after cataract extraction

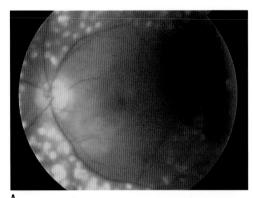

A

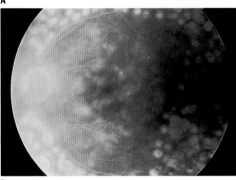

B

Figure 9-6 *(A) Fundus photograph of left eye of 62-year-old woman with quiescent PDR following phacoemulsification cataract extraction with implantation of posterior chamber IOL. Visual acuity was 20/200. (B) Intravenous fluorescein angiography reveals diffuse leakage of fluorescein in fovea. Note paucity of microaneurysms. About 6 months later, visual acuity had improved to 20/25 without laser treatment.*

in diabetic eyes results from a surgically induced inflammatory insult to an already compromised blood–retina barrier.

The development of CME following ECCE with IOL implantation occurs more frequently in diabetic eyes.[81] Postoperative angiographic or clinical CME develops in 8% of normal eyes, in 32% of diabetic eyes with no retinopathy, and in 81% of eyes with retinopathy. Persistence of the CME at 1 year following cataract surgery is present in 56% of eyes with preoperative retinopathy. Persistent clinical CME (not angiographic CME) at 1 year following cataract extraction is associated with the presence of preoperative retinopathy, progression of retinopathy, and a final visual acuity worse than 20/40. Although angiographic CME following cataract extraction is more common and persists longer in diabetic eyes, in the absence of retinopathy, it does not appear to impact the final visual acuity adversely.[82]

Because of the many overlapping clinical manifestations of pseudophakic CME and diabetic macular edema, subtle clinical features or fluorescein angiography may help to distinguish between the two.[23,26,81] In the treatment of CME, topical corticosteroids and nonsteroidal anti-inflammatory agents are used.[83,84] In eyes with macular edema thought to be primarily due to diabetic retinopathy, light laser photocoagulation to visible leaks is usually recommended. To allow the Irvine-Gass component of the edema to regress, the recommendation to delay laser treatment is supported by the observation that some eyes with a significant decrease in visual acuity secondary to macular edema spontaneously improve to 20/40 or better (Figure 9-6).[31] A reasonable option is to treat with topical medications for 3 to 6 months after cataract surgery before treating with macular laser photocoagulation, to allow time for the CME component to resolve.

CHOICE OF INTRAOCULAR LENS

The choice of IOL type in a diabetic patient depends on the likelihood that the patient will require macular laser photocoagulation, PRP, or vitreoretinal surgery in the future. It is generally recommended that patients with significant retinopathy have large-diameter (6.5- to 7.0-mm), all-PMMA implants without positioning holes.[26,85,86] A 7-mm IOL provides 36% more optical area than does a 6-mm IOL, enabling the vitreoretinal specialist to view the retinal periphery and provide laser treatment with less difficulty.[85] In addition, other potential problems involving secondary posterior capsulotomy and incarceration of the iris or lens capsule are avoided with the use of these lenses. A large anterior capsulorhexis is also important because a small opening in the anterior lens capsule may negate the advantages of a large IOL.

The shape of the IOL may also be an important factor for those eyes that may ultimately require vitreous substitutes with refractive indexes different from vitreous (that is, air, gas, or silicone). Both planoconvex[85] and convexoconcave[86] posterior chamber IOLs have been recommended for eyes that may require a future vitrectomy. These lens designs minimize refractive consequences caused by changes in the refractive index of the vitreous cavity when the vitreous gel is replaced with gas during vitrectomy.[85] There is considerably less minifi-

cation during air–fluid exchange, and a standard contact lens, rather than a high-minus lens, can be used to visualize the retina. Further, postoperative slit-lamp photocoagulation is made easier, and there is less refractive error if the eye is filled with silicone oil.

Silicone posterior chamber IOLs should be avoided for several reasons:

1. Deposition of precipitates on the anterior surface of silicone lenses is much more common than with other lenses.[87]

2. During the fluid–air exchange (if vitrectomy is required later), the view of the posterior segment is markedly compromised if the posterior capsule is not intact, because liquid droplets form on the posterior surface of the silicone IOL implant.[88] This may limit achieving vitrectomy objectives.

3. If the vitreous cavity is filled with silicone oil, the oil will adhere to the silicone IOL and may cause reduced visual acuity when the majority of the silicone oil has been removed.[89,90]

CONCLUSION

Although the majority of patients with diabetes benefit from cataract surgery, caution must be exercised when considering cataract surgery in patients who have retinopathy. Patients should be informed of the potential postoperative complications, especially progression of pre-existing retinopathy. Frequent postoperative evaluations

Figure 9-7 *Visual acuity outcomes and management decisions for diabetic patients with visually significant cataracts and no or mild retinopathy or NPDR with or without macular edema.*

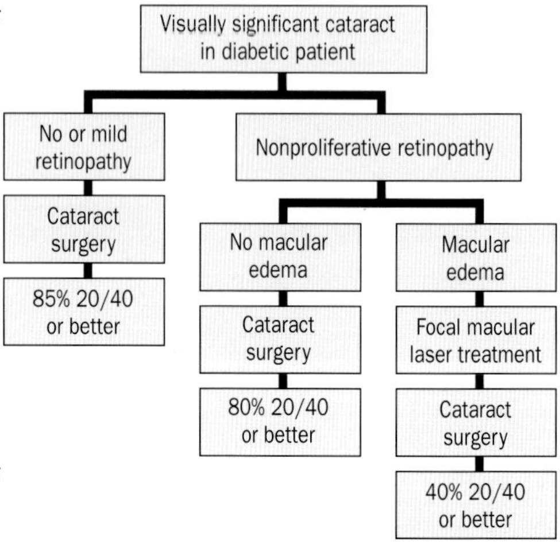

Figure 9-8 *Visual acuity outcomes and management decisions for diabetic patients with visually significant cataracts and active or quiescent PDR with or without macular edema.*

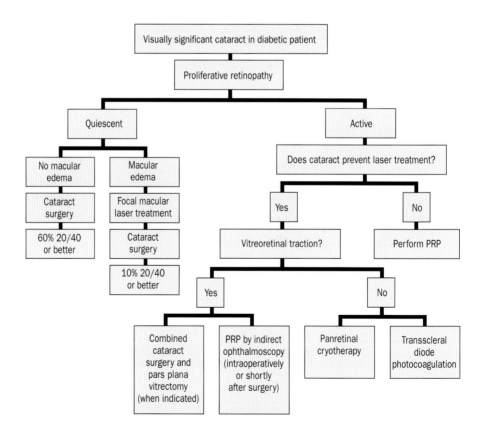

are recommended, with special attention to examining for NVI and macular edema or progression of retinopathy. After removal of the opaque lens, appropriate evaluation and management of active retinopathy with macular focal photocoagulation or PRP should be performed. The visual acuity outcomes and management decisions for diabetic patients with visually significant cataracts are summarized in Figures 9-7 and 9-8.

REFERENCES

1. Klein BE, Klein R, Moss SE: Incidence of cataract surgery in the Wisconsin Epidemiologic Study of Diabetic Retinopathy. *Am J Ophthalmol* 1995;119:295–300.

2. Klein BE, Klein R, Moss SE: Prevalence of cataracts in a population-based study of persons with diabetes mellitus. *Ophthalmology* 1985;92: 1191–1196.

3. Bron AJ, Sparrow J, Brown NA, et al: The lens in diabetes. *Eye* 1993;7:260–275.

4. Harding JJ, Egerton M, van Heyningen R, Harding RS: Diabetes, glaucoma, sex, and cataract: analysis of combined data from two case control studies. *Br J Ophthalmol* 1993;77:2–6.

5. Harris MI, Eastman RC, Cowie CC, et al: Comparison of diabetes diagnostic categories in the U.S. population according to the 1997 American Diabetes Association and 1980–1985 World Health Organization diagnostic criteria. *Diabetes Care* 1997;20:1859–1862.

6. Harris MI, Robbins DC: Prevalence of adult-onset IDDM in the U.S. population. *Diabetes Care* 1994;17:1337–1340.

7. Nielsen NV, Vinding T: The prevalence of cataract in insulin-dependent and non–insulin-dependent diabetes mellitus. *Acta Ophthalmologica* 1984;62:595–602.

8. Klein R, Klein BE, Moss SE: Visual impairment in diabetes. *Ophthalmology* 1984;91:1–9.

9. Edwards MG, Schachat AP, Bressler SB, Bressler NM: Outcome of cataract operations performed to permit diagnosis, to determine eligibility for laser therapy, or to perform laser therapy of retinal disorders. *Am J Ophthalmol* 1994;118:440–444.

10. Minckler D, Astorino A, Hamilton AM: Cataract surgery in patients with diabetes. *Ophthalmology* 1998;105:949–950.

11. Aiello LM, Wand M, Liang G: Neovascular glaucoma and vitreous hemorrhage following cataract surgery in patients with diabetes mellitus. *Ophthalmology* 1983;90:814–820.

12. Poliner LS, Christianson DJ, Escoffery RF, et al: Neovascular glaucoma after intracapsular and extracapsular cataract extraction in diabetic patients. *Am J Ophthalmol* 1985;100:637–643.

13. Pavese T, Insler MS: Effects of extracapsular cataract extraction with posterior chamber lens implantation on the development of neovascular glaucoma in diabetics. *J Cataract Refract Surg* 1987;13:197–201.

14. Prasad P, Setna PH, Dunne JA: Accelerated ocular neovascularisation in diabetics following posterior chamber lens implantation. *Br J Ophthalmol* 1990;74:313–314.

15. Sadiq SA, Chatterjee A, Vernon SA: Progression of diabetic retinopathy and rubeotic glaucoma following cataract surgery. *Eye* 1995;9: 728–738.

16. Suzuki Y, Ohtsuki K, Goto T, Sumiya Y: [Comparative study of postoperative complications in primary and secondary implantation of posterior chamber intraocular lens in cataract surgery for diabetic patients.] *Nippon Ganka Gakkai Zasshi* 1992;96:359–363.

17. Krupsky S, Zalish M, Oliver M, Pollack A: Anterior segment complications in diabetic patients following extracapsular cataract extraction and posterior chamber intraocular lens implantation. *Ophthalmic Surg* 1991;22:526–530.

18. Hykin PG, Gregson RM, Hamilton AM: Extracapsular cataract extraction in diabetics with rubeosis iridis. *Eye* 1992;6:296–299.

19. Weinreb RN, Wasserstrom JP, Forman JS, Ritch R: Pseudophakic pupillary block with angle-closure glaucoma in diabetic patients. *Am J Ophthalmol* 1986;102:325–328.

20. Ionides A, Dowler JG, Hykin PG, et al: Posterior capsule opacification following diabetic extracapsular cataract extraction. *Eye* 1994;8:535–537.

21. Helbig H, Kellner U, Bornfeld N, Foerster MH: Cataract surgery and YAG-laser capsulotomy following vitrectomy for diabetic retinopathy. *Ger J Ophthalmol* 1996;5:408–414.

22. Jaffe GJ, Burton TC: Progression of nonproliferative diabetic retinopathy following cataract extraction. *Arch Ophthalmol* 1988;106:745–749.

23. Pollack A, Dotan S, Oliver M: Course of diabetic retinopathy following cataract surgery. *Br J Ophthalmol* 1991;75:2–8.

24. Pollack A, Dotan S, Oliver M: Progression of diabetic retinopathy after cataract extraction. *Br J Ophthalmol* 1991;75:547–551.

25. Cunliffe IA, Flanagan DW, George ND, et al: Extracapsular cataract surgery with lens implantation in diabetics with and without proliferative retinopathy. *Br J Ophthalmol* 1991;75:9–12.

26. Jaffe GJ, Burton TC, Kuhn E, et al: Progression of nonproliferative diabetic retinopathy and visual outcome after extracapsular cataract extraction and intraocular lens implantation. *Am J Ophthalmol* 1992;114:448–456.

27. Dureau P, Massin P, Chaine G, et al: [Extracapsular extraction and posterior chamber implantation in diabetics: prospective study of 198 eyes.] *J Fr Ophtalmol* 1997;20:117–123.

28. Vignanelli M: [Progression of diabetic retinopathy following cataract extraction.] *Klin Monatsbl Augenheilkd* 1990;196:334–337.

29. Raniel Y, Teichner Y, Friedman Z: The course of nonproliferative diabetic retinopathy following ECCE with posterior chamber IOL implantation. *Metab Pediatr Syst Ophthalmol* 1994;17:10–13.

30. Ruiz RS, Saatci OA: Posterior chamber intraocular lens implantation in eyes with inactive and active proliferative diabetic retinopathy. *Am J Ophthalmol* 1991;111:158–162.

31. Benson WE, Brown GC, Tasman W, et al: Extracapsular cataract extraction with placement of a posterior chamber lens in patients with diabetic retinopathy. *Ophthalmology* 1993;100:730–738.

32. Henricsson M, Heijl A, Janzon L: Diabetic retinopathy before and after cataract surgery. *Br J Ophthalmol* 1996;80:789–793.

33. Kodama T, Hayasaka S, Setogawa T: Plasma glucose levels, postoperative complications, and progression of retinopathy in diabetic patients undergoing intraocular lens implantation. *Graefes Arch Klin Exp Ophthalmol* 1993;231:439–443.

34. Pollack A, Leiba H, Bukelman A, et al: The course of diabetic retinopathy following cataract surgery in eyes previously treated by laser photocoagulation. *Br J Ophthalmol* 1992;76:228–231.

35. Hutton WL, Pesicka GA, Fuller DG: Cataract extraction in the diabetic eye after vitrectomy. *Am J Ophthalmol* 1987;104:1–4.

36. Sebestyen JG: Intraocular lenses and diabetes mellitus. *Am J Ophthalmol* 1986;101:425–428.

37. Straatsma BR, Pettit TH, Wheeler N, Miyamasu W: Diabetes mellitus and intraocular lens implantation. *Ophthalmology* 1983;90:336–343.

38. Cheng H, Franklin SL: Treatment of cataract in diabetics with and without retinopathy. *Eye* 1988;2:607–614.

39. Ngui MS, Lim AS, Chong AB: Posterior chamber intraocular lenses in diabetics: review of 63 patients. *Int Ophthalmol* 1985;8:257–259.

40. Dowler JG, Hykin PG, Lightman SL, Hamilton AM: Visual acuity following extracapsular cataract extraction in diabetes: a meta-analysis. *Eye* 1995;9:313–317.

41. Wagner T, Knaflic D, Rauber M, Mester U: Influence of cataract surgery on the diabetic eye: a prospective study. *Ger J Ophthalmol* 1996;5: 79–83.

42. Early Treatment Diabetic Retinopathy Study Research Group: Results after lens extraction in patients with diabetic retinopathy. ETDRS Report Number 25. *Arch Ophthalmol* 1999;117: 1600–1606.

43. Early Treatment Diabetic Retinopathy Study Research Group: Photocoagulation for diabetic macular edema. ETDRS Report Number 1. *Arch Ophthalmol* 1985;103:1796–1806.

44. Klein R, Klein BE, Moss SE, et al: The Wisconsin epidemiologic study of diabetic retinopathy, IV: diabetic macular edema. *Ophthalmology* 1984;91:1464–1474.

45. Hykin PG, Gregson RM, Stevens JD, Hamilton PA: Extracapsular cataract extraction in proliferative diabetic retinopathy. *Ophthalmology* 1993;100:394–399.

46. Antcliff RJ, Poulson A, Flanagan DW: Phacoemulsification in diabetics. *Eye* 1996;10: 737–741.

47. Benson WE, Brown GC, Tasman W, McNamara JA: Extracapsular cataract extraction, posterior chamber lens insertion, and pars plana vitrectomy in one operation. *Ophthalmology* 1990; 97:918–921.

48. Senn P, Schipper I, Perren B: Combined pars plana vitrectomy, phacoemulsification, and intraocular lens implantation in the capsular bag: a comparison to vitrectomy and subsequent cataract surgery as a two-step procedure. *Ophthalmic Surg Lasers* 1995;26:420–428.

49. Blankenship GW, Flynn HW Jr, Kokame GT: Posterior chamber intraocular lens insertion during pars plana lensectomy and vitrectomy for complications of proliferative diabetic retinopathy. *Am J Ophthalmol* 1989;108:1–5.

50. Kokame GT, Flynn HW Jr, Blankenship GW: Posterior chamber intraocular lens implantation during diabetic pars plana vitrectomy. *Ophthalmology* 1989;96:603–610.

51. McElvanney AM, Talbot EM: Posterior chamber lens implantation combined with pars plana vitrectomy. *J Cataract Refract Surg* 1997; 23:106–110.

52. Ullern M, Nicol JL, Ruellan YM, et al: [Phacoemulsification by the anterior approach combined with vitreoretinal surgery.] *J Fr Ophtalmol* 1993;16:320–324.

53. Menchini U, Azzolini C, Camesasca FI, Brancato R: Combined vitrectomy, cataract extraction, and posterior chamber intraocular lens implantation in diabetic patients. *Ophthalmic Surg* 1991;22:69–73.

54. Koenig SB, Mieler WF, Han DP, Abrams GW: Combined phacoemulsification, pars plana vitrectomy, and posterior chamber intraocular lens insertion. *Arch Ophthalmol* 1992;110: 1101–1104.

55. Pagot V, Gazagne C, Galiana A, et al: [Extracapsular cataract extraction and implantation in the capsular sac during vitrectomy in diabetics.] *J Fr Ophtalmol* 1991;14:523–528.

56. Mamalis N, Teske MP, Kreisler KR, et al: Phacoemulsification combined with pars plana vitrectomy. *Ophthalmic Surg* 1991;22:194–198.

57. Mackool RJ: Pars plana vitrectomy and posterior chamber intraocular lens implantation in diabetic patients. *Ophthalmology* 1989;96: 1679–1680.

58. de Ortueta Hilberath D, Losche CC: Choice of surgical technique in the management of cataract combined with vitreous surgery. *Eur J Ophthalmol* 1997;7:245–250.

59. Rice TA, Michels RG, Maguire MG, Rice EF: The effect of lensectomy on the incidence of iris neovascularization and neovascular glaucoma after vitrectomy for diabetic retinopathy. *Am J Ophthalmol* 1983;95:1–11.

60. Wand M, Madigan JC, Gaudio AR, Sorokanich S: Neovascular glaucoma following pars plana vitrectomy for complications of diabetic retinopathy. *Ophthalmic Surg* 1990;21:113–118.

61. Shioya M, Ogino N, Shinjo U: Change in postoperative refractive error when vitrectomy is added to intraocular lens implantation. *J Cataract Refract Surg* 1997;23:1217–1220.

62. Sneed S, Parrish RK II, Mandelbaum S, O'Grady G: Technical problems of extracapsular cataract extractions after vitrectomy. *Arch Ophthalmol* 1986;104:1126–1127.

63. Smiddy WE, Stark WJ, Michels RG, et al: Cataract extraction after vitrectomy. *Ophthalmology* 1987;94:483–487.

64. Saunders DC, Brown A, Jones NP: Extracapsular cataract extraction after vitrectomy. *J Cataract Refract Surg* 1996;22:218–221.

65. McDermott ML, Puklin JE, Abrams GW, Eliott D. Phacoemulsification for cataract following pars plana vitrectomy. *Ophthalmic Surg Lasers* 1997;28:558–564.

66. Charles S: Endophotocoagulation. *Retina* 1981;1:117–120.

67. Peyman GA, Grisolano JM, Palacio MN: Intraocular photocoagulation with the argon-krypton laser. *Arch Ophthalmol* 1980;98:2061–2064.

68. Fleischman JA, Swartz M, Dixon JA: Argon laser endophotocoagulation: an intraoperative trans–pars plana technique. *Arch Ophthalmol* 1981;99:1610–1612.

69. Federman JL, Boyer D, Lanning R, Breit P: An objective analysis of proliferative diabetic retinopathy before and after pars plana vitrectomy. *Ophthalmology* 1979;86:276–282.

70. Nasrallah FP, Jalkh AE, Van Coppenolle F, et al: The role of the vitreous in diabetic macular edema. *Ophthalmology* 1988;95:1335–1339.

71. Nasrallah FP, Van de Velde F, Jalkh AE, et al: Importance of the vitreous in young diabetics with macular edema. *Ophthalmology* 1989;96: 1511–1516; discussion 1516–1517.

72. Weinreb RN, Wasserstrom JP, Parker W: Neovascular glaucoma following neodymium-YAG laser posterior capsulotomy. *Arch Ophthalmol* 1986;104:730–731.

73. Glaser BM: Extracellular modulating factors and the control of intraocular neovascularization. *Arch Ophthalmol* 1988;106:603–607.

74. Stefansson E, Landers MB III, Wolbarsht ML: Increased retinal oxygen supply following pan-retinal photocoagulation and vitrectomy and lensectomy. *Trans Am Ophthalmol Soc* 1981;79: 307–334.

75. Miyake K: Fluorophotometric evaluation of the blood–ocular barrier function following cataract surgery and intraocular lens implantation. *J Cataract Refract Surg* 1988;14:560–568.

76. Cunha-Vaz JG: Studies on the pathophysiology of diabetic retinopathy: the blood–retinal barrier in diabetes. *Diabetes* 1983;32:20–27.

77. Boot JP, van Gerven JM, van Best JA, et al: Blood retinal and blood aqueous barriers in diabetics by fluorophotometry. *Doc Ophthalmol* 1989;71:19–27.

78. Bordat B, Arnaud C, Guirguis IR, Laudeho A: Fluorophotometric study of lens autofluorescence and the blood–retinal barrier in 56 diabetic patients. *Eur J Ophthalmol* 1995;5:13–18.

79. Schalnus R, Ohrloff C, Jungmann E, et al: Permeability of the blood–retinal barrier and the blood–aqueous barrier in type I diabetes without diabetic retinopathy: simultaneous evaluation with fluorophotometry. *Ger J Ophthalmol* 1993; 2:202–206.

80. Schalnus R, Ohrloff C: The blood–ocular barrier in type I diabetes without diabetic retinopathy: permeability measurements using fluorophotometry. *Ophthalmic Res* 1995; 27:116–123.

81. Pollack A, Leiba H, Bukelman A, Oliver M: Cystoid macular oedema following cataract extraction in patients with diabetes. *Br J Ophthalmol* 1992;76:221–224.

82. Menchini U, Bandello F, Brancato R, et al: Cystoid macular oedema after extracapsular cataract extraction and intraocular lens implantation in diabetic patients without retinopathy. *Br J Ophthalmol* 1993;77:208–211.

83. Jampol LM: Pharmacologic therapy of aphakic and pseudophakic cystoid macular edema: 1985 update. *Ophthalmology* 1985;92:807–810.

84. Jampol LM: Aphakic cystoid macular edema: a hypothesis. *Arch Ophthalmol* 1985; 103:1134–1135.

85. McCuen BW II, Klombers L: The choice of posterior chamber intraocular lens style in patients with diabetic retinopathy. *Arch Ophthalmol* 1990;108:1376–1377.

86. McCartney DL, Guyton DL: The choice of posterior chamber intraocular lens style in patients with diabetic retinopathy. *Arch Ophthalmol* 1991;109:615.

87. Apple DJ, Mamalis N, Loftfield K, et al: Complications of intraocular lenses: a historical and histopathological review. *Surv Ophthalmol* 1984;29:1–54.

88. Eaton AM, Jaffe GJ, McCuen BW II, Mincey GJ: Condensation on the posterior surface of silicone intraocular lenses during fluid–air exchange. *Ophthalmology* 1995;102:733–736.

89. Apple DJ, Federman JL, Krolicki TJ, et al: Irreversible silicone oil adhesion to silicone intraocular lenses: a clinicopathologic analysis. *Ophthalmology* 1996;103:1555–1561; discussion 1561–1562.

90. Kusaka S, Kodama T, Ohashi Y: Condensation of silicone oil on the posterior surface of a silicone intraocular lens during vitrectomy. *Am J Ophthalmol* 1996;121:574–575.

Nonretinal Abnormalities in Diabetes

Ingrid U. Scott, MD, MPH

Harry W. Flynn, Jr, MD

While most diabetes-associated blindness is due to complications of diabetic retinopathy, many nonretinal ophthalmic abnormalities may contribute to visual loss and must be considered in the management of diabetic patients. This chapter reviews the various ophthalmic conditions associated with diabetes that are listed in Table 10-1.

10-1

CORNEAL DISEASES

Diabetic patients often have significantly decreased corneal sensitivity, and the severity of the decreased sensitivity usually shows a positive correlation with the severity of retinopathy.[1,2] This abnormality may account for the increased incidence of contact lens–associated bacterial corneal ulcers[3] and neurotrophic ulcers[4] in diabetic patients compared with nondiabetic persons (Figure 10-1).

Intrinsic abnormalities of the epithelial basement membrane complexes[5,6] and impaired epithelial barrier function[7] predispose to superficial punctate keratitis, poor epithelial wound healing after trauma, and persistent epithelial defects.[4] The latter are seen frequently in diabetic patients whose corneal epithelium was removed during vitreoretinal surgery (Figure 10-2).[8]

Diabetic patients are prone to recurrent corneal erosions, especially after photocoagulation and vitrectomy.[9] In a 1976 study of 100 vitrectomies performed for advanced diabetic retinopathy with vitreous hemorrhage, persistent corneal epithelial defects or recurrent corneal erosions occurred in 25% of patients.[10] When the epithelium of the diabetic cornea is removed, it often comes off as an intact epithelial sheet, with the basement membrane attached to basal epithelial cells. In the nondiabetic eye, scraping of the epithelium removes only the epithelium and usually leaves the basement membrane intact and adherent to the stroma.[8,11,12] Ultrastructural abnormalities of the diabetic corneal epithelial basement

TABLE 10-1

Nonretinal Abnormalities in Diabetes

Corneal Diseases

Decreased corneal sensitivity

Bacterial keratitis

Neurotrophic ulcers

Persistent epithelial defects

Recurrent epithelial erosions

Glaucoma

Primary open-angle glaucoma

Angle-closure glaucoma

Neovascular glaucoma

Blood-associated glaucoma

Lens Abnormalities

Refractive error

Cataract

Optic Nerve Abnormalities

Acute optic disc edema

Wolfram syndrome

Optic nerve hypoplasia

Optic atrophy

Cranial Nerve Abnormalities

Cranial nerve III, IV, and VI palsies

Infectious Diseases

Endophthalmitis

Mucormycosis

membrane complex mimic findings in epithelial basement membrane dystrophies[13] and include thickening of the multilaminar basement membrane,[5] decreased hemidesmosome frequency,[14] and decreased penetration of anchoring fibrils.[15]

The poor adhesiveness of the diabetic corneal basement membrane may be related to changes in biochemical composition induced by increased sorbitol and fructose produced by the aldose reductase pathway.[8,16] While topical aldose-reductase inhibitors may promote epithelial regeneration,[17–20] most studies have been performed in rats[17–19] and the efficacy of these agents in humans is unproven. In contrast, lubricants, limited epithelial debridement, and bandage contact lenses have proven to be effective in avoiding major ocular surface problems.

10-2

GLAUCOMA

10-2-1 Primary Open-Angle Glaucoma

The association between diabetes and primary open-angle glaucoma (POAG) is unclear. Several studies have demonstrated a higher prevalence of elevated mean intraocular pressure (IOP) and POAG among diabetic patients compared with nondiabetic persons.[21–27] Case-control studies support an association between diabetes and POAG, with the relative odds of having glaucoma among diabetic patients versus controls ranging from 1.6 to 4.7.[28–31] Other studies, including population-based surveys, demonstrated no association between diabetes and POAG.[32–34] The Baltimore Eye Survey found little evidence of an association between glaucoma and diabetes.[35] In the Beaver Dam Eye Study, older-onset diabetes (≥30 years of age) was associated with a modest increase in the risk of glaucoma.[27]

When patients are treated medically for POAG, it is important to recognize that the potential side effects of beta-adrenergic antagonists include reduced glucose tolerance and masking of hypoglycemic signs. Therefore, although the relatively cardioselective beta-1-adrenergic antagonist betaxolol is somewhat less effective than other beta blockers in lowering IOP,[36–39] it may be a safer alternative in diabetic patients.

10-2-2 Angle-Closure Glaucoma

Several observations suggest an association between diabetes and angle-closure glaucoma (ACG). One study found that patients with ACG had a higher prevalence of abnormal glucose tolerance test results compared with POAG patients and controls.[40] Patients with ACG also have a high prevalence of non–insulin-dependent diabetes.[41] It has been hypothesized that, in some cases, ACG may be a symptom of diabetes, perhaps due to autonomic dysfunction.[42] Finally, lens swelling related to hyperglycemia may precipitate ACG.[43]

Hyperosmotic agents are commonly included in the medical treatment of acute episodes of elevated IOP. In diabetic patients, isosorbide is preferred to glycerol because isosorbide is not metabolized into sugar, while glycerol is metabolized into sugar and ketone bodies. Glycerol, therefore, can produce hyperglycemia and, rarely, ketoacidosis in diabetic patients.

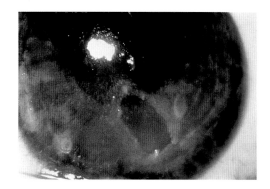

Figure 10-1 *Neurotrophic corneal ulcer in diabetic patient with decreased corneal sensitivity.*

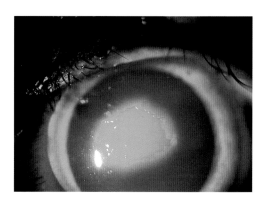

Figure 10-2 *Persistent corneal epithelial defect in diabetic patient after vitreoretinal surgery.*

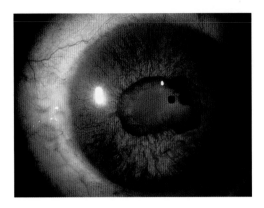

Figure 10-3 *Extensive neovascularization of iris in patient with PDR.*

10-2-3 Neovascular Glaucoma

Despite the widespread use of panretinal photocoagulation (PRP), proliferative diabetic retinopathy (PDR) remains a leading cause of neovascular glaucoma. In a 1973 report of 56 patients with neovascular glaucoma, 43% were attributed to diabetic retinopathy, 37% to central retinal vein occlusion, and the rest to miscellaneous causes.[44] In 1984, Brown and associates reviewed 208 cases of neovascular glaucoma and reported that 36% were caused by central retinal vein occlusion, 32% by diabetic retinopathy, and 13% by carotid occlusive disease.[45]

The reported incidence of any neovascularization of the iris (NVI) among diabetic patients ranges from 1%[46] to 17%.[47] In eyes with PDR, the reported incidence in one study was 65%.[48] In the early stages, NVI usually appears as small vascular tufts either at the pupillary margin or in the anterior chamber angle. As these vessels later spread across the iris surface, they are frequently accompanied by fibrous tissue, which contracts and may cause ectropion uveae (Figure 10-3) and peripheral anterior synechiae. While angle closure can cause severe glaucoma, IOP may be elevated even before any angle is closed, probably because of leakage of protein and cells from the new iris vessels.[49]

It is generally well accepted that NVI is associated with retinal hypoxia and PDR,[50] and many authors have reported regression of early NVI following PRP.[51-54] In goniophotocoagulation, argon laser treatment is applied directly to new vessels in the anterior chamber angle. Although performed infrequently, goniophotocoagulation has been proposed as a treatment in the early stages of neovascular glaucoma to prevent progressive angle closure, while PRP facilitates regression of the anterior segment neovascularization.

Use of adjunctive 5-fluorouracil or mitomycin C has been shown to increase the success rate of filtering surgery in eyes with neovascular glaucoma.[55–59] Glaucoma drainage devices have gained increasing popularity in recent years to achieve IOP control in various refractory glaucomas, including neovascular glaucoma.[60–66] A traditional approach to the management of patients with neovascular glaucoma is as follows:

1. PRP is performed to induce regression of NVI.

2. If NVI regresses and IOP is not controlled medically, filtering surgery with an adjunctive antimetabolite is performed.

3. If NVI fails to regress and the eye has visual potential, a drainage device may be considered.

4. If NVI fails to regress and the eye has limited visual potential, a cyclodestructive procedure may be considered as a last resort.

For eyes with NVI and opaque media, an alternative approach is combined pars plana vitrectomy, lensectomy with or without intraocular lens implantation, and implantation of a glaucoma drainage device.[66] Medical management of IOP elevation in neovascular glaucoma principally involves aqueous suppressants, such as alpha-2 agonists, beta blockers, and topical and oral carbonic anhydrase inhibitors. Miotics are not beneficial when the anterior chamber angle is closed and are avoided, as they can exacerbate intraocular inflammation and may hamper access to the posterior segment. Topical corticosteroids are often useful in treating intraocular inflammation and pain.

10-2-4 Blood-Associated Glaucoma

Glaucoma associated with degenerated intraocular blood is not unique to diabetic patients. Ghost-cell glaucoma may occur after vitreous hemorrhage of any cause in an eye with a communication between the vitreous and the anterior segment through a disrupted anterior hyaloid face. Ghost-cell glaucoma was originally observed after early attempts at vitrectomy, when only a core vitrectomy was performed. Blood products in the peripheral vitreous leach out, and degenerated erythrocytes (ghost cells) travel around lens zonules and into the anterior chamber, obstructing the trabecular meshwork and causing elevated IOP within days to weeks postvitrectomy.[67]

Slit-lamp examination usually permits differentiation of white inflammatory cells associated with anterior uveitis from khaki-colored ghost cells. In severe cases, it is important to distinguish the white color of a hypopyon due to uveitis or endophthalmitis from the khaki-colored pseudohypopyon characteristic of ghost-cell glaucoma. In questionable cases, anterior chamber aspiration, combined with phase-contrast microscopy, may be performed. In ghost-cell glaucoma, degenerated erythrocytes with precipitated hemoglobin (Heinz bodies) adherent to the inner walls of the cells may be evident.[68–70]

Medical treatment focuses on agents that decrease aqueous production—for example, alpha-2 agonists, beta-adrenergic blocking agents, and carbonic anhydrase inhibitors. Because the trabecular meshwork is obstructed by ghost cells, miotics may be unsuccessful in increasing aqueous outflow. In severe cases or if medical therapy is unsuccessful or not tolerated, surgical management may be limited to anterior chamber washout or may include a pars plana vitrectomy.

Hemolytic glaucoma results when macrophages ingest contents of red blood cells and then accumulate in the trabecular meshwork, where they obstruct aqueous outflow.[71] Examination reveals red-tinted blood cells floating in the aqueous, and the anterior chamber angle is usually open, with the trabecular meshwork covered with reddish brown pigment.[72] As the condition is typically self-limited, it is generally managed medically. Occasionally, anterior chamber lavage is required.[72]

First described in 1960, hemosiderotic glaucoma is thought to result from obstruction of the aqueous outflow channels by iron deposition, with subsequent degenerative and inflammatory changes.[73] Hemosiderotic glaucoma is reported to have a later onset than that of ghost-cell glaucoma (patients with hemosiderotic glaucoma typically present with elevated IOP years after the initial intraocular hemorrhage), and ghost cells are not present.[74]

Because treatment is similar to that of ghost-cell glaucoma, these two entities (hemolytic glaucoma and hemosiderotic glaucome) may represent part of the broad spectrum of blood-associated glaucoma.

LENS ABNORMALITIES

10-3-1 Refractive Error

Reversible swelling in lenses of diabetic patients causes "fluctuating myopia," which may be a presenting sign of diabetes. It is thought that accumulation of the sugar alcohol sorbitol, an end product of glucose reduction by aldose reductase, exerts an osmotic effect in lens cells.[75] Because lens shape, and thus refractive error, may fluctuate with blood glucose levels, it is best to prescribe glasses when the blood glucose level is relatively stable. Prior to prescribing glasses in patients with labile blood glucose levels, the clinician may need to evaluate the refractive error on several visits to confirm a stable refractive error.

10-3-2 Cataract

The risk of cataract formation is 2 to 4 times higher in diabetic patients than in nondiabetic persons.[76,77] The risk of cataract increases with duration of diabetes and with poor metabolic control.[75,78] Cataract in diabetic patients usually does not differ morphologically from age-related cataract, but may occur 20 to 30 years earlier than in nondiabetic persons. In young diabetic patients, a rare "snowflake" cataract may develop, with superficial vacuoles and white snowflake opacities (Figure 10-4) in the subcapsular region, and rapidly progress to a mature cataract.

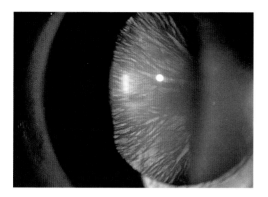

Figure 10-4 *"Snowflake" cataract in patient with type 1 diabetes.*

10-4

OPTIC NERVE ABNORMALITIES

10-4-1 Acute Optic Disc Edema

Acute optic disc edema associated with diabetes, or diabetic papillopathy, usually occurs in the second to fourth decades of life and generally shows no correlation with the severity of diabetic retinopathy. It is typically associated with mild loss of vision (≥20/50),[79–81] and the visual field may be normal or may show defects, such as an increased blind spot, arcuate scotoma, or altitudinal scotoma. Fluorescein angiography usually demonstrates diffuse leakage on the disc. The condition presents bilaterally in approximately 50% of cases, while in other cases the second eye may be affected as late as 3 years after initial presentation.[80] The visual prognosis is usually good, with nearly all younger patients recovering to a visual acuity of ≥20/30 (Figure 10-5). Visual field defects infrequently persist.[80,82,83]

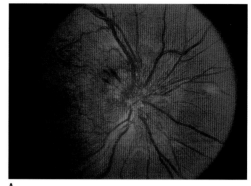

A

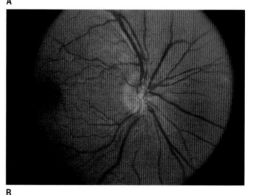

B

Figure 10-5 *Diabetic papillopathy with good visual prognosis. (A) Disc edema, telangiectasia, and splinter hemorrhages in 20-year-old patient. Visual acuity is 20/30⁻². (B) About 7 months later, disc edema has resolved and there is gliosis on disc. Visual acuity is 20/25.*

While the optic disc appearance usually returns to normal, occasionally diffuse or segmental atrophy may result (Figure 10-6).

In diabetic papillopathy, diffuse disc swelling may mimic papilledema.[84] However, careful visual field testing may demonstrate an arcuate or altitudinal defect, which would be unusual in papilledema. To avoid unnecessary PRP, it is important to differentiate the prominent telangiectasia of disc vessels often seen in diabetic papillopathy from neovascularization of the disc.

Diabetic papillopathy may be a mild form of acute anterior ischemic optic neuropathy, which differs from typical anterior ischemic optic neuropathy. Typical AION is generally seen in middle-aged persons with or without diabetes and is characterized by unilateral marked loss of vision, pale swelling of the optic disc, segmental areas of nonperfusion on fluorescein angiography, poor prognosis for visual recovery, and late optic disc pallor.[81,85]

10-4-2 Wolfram Syndrome

Wolfram syndrome refers to type 1 diabetes mellitus and progressive optic atrophy. The clinical spectrum includes multiple other neurologic and systemic abnormalities, such as neurosensory hearing loss, neurogenic bladder, diabetes insipidus, nystagmus, anosmia, and gonadal dysfunction.[86] The inheritance is autosomal recessive or sporadic. In a series of nine patients reported by Lessell and Rosman, diabetes was diagnosed between the ages of 2 and 11 years, and progressive loss of vision to ≤20/200 occurred within several years.[86]

10-4-3 Optic Nerve Hypoplasia

Optic nerve hypoplasia is a congenital anomaly associated with a decreased complement of axons in the optic nerve but relatively normal vessels.[87,88] Examination may reveal a double-ring sign caused by concentric chorioretinal pigment changes.[88] Optic nerve hypoplasia occurs most often in children born to mothers exposed to anticonvulsants, quinine, excessive alcohol, or lysergic acid diethylamide (LSD) and in children born to mothers with diabetes, but may also be seen in children with congenital intracranial tumors or basal encephaloceles.[87–89] The optic nerve hypoplasia seen in children of diabetic mothers is often superior and segmental, with a corresponding inferior semialtitudinal visual field defect; central acuity is usually normal.[88]

10-4-4 Optic Atrophy

Optic atrophy in diabetic patients may be due to such causes as prior diabetic papillitis or nonarteritic anterior ischemic optic neuropathy. Further, at least two mild forms of optic atrophy are due to diabetic retinopathy[87]:

1. Multiple nerve fiber layer infarcts, which accumulate over time, may cause temporal or diffuse optic atrophy.

2. PRP destroys many retinal ganglion cells.

A

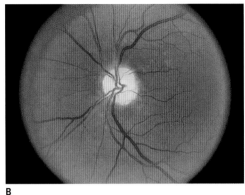

B

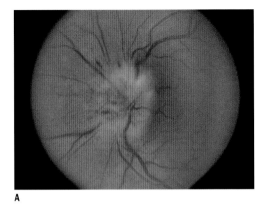

10-5

CRANIAL NERVE ABNORMALITIES

Diabetic patients may have an isolated cranial nerve (III, IV, or VI) palsy due to focal small-vessel occlusion with ischemic demyelination. The differential diagnosis includes microvascular infarction, vasculitic infarction, a compressive lesion, trauma, inflammation, and, in young patients, ophthalmoplegic migraine.[87,90] Trauma is a frequent cause of nerve IV palsy. A nerve VI palsy may be nonlocalizing and may be a sign of increased intracranial pressure.[91] The risk of a compressive lesion is higher for an isolated nerve III palsy, but is almost always accompanied by pupillary dilation. If nerve III is involved due to microvascular infarction, the pupil is almost always spared (Figure 10-7). When present, pupillary involvement generally consists of anisocoria of ≤1 mm rather than a fully dilated unreactive pupil,[92] and internal ophthalmoplegia is incomplete.[93] Despite what is often reported, cranial nerve palsies caused by mi-

Figure 10-6 *Diabetic papillopathy with eventual optic atrophy. (A) Disc edema, hemorrhages, and cotton-wool spots in 52-year-old patient with 6-year history of diabetes. Visual acuity is 20/25. (B) About 3 years later, diffuse optic atrophy is present. Visual acuity is 20/100.*

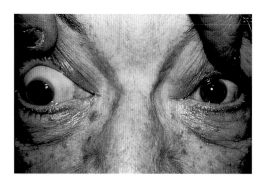

Figure 10-7 *Right cranial nerve III palsy in 71-year-old patient with type 2 diabetes.*

crovascular disease may present with orbital pain in up to 20% of cases,[91] and pain may precede the palsy by a few days.

Workup for causes other than microvascular disease is indicated if examination reveals involvement of more than one cranial nerve, other neurologic signs, progressive deterioration, or lack of complete recovery within 3 months. Patients under the age of 45 years with an isolated cranial nerve palsy usually do not have a microvascular infarct even if they have long-standing diabetes.[87] Recurrences are not rare and may involve the same or another cranial nerve on either side.

10-6

INFECTIOUS DISEASES

10-6-1 Endophthalmitis

Several studies suggest that patients with diabetes may have an increased risk of developing postoperative endophthalmitis (Figure 10-8) compared to nondiabetic persons.[94–96] In a 1991 report of the 5-year incidence rates of endophthalmitis following intraocular surgery, a statistically significant increased incidence of endophthalmitis occurred in diabetic patients (0.163%) compared with nondiabetic patients (0.055%) who underwent extracapsular cataract extraction with or without intraocular lens implantation.[94] In a 1995 case-control study of endophthalmitis following secondary intraocular lens implantation, 50% of patients had a history of diabetes compared with 5.9% of control patients.[96] In a 1994 report of 162 consecutive patients treated for acute postoperative endophthalmitis, 21% had diabetes.[95]

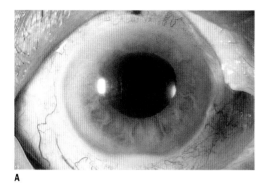

A

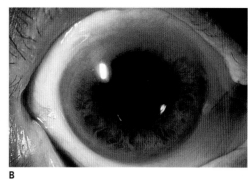

B

The increased risk of postoperative en-dophthalmitis among diabetic patients is not surprising, because patients with diabetes have been demonstrated to have impaired cellular and humoral immune responses, as well as altered phagocytic capabilities.[97–100] Further, it is well known that diabetic patients are more likely than nondiabetic patients to experience delayed wound healing.[101] Thus, diabetic patients may be predisposed to wound breakdown or persistent wound defects or both, which, in turn, may increase their risk of developing endophthalmitis. Finally, vitrectomy for complications of PDR often requires longer surgical time and more instrument changes passing through the pars plana sclerotomies compared with vitrectomy for other diseases.

10-6-2 Mucormycosis

Mucormycosis is a rare orbital infection that affects diabetic patients, especially those with ketoacidosis. In fact, it is estimated that 50% of mucormycosis cases occur in diabetic patients.[102,103] The diagnosis should be suspected in any diabetic, immunosuppressed, or debilitated patient who develops facial or orbital pain, diplopia, or other

Figure 10-8 *(A)* Staphylococcus epidermidis *endophthalmitis in 86-year-old diabetic man 1 week after small-incision phacoemulsification with posterior chamber intraocular lens implantation. Visual acuity is hand motions at 1 ft. (B) About 5 months later and after pars plana vitrectomy with intraocular antibiotics, visual acuity is 20/40.*

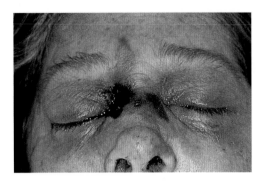

Figure 10-9 *Mucormycosis with characteristic black eschar in patient with uncontrolled diabetes.*

neurologic signs and symptoms, and in diabetic patients with ketoacidosis who remain obtunded after correction of the underlying ketoacidosis.

Orbital mucormycosis usually originates in adjacent sinuses and presents with complete internal and external ophthalmoplegia, decreased vision, proptosis, ptosis, and chemosis. Histopathologic hallmarks of the disease are vascular invasion and tissue necrosis. Clinically, affected areas are characterized by black eschars (Figure 10-9) and discharge, although this may be a late finding. Even today, the overall mortality rate in mucormycosis exceeds 50%[104] and underscores the importance of prompt diagnosis and treatment with tissue debridement and amphotericin B.

10-7

CONCLUSION

Diabetes is associated with a myriad of nonretinal ophthalmic abnormalities. The most common of these include corneal diseases (decreased corneal sensitivity, infectious and neurotrophic ulcers, and epithelial defects and erosions), glaucoma (open-angle, angle-closure, neovascular, and blood-associated), refractive changes, and cataract. Optic and cranial nerve abnormalities are not rare. Endophthalmitis and mucormycosis occur less frequently and are associated with a guarded prognosis, especially if not detected and treated promptly. Care of the diabetic patient usually includes referral to an appropriate primary care physician to ensure optimal glucose control, with the goal of reducing the rates of ocular and systemic complications from diabetes.

REFERENCES

1. Schwartz DE: Corneal sensitivity in diabetics. *Arch Ophthalmol* 1974;91:174–178.

2. Rogell GD: Corneal hypesthesia and retinopathy in diabetes mellitus. *Ophthalmology* 1980; 87:229–233.

3. Eichenbaum JW, Feldstein M, Podos SM: Extended-wear soft contact lenses and corneal ulcers. *Br J Ophthalmol* 1982;66:663–666.

4. Hyndiuk RA, Kazarian EL, Schultz RO, Seideman S: Neurotrophic corneal ulcers in diabetes mellitus. *Arch Ophthalmol* 1977;95: 2193–2196.

5. Kenyon KR: Anatomy and pathology of the ocular surface. *Int Ophthalmol Clin* 1979;19:3–35.

6. Azar DT, Spurr-Michaud SJ, Tisdale AS, Gipson IK: Altered epithelial-basement membrane interactions in diabetic corneas. *Arch Ophthalmol* 1992;110:537–540.

7. Gobbels M, Spitznas M, Oldendoerp J: Impairment of corneal epithelial barrier function in diabetics. *Graefes Arch Klin Exp Ophthalmol* 1989; 227:142–144.

8. Foulks GN, Thoft RA, Perry HD, Tolentino FI: Factors related to corneal epithelial complications after closed vitrectomy in diabetics. *Arch Ophthalmol* 1979;97:1076–1078.

9. Arentsen J, Tasman W: Using a bandage contact lens to prevent recurrent corneal erosion during photocoagulation in patients with diabetes. *Am J Ophthalmol* 1981;92:714–716.

10. Mandelcorn MS, Blankenship G, Machemer R: Pars plana vitrectomy for the management of severe diabetic retinopathy. *Am J Ophthalmol* 1976;81:561–570.

11. Perry HD, Foulks GN, Thoft RA, Tolentino FI: Corneal complications after closed vitrectomy through the pars plana. *Arch Ophthalmol* 1978;96:1401–1403.

12. Kenyon KR: Recurrent corneal erosion: pathogenesis and therapy. *Int Ophthalmol Clin* 1979;19:169–195.

13. Fogle JA, Kenyon KR, Stark WJ, Green WR: Defective epithelial adhesion in anterior corneal dystrophies. *Am J Ophthalmol* 1975;79:925–940.

14. Tabatabay CA, Bumbacher M, Baumgartner B, Leuenberger PM: Reduced number of hemidesmosomes in the corneal epithelium of diabetics with proliferative vitreoretinopathy. *Graefes Arch Klin Exp Ophthalmol* 1988;226:389–392.

15. Azar DT, Spurr-Michaud SJ, Tisdale AS, Gipson IK: Decreased penetration of anchoring fibrils into the diabetic stroma: a morphometric analysis. *Arch Ophthalmol* 1989;107:1520–1523.

16. Friend J, Snip RC, Kiorpes TC, et al: Metabolic effects of diabetes mellitus on rabbit corneal epithelium. *Invest Ophthalmol Vis Sci* 1980; 19:913–916.

17. Kinoshita JH, Fukushi S, Kador P, Merola LO: Aldose reductase in diabetic complications of the eye. *Metabolism* 1979;28:462–469.

18. Datiles MB, Kador PF, Fukui HN, et al: Corneal re-epithelialization in galactosemic rats. *Invest Ophthalmol Vis Sci* 1983;24:563–569.

19. Matsuda M, Awata T, Ohashi Y, et al: The effects of aldose reductase inhibitor on the corneal endothelial morphology in diabetic rats. *Curr Eye Res* 1987;6:391–397.

20. Ohashi Y, Matsuda M, Hosotani H, et al: Aldose reductase inhibitor (CT-112) eyedrops for diabetic corneal epitheliopathy. *Am J Ophthalmol* 1988;105:233–238.

21. Armstrong JR, Daily RK, Dobson HL, Girard LJ: The incidence of glaucoma in diabetes mellitus: a comparison with the incidence of glaucoma in the general population. *Am J Ophthalmol* 1960;50:55–63.

22. Lieb WA, Stark N, Jelinek MB, Malzi R: Diabetes mellitus and glaucoma. *Acta Ophthalmol (Copenh)* 1967;suppl 94:3–62.

23. Becker B: Diabetes mellitus and primary open-angle glaucoma. The XXVII Edward Jackson Memorial Lecture. *Am J Ophthalmol* 1971;1: 1–16.

24. Leske MC, Podgor MJ: Intraocular pressure, cardiovascular risk variables, and visual field defects. *Am J Epidemiol* 1983;118:280–287.

25. Nielsen NV: The prevalence of glaucoma and ocular hypertension in type 1 and 2 diabetes mellitus: an epidemiological study of diabetes mellitus on the island of Falster, Denmark. *Acta Ophthalmol (Copenh)* 1983;61:662–672.

26. Klein BE, Klein R, Moss SE: Intraocular pressure in diabetic persons. *Ophthalmology* 1984;91:1356–1360.

27. Klein BE, Klein R, Jensen SC: Open-angle glaucoma and older-onset diabetes: the Beaver Dam Eye Study. *Ophthalmology* 1994;101: 1173–1177.

28. Morgan RW, Drance SM: Chronic open-angle glaucoma and ocular hypertension: an epidemiological study. *Br J Ophthalmol* 1975; 59:211–215.

29. Reynolds DC: Relative risk factors in chronic open-angle glaucoma: an epidemiological study. *Am J Optom Physiol Opt* 1977;54:116–120.

30. Wilson MR, Hertzmark E, Walker AM, et al: A case-control study of risk factors in open angle glaucoma. *Arch Ophthalmol* 1987;105:1066–1071.

31. Katz J, Sommer A: Risk factors for primary open angle glaucoma. *Am J Prev Med* 1988;4: 110–114.

32. Kahn HA, Leibowitz HM, Ganley JP, et al: The Framingham Eye Study, II: association of ophthalmic pathology with single variables previously measured in the Framingham Heart Study. *Am J Epidemiol* 1977;106:33–41.

33. Armaly MF, Krueger DE, Maunder L, et al: Biostatistical analysis of the collaborative glaucoma study, I: summary report of the risk factors for glaucomatous visual-field defects. *Arch Ophthalmol* 1980;98:2163–2171.

34. Bengtsson B: The prevalence of glaucoma. *Br J Ophthalmol* 1981;65:46–49.

35. Tielsch JM, Katz J, Quigley HA, et al: Diabetes, intraocular pressure, and primary open-angle glaucoma in the Baltimore Eye Survey. *Ophthalmology* 1995;102:48–53.

36. Fry LL: Comparison of the postoperative intraocular pressure with Betagan, Betoptic, Timoptic, Iopidine, Diamox, Pilopine Gel, and Miostat. *J Cataract Refract Surg* 1992;18:14–19.

37. Vuori ML, Ali-Melkkila T: The effect of betaxolol and timolol on postoperative intraocular pressure. *Acta Ophthalmol (Copenh)* 1993;71: 458–462.

38. Strahlman E, Tipping R, Vogel R: A double-masked, randomized 1-year study comparing dorzolamide (Trusopt), timolol, and betaxolol. International Dorzolamide Study Group. *Arch Ophthalmol* 1995;113:1009–1016.

39. Sorensen SJ, Abel SR: Comparison of the ocular beta-blockers. *Ann Pharmacother* 1996;30: 43–54.

40. Mapstone R, Clark CV: Prevalence of type 2 diabetes in glaucoma. *Br Med J* 1985;291:93–95.

41. Clark CV, Mapstone R: The prevalence of diabetes mellitus in the family history of patients with primary glaucoma. *Doc Ophthalmol* 1986;62:161–163.

42. Mapstone R, Clark CV: The prevalence of autonomic neuropathy in glaucoma. *Trans Ophthalmol Soc UK* 1985;104:265–269.

43. Sorokanich S, Wand M, Nix HR: Angle closure glaucoma and acute hyperglycemia. *Arch Ophthalmol* 1986;104:1434.

44. Madsen PH: Experiences in surgical treatment of haemorrhagic glaucoma. *Acta Ophthalmol (Copenh)* 1973;120(suppl):88–91.

45. Brown GC, Magargal LE, Schachat A, Shah H: Neovascular glaucoma: etiologic considerations. *Ophthalmology* 1984;91:315–320.

46. Armaly MF, Baloglou PJ: Diabetes mellitus and the eye, I: changes in the anterior segment. *Arch Ophthalmol* 1967;77:485–492.

47. Madsen PH: Haemorrhagic glaucoma: comparative study in diabetic and nondiabetic patients. *Br J Ophthalmol* 1971;55:444–450.

48. Ohrt V: The frequency of rubeosis iridis in diabetic patients. *Acta Ophthalmol (Copenh)* 1971;49:301–307.

49. Zirm M: Protein glaucoma—overtaxing of flow mechanisms? Preliminary report. *Ophthalmologica* 1982;184:155–161.

50. Hohl RD, Barnett DM: Diabetic hemorrhagic glaucoma. *Diabetes* 1970;19:994–997.

51. Callahan MA: Photocoagulation and rubeosis iridis [letter]. *Am J Ophthalmol* 1974;78:873–874.

52. Little HL, Rosenthal AR, Dellaporta A, Jacobson DR: The effect of pan-retinal photocoagulation on rubeosis iridis. *Am J Ophthalmol* 1976;81:804–809.

53. Laatikainen L: Preliminary report on effect of retinal panphotocoagulation on rubeosis iridis and neovascular glaucoma. *Br J Ophthalmol* 1977;61:278–284.

54. Pavan PR, Folk JC, Weingeist TA, et al: Diabetic rubeosis and panretinal photocoagulation. *Arch Ophthalmol* 1983;101:882–884.

55. Heuer DK, Parrish RK II, Gressel MG, et al: 5-Fluorouracil and glaucoma filtering surgery, II: a pilot study. *Ophthalmology* 1984;91:384–394.

56. Heuer DK, Parrish RK II, Gressel MG, et al: 5-Fluorouracil and glaucoma filtering surgery, III: intermediate follow-up of a pilot study. *Ophthalmology* 1986;93:1537–1546.

57. Rockwood EJ, Parrish RK II, Heuer DK, et al: Glaucoma filtering surgery with 5-fluorouracil. *Ophthalmology* 1987;94:1071–1078.

58. Kitazawa Y, Kawase K, Matsushita H, Minobe M: Trabeculectomy with mitomycin: a comparative study with fluorouracil. *Arch Ophthalmol* 1991;109:1693–1698.

59. Skuta GL, Beeson CC, Higginbotham EJ, et al: Intraoperative mitomycin versus postoperative 5-fluorouracil in high-risk glaucoma filtering surgery. *Ophthalmology* 1992;99:438–444.

60. Krupin T, Kaufman P, Mandell AI, et al: Long-term results of valve implants in filtering surgery for eyes with neovascular glaucoma. *Am J Ophthalmol* 1983;95:775–782.

61. Honrubia FM, Gomez ML, Hernandez A, Grijalbo MP: Long-term results of silicone tube filtering surgery for eyes with neovascular glaucoma. *Am J Ophthalmol* 1984;97:501–504.

62. Molteno AC, Haddad PJ: The visual outcome in cases of neovascular glaucoma. *Aust N Z J Ophthalmol* 1985;13:329–335.

63. Forestier F, Salvanet-Bouccara A: An evaluation of the Krupin-Denver valve implant in glaucoma. *Glaucoma* 1986;8:92–99.

64. Krupin T, Ritch R, Camras CB, et al: A long Krupin-Denver valve implant attached to a 180 degree scleral explant for glaucoma surgery. *Ophthalmology* 1988;95:1174–1180.

65. Minckler DS, Heuer DK, Hasty B, et al: Clinical experience with the single-plate Molteno implant in complicated glaucomas. *Ophthalmology* 1988;95:1181–1188.

66. Lloyd MA, Heuer DK, Baerveldt G, et al: Combined Molteno implantation and pars plana vitrectomy for neovascular glaucomas. *Ophthalmology* 1991;98:1401–1405.

67. Campbell DG, Simmons RJ, Tolentino FI, McMeel JW: Glaucoma occurring after closed vitrectomy. *Am J Ophthalmol* 1977;83:63–69.

68. Cameron JD, Havener VR: Histologic confirmation of ghost cell glaucoma by routine light microscopy. *Am J Ophthalmol* 1983;96:251–252.

69. Campbell DG, Essigmann EM: Hemolytic ghost cell glaucoma: further studies. *Arch Ophthalmol* 1979;97:2141–2146.

70. Summers CG, Lindstrom RL, Cameron JD: Phase contrast microscopy: diagnosis of ghost cell glaucoma following cataract extraction. *Surv Ophthalmol* 1984;28:342–344.

71. Fenton RH, Zimmerman LE: Hemolytic glaucoma: an unusual cause of acute open-angle secondary glaucoma. *Arch Ophthalmol* 1963;70:236–239.

72. Phelps CD, Watzke RC: Hemolytic glaucoma. *Am J Ophthalmol* 1975;80:690–695.

73. Vannas M, Teir H: Hemosiderosis in eyes with secondary glaucoma after delayed intraocular hemorrhages. *Acta Ophthalmol (Copenh)* 1960;38:254–267.

74. Campbell DG, Schertzer RM: Ghost cell glaucoma. In: Ritch R, Shields MB, Krupin T, eds: *The Glaucomas*. 2nd ed. St Louis: CV Mosby Co; 1996:1277–1285.

75. Benson WE, Brown GC, Tasman W: *Diabetes and Its Ocular Complications*. Philadelphia: WB Saunders Co; 1988:27–34.

76. Klein BE, Klein R, Moss SE: Prevalence of cataracts in a population-based study of persons with diabetes mellitus. *Ophthalmology* 1985;92:1191–1196.

77. Nielsen NV, Vinding T: The prevalence of cataract in insulin-independent and non–insulin-dependent diabetes mellitus. *Acta Ophthalmol (Copenh)* 1984;62:595–602.

78. Schwab IR, Dawson CR, Hoshiwara I, et al: Incidence of cataract extraction in Pima Indians: diabetes as a risk factor. *Arch Ophthalmol* 1985;103:208–212.

79. Skillern PG, Lockhart G: Optic neuritis and uncontrolled diabetes mellitus in 14 patients. *Ann Intern Med* 1959;51:468–475.

80. Barr CC, Glaser JS, Blankenship G: Acute disc swelling in juvenile diabetes: clinical profile and natural history of 12 cases. *Arch Ophthalmol* 1980;98:2185–2192.

81. Benson WE, Brown GC, Tasman W: *Diabetes and Its Ocular Complications*. Philadelphia: WB Saunders Co; 1988:116–117.

82. Appen RE, Chandra SR, Klein R, Myers FL: Diabetic papillopathy. *Am J Ophthalmol* 1980;90:203–209.

83. Pavan PR, Aiello LM, Wafai MZ, et al: Optic disc edema in juvenile-onset diabetes. *Arch Ophthalmol* 1980;98:2193–2195.

84. Lubow M, Makley TA Jr: Pseudopapilledema of juvenile diabetes mellitus. *Arch Ophthalmol* 1971;85:417–422.

85. Hayreh SS, Zahoruk RM: Anterior ischemic optic neuropathy, VI: in juvenile diabetics. *Ophthalmologica* 1981;182:13–28.

86. Lessell S, Rosman NP: Juvenile diabetes mellitus and optic atrophy. *Arch Neurol* 1977;34:759–765.

87. Sadun AA: Neuro-ophthalmic manifestations of diabetes. *Ophthalmology* 1999;106:1047–1048.

88. *Neuro-Ophthalmology*. Basic and Clinical Science Course, Section 5. San Francisco: American Academy of Ophthalmology; 1998–1999:92–93.

89. Nelson M, Lessell S, Sadun AA: Optic nerve hypoplasia and maternal diabetes mellitus. *Arch Neurol* 1986;43:20–25.

90. Regillo CD, Brown GC, Savino PJ, et al: Diabetic papillopathy: patient characteristics and fundus findings. *Arch Ophthalmol* 1995;113: 889–895.

91. Moster M: Paresis of isolated and multiple cranial nerves and painful ophthalmoplegia. In: Yanoff M, Duker JS, Augsburger JJ, et al, eds: *Ophthalmology.* Philadelphia: CV Mosby Co; 1998:16.1–16.12.

92. Jacobson DM: Pupil involvement in patients with diabetes-associated oculomotor nerve palsy. *Arch Ophthalmol* 1998;116:723–727.

93. Glaser JS, Bachynski B: Infranuclear disorders of eye movement. In: Glaser JS, ed: *Neuro-ophthalmology.* 2nd ed. Philadelphia: JB Lippincott Co; 1990:376–377.

94. Kattan HM, Flynn HW Jr, Pflugfelder SC, et al: Nosocomial endophthalmitis survey: current incidence of infection after intraocular surgery. *Ophthalmology* 1991;98:227–228.

95. Phillips WB II, Tasman WS: Postoperative endophthalmitis in association with diabetes mellitus. *Ophthalmology* 1994;101:508–518.

96. Scott IU, Flynn HW Jr, Feuer W: Endophthalmitis after secondary intraocular lens implantation: a case-control study. *Ophthalmology* 1995; 102:1925–1931.

97. Carnazzo G, Mirone G, Turturici A, et al: Pathophysiology of the immune system in elderly subjects with or without diabetes and variations after recombinant interleukin-2. *Arch Gerontol Geriatr* 1989;9:163–180.

98. al-Kassab AS, Raziuddin S: Immune activation and T cell subset abnormalities in circulation of patients with recently diagnosed type I diabetes mellitus. *Clin Exp Immunol* 1990;81: 267–271.

99. Abrass CK: Fc-receptor-mediated phagocytosis: abnormalities associated with diabetes mellitus. *Clin Immunol Immunopathol* 1991;58: 1–17.

100. Moutschen MP, Scheen AJ, Lefebvre PJ: Impaired immune responses in diabetes mellitus: analysis of the factors and mechanisms involved—relevance to the increased susceptibility of diabetic patients to specific infections. *Diabetes Metab* 1992;18:187–201.

101. Morain WD, Colen LB: Wound healing in diabetes mellitus. *Clin Plast Surg* 1990;17: 493–501.

102. Benson WE, Brown GC, Tasman W: *Diabetes and Its Ocular Complications.* Philadelphia: WB Saunders Co; 1988:117–118.

103. Behlau I, Baker AS: Fungal infections of the eye. In: Albert DM, Jakobiec FA, eds: *Principles and Practice of Ophthalmology: Clinical Practice.* Philadelphia: WB Saunders Co; 1994:3041–3043.

104. Parfrey NA: Improved diagnosis and prognosis of mucormycosis: a clinicopathologic study of 33 cases. *Medicine* 1986;65:113–123.

Future Therapies for Diabetic Retinopathy

Lloyd Paul Aiello, MD, PhD

Thomas W. Gardner, MD, MS

Diabetic retinopathy is the leading cause of new blindness among working-age Americans.[1] Although this remains true today, over the preceding three decades dramatic advances have been made in our understanding of the natural history of the disease and in the development and validation of therapeutic modalities. Current therapeutic approaches permit remarkable reductions in diabetes-associated visual loss if timely and appropriate ocular care is provided to all patients with diabetes.[2] Nevertheless, laser photocoagulation, the mainstay of current therapy, is an inherently destructive procedure that obliterates areas of retina in an effort to retain greater visual function than would be achieved without such intervention. Thus, the treatment itself can be associated with significant side effects, and visual loss can progress despite timely and appropriate treatment.

The prospect of novel therapies with equivalent or improved efficacy, but without the side effects inherent in current treatment modalities, has stimulated extensive and diverse investigations into the many models, mechanisms, and mediators of diabetic retinopathy. Numerous advances in

this rapidly evolving field have suggested novel interventional approaches that hold promise for the development of effective, noninvasive, nondestructive, and possibly orally administered treatments of diabetic retinopathy. Some of these approaches are already being evaluated in clinical trials. This chapter describes the rationale, supporting experimental data, and developmental status of these strategies and speculates on their future clinical implications.

11-1

HISTORICAL PERSPECTIVE

Diabetic retinopathy is a complex, multifactorial process that occurs as a result of the similarly highly complex systemic disease diabetes mellitus. Numerous hypotheses explaining the clinical manifestations of diabetic retinopathy have been investigated, including evaluation of the polyol

TABLE 11-1

Selected Disorders Associated With Intraocular Neovascularization

Ischemic Retinopathies

Diabetic retinopathy

Retinopathy of prematurity

Retinal vein occlusion

Sickle cell retinopathy

Radiation retinopathy

Carotid occlusive disease

Chronic retinal detachment

Eales disease

Other Neovascular Disorders

Age-related macular degeneration (ARMD), (wet)

Ocular histoplasmosis syndrome

Myopic degeneration

pathway,[3] advanced glycosylated end products,[4] oxidative stress,[5] protein kinase C signaling,[6] cell–matrix and cell–cell interactions,[7] retinal blood flow abnormalities,[8] and the role of protein factors with angiogenic and vasopermeability characteristics. A comprehensive discussion of each of these areas is beyond the scope of this chapter, although inhibition of any of these pathways would be expected to at least partly ameliorate the ocular complications of diabetes.

Diabetic retinopathy, however, is the prototypical example of a group of disorders, known as *ischemic retinopathies*, that are characterized by areas of capillary nonperfusion and the development of intraocular angiogenesis. A large number of scientific discoveries have improved our understanding of the angiogenic factors and molecular mechanisms that mediate the growth and excessive permeability of these pathologic new vessels. As a result, numerous novel targets for the pharmacologic inhibition of diabetic retinopathy have become apparent, many of which are now being investigated in late-preclinical and early-stage clinical trials. The development of growth-factor inhibitors serves as a useful paradigm for the discussion of future therapies for diabetic retinopathy and is the principal focus of this chapter.

Table 11-1 presents a partial list of the ischemic retinopathies and several other disorders associated with intraocular neovascularization. These conditions share numerous clinical features (Figure 11-1). Neovascularization is often preceded by, and spatially associated with, retinal capillary nonperfusion (Figure 11-1A).[9,10] Retinal neovascularization commonly arises at the

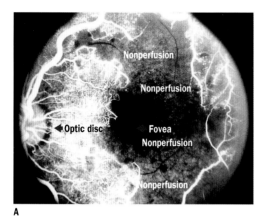

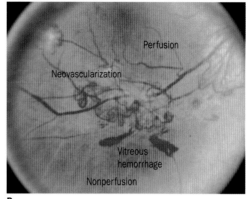

A

B

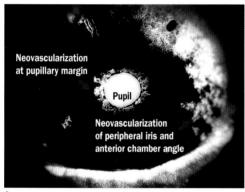

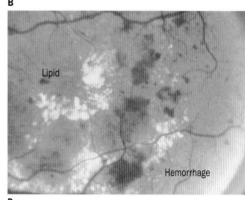

C

D

Figure 11-1 *Ischemic retinopathies share numerous clinical features. (A) Neovascularization is often preceded by areas of nonperfusion, as demonstrated in this fluorescein angiogram of patient with diabetes. (B) Retinal neovascularization often occurs at border of perfused and nonperfused zones. These vessels are fragile and often bleed, resulting in vitreous hemorrhage. Neovascularization can also occur at distant sites in retina or anteriorly at pupillary margin and anterior chamber angle. (C) Iris angiogram of diabetic patient with neovascularization of iris at both pupillary margin and anterior chamber angle. (D) Retinal vessels often exhibit increased vascular permeability, with transudation of serum components and deposition of lipid.*

Parts A, C, and D reproduced with permission from Aiello LP: Eye complications of diabetes. In: Kahn CR, ed: Diabetes. *Vol 2 of Korenman SG, ed:* Atlas of Clinical Endocrinology. *Philadelphia: Current Medicine; 2000:135–150. Part B is ETDRS standard photograph 7 and is reproduced with permission from Early Treatment Diabetic Retinopathy Study Research Group: Grading diabetic retinopathy from stereoscopic color fundus photographs—an extension of the modified Airlie House classification. ETDRS Report Number 10.* Ophthalmology *1991;98:786–806.*

border of perfused and nonperfused zones and is universally associated with increased vessel permeability (Figures 11-1B,D).[11,12] The extent of capillary nonperfusion is correlated with the risk of retinal neovascularization,[13] and the risk of neovascularization of the iris (NVI) (Figure 11-1C) is increased following cataract surgery in patients with diabetic retinopathy, presumably due to removal of the lens and its barrier function.[14] More than a half century ago, it was recognized that these shared clinical attributes suggested a common mechanism for the development of the neovascular and permeability complications in conditions such as diabetic retinopathy.[15]

11-2

GROWTH-FACTOR HYPOTHESIS OF NEOVASCULARIZATION

Based on these observations, Michaelson proposed the growth-factor hypothesis of intraocular neovascularization in 1948.[15] This theory was later refined by his student Ashton and others.[16] In essence, the hypothesis states that ischemia of the retina induces a factor or factors capable of stimulating the growth of new vessels (Figure 11-2). These factors must meet several criteria to completely account for the classic clinical observations (Table 11-2). The postulated factors would be freely diffusible within the eye to account for neovascularization of

both retinal tissue adjacent to areas of nonperfusion and distant retina or iris. The molecule should be an endothelial mitogen to induce proliferation of new vessels, expression should be induced by retinal hypoxia, and retinal endothelial cells should possess receptors to permit cellular responses. Intraocular concentrations that progressively decline more anteriorly within the eye would account for diffusion of a retina-produced growth factor to the trabecular meshwork for clearance and for neovascularization arising at the iris and anterior chamber angle. Finally, the growth factor would be expected to increase during periods of active intraocular neovascularization and diminish when neovascularization becomes quiescent due to either natural progression of the disease or successful therapy.

The process of growth-factor stimulation of intraocular neovascularization can be broken down into a series of stages, as presented in Figure 11-3. Diabetes mellitus induces vascular damage to the retina through a variety of mechanisms resulting in vascular nonperfusion and retinal ischemia (Figure 11-3A). These changes stimulate expression and secretion of the growth factors from a variety of retinal cells (Figure 11-3B). The growth factors diffuse within the retina and eye, eventually binding to high-affinity receptors on retinal endothelial cells (Figure 11-3C). Receptor binding induces a series of intracellular biochemical reactions that transmit the signals for cell replication and increased permeability (Figure 11-3D). Each of these steps is a potential target site for therapeutic intervention. The regulation of cell proliferation, once the intracellular signal is transmitted, involves numerous non–

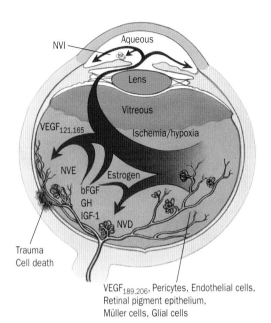

Figure 11-2 *Growth factors such as vascular endothelial growth factor (VEGF), produced by retinal cells, act locally or diffuse through vitreous down concentration gradients, represented by arrow width in figure. Larger VEGF isoforms ($VEGF_{189,206}$) tend to be nondiffusible and act locally, while shorter isoforms ($VEGF_{121,165}$) are diffusible. Growth factors can therefore elicit neovascularization at distant sites in retina or at iris and anterior chamber angle, where they are eventually cleared through trabecular meshwork. Other factors, such as growth hormone (GH), basic fibroblast growth factor (bFGF), and insulin-like growth factor (IGF-1), probably act as synergistic or mediating factors. Release of bFGF is increased by trauma and cell death. NVE = neovascularization elsewhere. NVD = neovascularization of disc.*
Redrawn with permission from Aiello LP, Northrup JM, Keyt BA, et al: Hypoxic regulation of vascular endothelial growth factor in retinal cells. Arch Ophthalmol *1995; 113:1538–1544. Copyrighted 1995, American Medical Association.*

TABLE 11-2

Expected Attributes of Major Growth-Factor Mediator of Neovascularization in Diabetic Retinopathy

Attribute	Rationale
Induced by ischemia	Accounts for association of neovascularization with areas of retinal ischemia
Produced by retinal cells	Accounts for factor production from ischemic area
Secreted and diffusible	Accounts for local factor effect and effects distant to areas of retinal ischemia
Stimulates endothelial cell growth	Accounts for endothelial cell growth during vasculogenesis
Specific receptors on endothelial cells	Accounts for mechanism by which factors can induce action in endothelial cells
Elevated with or before onset of neovascularization	Necessary if factor is actually inducing neovascularization
Diminished with treated or quiescent neovascularization	Expected if reduction of growth-factor stimulus is responsible for neovascular regression
Intraocular concentration is greater posteriorly than anteriorly	Accounts for clearance of retina-produced factor by diffusion down concentration gradient to be cleared through trabecular meshwork; also accounts for neovascularization at iris and anterior chamber angle

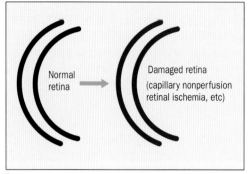

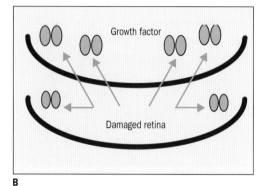

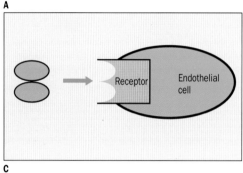

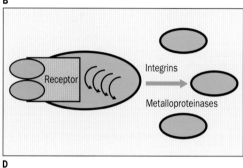

Figure 11-3 *(A) Diabetes results in retinal damage by diverse array of mechanisms, eventually leading to capillary nonperfusion and retinal ischemia. (B) Damaged retina induces production of growth factors, such as vascular endothelial growth factor (VEGF), partly as result of retinal ischemia. (C) Factors act within retina or diffuse into vitreous. Growth factors specifically bind to high-affinity receptors on retinal endothelial cells. (D) Receptor binding induces series of intracellular reactions (arrows),* termed *intracellular signal transduction cascade, which ultimately results in endothelial cell proliferation via complex mechanism probably involving numerous mediators, such as integrins and metalloproteinases.*

Redrawn with permission from Aiello LP: Vascular endothelial growth factor: 20th-century mechanisms, 21st-century therapies. Invest Ophthalmol Vis Sci *1997;38: 1647–1652. Copyright 1977, Association for Research in Vision and Ophthalmology.*

growth-factor molecules, such as the integrins,[7,17] angiostatin,[18] endostatin,[19] and metalloproteinases,[20–22] all of which might also be exploited for therapeutic indications.

11-3

CANDIDATE MEDIATORS OF NEOVASCULARIZATION

Numerous growth factors have been evaluated as possible mediators of intraocular neovascularization. Some of those that have received the most extensive investigation with regard to diabetic retinopathy are listed in Table 11-3 and include growth hormone (GH), basic fibroblast growth factor (bFGF), insulin-like growth factor 1 (IGF-1), and vascular endothelial growth factor (VEGF).

TABLE 11-3

Candidate Mediators of Diabetic Retinopathy

Growth Factor or Mediating Molecule	Principal Effect on Angiogenesis in Diabetic Retinopathy		
	Primary	Permissive	Synergistic*
Growth hormone (GH)	Unlikely	Probable	Unlikely
Basic fibroblast growth factor (bFGF)	Unlikely	Probable	Probable
Vascular endothelial growth factor (VEGF)	Probable	Unknown	Probable
Hepatocyte growth factor (HGF)	Possible	Unknown	Possible
Integrins	Unlikely	Probable	Unlikely
Angiostatin Endostatin	Unlikely	Possible Inhibitor	Unlikely

Synergy with regard to action of other growth factors. Therapies combining inhibitors of multiple factors would be expected to have increased effectiveness over single agents in most cases.

There are three main actions by which growth factors could influence the development of diabetic retinopathy:

1. Primary stimulator of angiogenesis

2. Permissive factor, allowing primary stimulators to induce neovascularization but not primarily stimulating the neovascularization themselves

3. Synergistically increase the action of other factors

The current understanding of the relative role of these actions for each growth factor is also indicated in Table 11-3.

The growth factor bFGF is tightly associated with the extracellular matrix[23,24] and induces endothelial cell proliferation, migration, and vasculogenesis. However, bFGF is not secreted from cells by classical mechanisms.[25–27] Although bFGF has been located in the retina,[28] no causal relationship with neovascularization has been identified.[29] Studies using transgenic mice have demonstrated that bFGF is neither neces-

sary nor sufficient to induce retinal neovascularization.[30] However, bFGF is synergistic in its mitogenic activity with VEGF[31–33] and probably acts primarily as a potentiating factor in diabetic retinopathy.

GH and its biological mediator IGF-1[34] have been studied for many years as possible mediators of diabetic retinopathy,[35,36] leading to a brief period when hypophysectomy was employed as a treatment of diabetic retinopathy.[37] Although GH/IGF-1 reduction is modestly correlated with regression of proliferative diabetic retinopathy (PDR), this treatment was associated with extensive morbidity in diabetic patients and was abandoned with the advent of laser photocoagulation.

Studies using an inhibitor of GH secretion and transgenic mice expressing a GH antagonist suggest that GH plays a permissive role in ischemia-induced retinopathy, rather than acting as the principal stimulating factor.[38] Inhibition of GH does reduce the extent of ischemia-induced retinal neovascularization and, consequently, GH antagonists may soon be entering early-phase clinical trials in adults to assess their effects on PDR.

Hepatocyte growth factor (HGF), a mitogenic and monogenic protein for many nonocular cells, has been found to be elevated in the vitreous of patients with PDR.[39] Concentrations were highest in patients with active PDR and were reduced if PDR was quiescent. The extent of HGF's role in mediating PDR remains unknown. Angiostatin[18] and endostatin[19] are endogenous inhibitors of angiogenesis known to be involved in tumor suppression; their significance in diabetic retinopathy is currently unknown.

The role of VEGF in the eye has been extensively evaluated over the past few years. Considerable evidence now suggests that VEGF mediates a significant portion of the retinal neovascularization and excessive vascular permeability that are characteristic of PDR. VEGF may even play a role in the development of nonproliferative diabetic retinopathy (NPDR), as discussed in Section 11-5-2. VEGF is a protein with potent vasopermeability[40] and angiogenic activities.[41,42] Four different forms of VEGF exist in the human,[43] with the smaller two forms being freely diffusible and the larger molecules being bound to cell surfaces and basement membranes (see Figure 11-2).

The general functions of VEGF in ocular disease have been extensively re-viewed[44-47] and are not described in detail here. However, it is important to note that VEGF possesses all of the attributes predicted for a major mediator of neovascularization in diabetic retinopathy, as detailed in Table 11-2. VEGF is an endothelial cell mitogen,[48] whose expression is increased up to 30-fold by hypoxia in various cultured ocular cells.[49] At least two types of high-affinity VEGF receptors exist,[48,50,51] and numerous retinal cells express VEGF, including pigment epithelial cells,[52] pericytes, endothelial cells, glial cells, Müller cells, and ganglion cells.[49,53] Thus, VEGF currently represents the classic paradigm for growth-factor mediation in diabetic retinopathy.

11-4

CLINICAL ASSOCIATIONS OF VEGF IN PROLIFERATIVE RETINOPATHY

The in vivo evidence associating VEGF with retinal neovascularization and NVI in PDR is extensive. Ischemia-induced retinal neovascularization that histologically resembles diabetic retinopathy is observed in neonatal rats,[54] cats,[55] and mice (Figures 11-4A,B).[56,57] Similar NVI is observed in the primate. VEGF expression is temporally correlated in these models, increasing just prior to the onset of neovascularization (Figures 11-4C,D)[54,55,57-60] and slowly declining as neovascularization regresses.

VEGF concentrations are elevated in the vitreous of patients with PDR as compared with concentrations in patients with NPDR or quiescent PDR or in nondiabetic patients without neovascularization (Figure 11-5).[61-63] Intravitreal VEGF is also elevated when neovascularization is present due to other

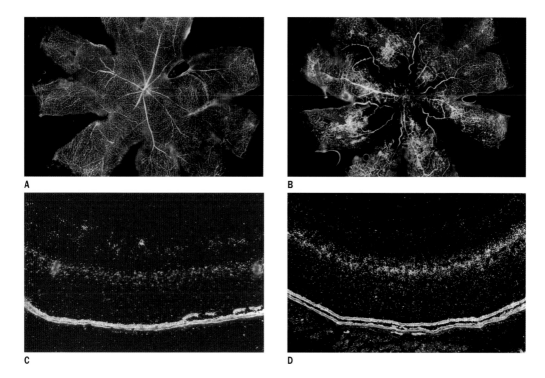

C   D

Figure 11-4 *When neonatal mice are exposed to alterations in oxygen concentration for several days, (A) normal vascularization pattern of retina is altered, resulting in (B) areas of nonperfusion (dark central areas) and retinal neovascularization (arrows), which closely resemble those observed in diabetic retinopathy. Production of VEGF is low under normal conditions (C) and markedly increased just prior to onset of retinal neovascularization (D). Parts A and B are retinal flat mounts from neonatal mice whose vasculature has been perfused with fluorescein-conjugated dextran for visualization purposes. Parts C and D are cross sectional in situ hybridization photomicrographs showing location of VEGF production.*

Reproduced with permission from Pierce EA, Avery RL, Foley ED, et al: Vascular endothelial growth factor/vascular permeability factor expression in a mouse model of retinal neovascularization. Proc Natl Acad Sci USA *1995;92: 905–909. Copyright 1995, National Academy of Sciences, U.S.A.*

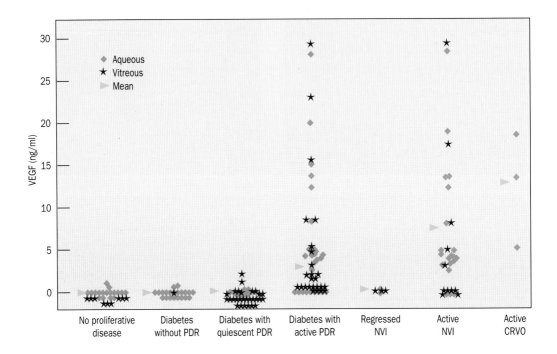

Figure 11-5 *Aqueous, vitreous, and mean VEGF concentrations are indicated for patients with particular clinical findings noted under each group of values. Values of 0 or below denote concentrations below detection limit of assay (50 ng/ml).*

Redrawn with permission from Aiello LP, Avery RL, Arrigg PG, et al: Vascular endothelial growth factor in ocular fluid of patients with diabetic retinopathy and other retinal disorders . N Engl J Med 1994;331:1480–1487. Copyright © 1994, Massachusetts Medical Society. All rights reserved.

ischemic retinal disorders, such as central retinal vein occlusion (CRVO). Neovascular membranes obtained from patients with PDR demonstrate near-universal VEGF expression (Figure 11-6).[64–70]

11-5

VEGF INDUCTION OF DIABETES-LIKE RETINAL PATHOLOGY

11-5-1 VEGF in Proliferative Retinopathy

Several findings support the conclusion that VEGF can induce intraocular neovascularization resembling that of PDR. Growth of retinal microvascular endothelial cells in culture is increased by concentrations of VEGF well below those found in active PDR (Figure 11-7).[48] Repetitive intravitreal

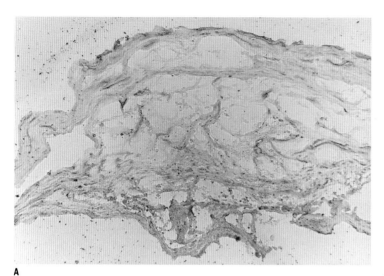

A

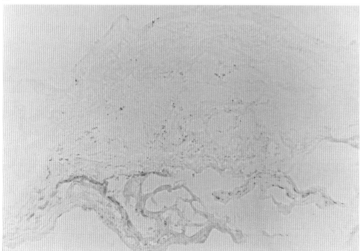

B

Figure 11-6 *(A) Immunohisto-chemical localization of VEGF protein in membranes derived from patients with PDR shows markedly increased VEGF expression. Cells lining portion of membrane at top of figure are immunopositive, as are cells, and, to lesser degree, extracellular matrices throughout tissue. (B) Negative control staining of adjacent serial section shows minimal nonspecific staining.*

Reproduced from Frank RN, Amin RH, Eliott D, et al: Basic fibroblast growth factor and vascular endothelial growth factor are present in epiretinal and choroidal neovascular membranes. Am J Ophthalmol *1996;122:393–403. Copyright 1996, with permission from Elsevier Science.*

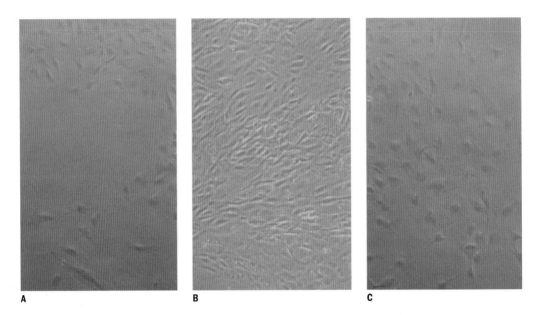

A   B   C

Figure 11-7 *Retinal microvascular endothelial cells in culture 4 days after plating each group at same density. (A) Control cells. (B) Cell number in presence of physiologic concentration of VEGF is markedly higher than in control cells. (C) Cells grown in presence of VEGF but with addition of PKC-β-isoform-selective inhibitor LY333531 proliferated at approximately same rate as control cells.*

Reproduced with permission from Thieme H, Aiello LP, Takagi H, et al: Comparative analysis of vascular endothelial growth factor receptors on retinal and aortic vascular endothelial cells. Diabetes 1995;44:98–103.

injections of recombinant human VEGF are sufficient to produce NVI in a nonhuman primate, leading to ectropion uveae and neovascular glaucoma (Figure 11-8).[71]

Similarly, transgenic mice constructed to overexpress VEGF in the photoreceptors develop extensive intraretinal neovascularization, as confirmed by light, confocal, and standard fluorescent microscopy (Figure 11-9).[72,73] Interestingly, the vessels originate from the retinal vasculature and grow toward the VEGF-producing photoreceptor layer—an inverted scenario from that observed in diabetic retinopathy.

Although increased permeability can occur in the absence of neovascularization, as is often observed with diabetic macular edema (DME)(see Figure 11-1D), a universal characteristic of retinal proliferation is an increase in vascular permeability. VEGF is a very effective inducer of permeability,

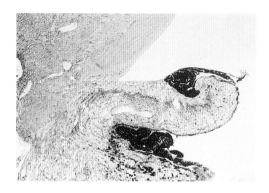

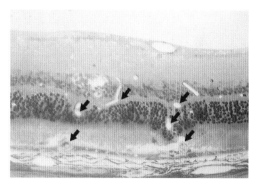

Figure 11-8 *Repetitive intravitreal injections of high concentrations of VEGF result in NVI, ectropion uveae, and trabecular meshwork scarring, findings similar to those of neovascular glaucoma from advanced PDR.*

Reproduced with permission from Tolentino MJ, Miller JW, Gragoudas ES, et al: Vascular endothelial growth factor is sufficient to produce iris neovascularization and neovascular glaucoma in a nonhuman primate. Arch Ophthalmol 1996;114:964–970. Copyrighted 1996, American Medical Association.

Figure 11-9 *Transgenic mice overexpressing VEGF in photoreceptors demonstrate marked intraretinal neovascularization (arrows), which appears to be proliferating toward site of VEGF expression in outer retina.*

Reproduced with permission from Okamoto N, Tobe T, Hackett SF, et al: Transgenic mice with increased expression of vascular endothelial growth factor in the retina: a new model of intraretinal and subretinal neovascularization. Am J Pathol 1997;151:281–291.

being 50,000 times more potent in the dermal microvasculature than is histamine.[74] In the eye, extravasated albumin and VEGF immunoreactivity colocalize.[75,76] Repeated injections of high concentrations of VEGF result in leakage of fluorescein dye from the retinal vessels.[77] Use of vitreous fluorophotometry and albumin-sized, fluorescein-conjugated dextrans has demonstrated that physiologic concentrations of VEGF administered intravitreally induce a rapid 3- to 5-fold increase in retinal vascular permeability in rats (Figure 11-10).[78] Recent data suggest that VEGF may exert its effects of retinal vascular permeability by altering tight-junction proteins, such as occludin and VE-cadherin.[79,80]

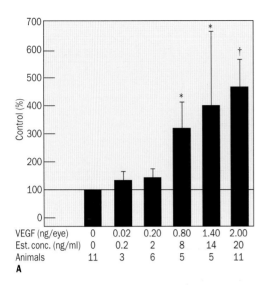

VEGF (ng/eye)	0	0.02	0.20	0.80	1.40	2.00
Est. conc. (ng/ml)	0	0.2	2	8	14	20
Animals	11	3	6	5	5	11

A

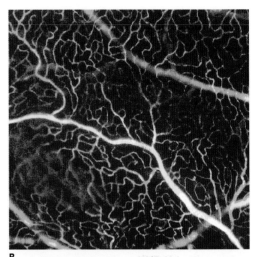

B

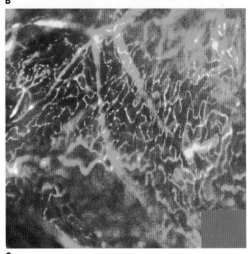

C

Figure 11-10 *(A) Ability of intravitreal injections of VEGF to induce retinal vascular permeability in rats was evaluated utilizing vitreous fluorophotometry. Dose-dependent 5-fold increase in retinal vascular permeability is evident with physiologic concentrations of VEGF that are consistent with those observed in patients with active PDR (see Figure 11-5). *P <0.050. †P <0.001. Retinal vasculature was also perfused with fluorescein-conjugated 70,000-MW dextran approximately same size as albumin, which should be retained within lumen of normal vessels. (B) Normal retinal vessel architecture for animal receiving control intravitreal injection. Note that dextran fluorescence is primarily retained within vasculature. (C) However, intravitreal VEGF injection induced readily apparent increase in vessel permeability to fluorescent compound.*

Part A redrawn and parts B and C reproduced with permission from Aiello LP, Bursell SE, Clermont A, et al: Vascular endothelial growth factor–induced retinal permeability is mediated by protein kinase C in vivo and suppressed by an orally effective beta-isoform-selective inhibitor. Diabetes *1997;46:1473–1480.*

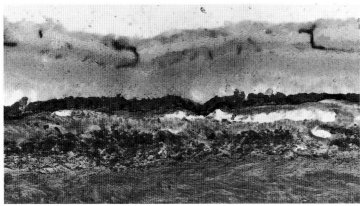

A

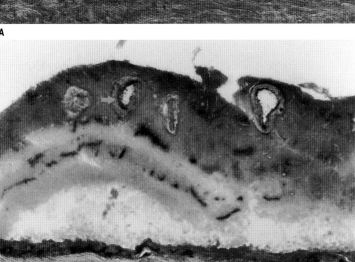

B

Figure 11-11 *Immunohistochemical evaluation of VEGF protein was performed in patients with NPDR, but without extensive areas of retinal nonperfusion. Increased VEGF expression (arrows) is observed in periphery (A) and macula (B).*

Reproduced with permission from Amin RH, Frank RN, Kennedy A, et al: Vascular endothelial growth factor is present in glial cells of the retina and optic nerve of human subjects with nonproliferative diabetic retinopathy. Invest Ophthalmol Vis Sci 1997;38:36–47. Copyright 1997, Association for Research in Vision and Ophthalmology.

11-5-2 VEGF in Nonproliferative Retinopathy

Although the role of VEGF in NPDR is less firmly established than in PDR, recent findings suggest that it may be an important factor in the development of early diabetic retinopathy. Immunohistochemical evaluation of postmortem human eyes with NPDR, but without extensive retinal nonperfusion, demonstrated increased VEGF expression as compared with nondiabetic controls (Figure 11-11).[81,82] However, one study observed VEGF expression in both normal and diabetic human retinas, but did not detect any difference in VEGF mRNA or protein.[83] Repeated injections of high concentrations of VEGF into the normal nonhuman primate eye produce retinal

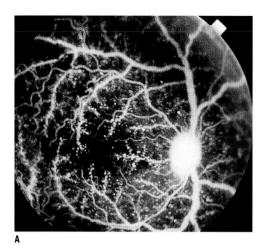

A

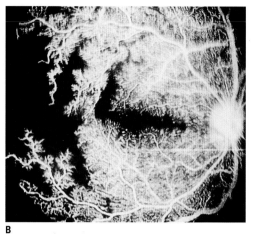

B

Figure 11-12 *(A) Repetitive intravitreal injections of VEGF into normal primate eye result in vascular tortuosity and capillary abnormalities resembling microaneurysms. (B) Increased VEGF dose results in capillary nonperfusion and retinal vascular leakage of fluorescein.*

Reproduced with permission from Tolentino MJ, Miller JW, Gragoudas ES, et al: Intravitreous injections of vascular endothelial growth factor produce retinal ischemia and microangiopathy in an adult primate. Ophthalmology *1996;103:1820–1828.*

changes resembling NPDR, including vascular tortuosity, capillary abnormalities resembling microaneurysms, and leakage of fluorescein (Figure 11-12).[77]

Intravitreal injections of physiologic concentrations of VEGF in the rat alter retinal blood flow and venous caliber in the same manner as observed in diabetic patients with increasingly severe retinopathy.[84] Furthermore, diabetes potentiates the retina's response to VEGF as compared with nondiabetic animals.

These data suggest that, even early in the course of diabetes, the retina may have both increased expression and accentuated response to VEGF (Figure 11-13). This could theoretically result in a positive feedback loop that may eventually induce enough retinal ischemia and VEGF expression to stimulate intraocular neovascularization. This hypothesis raises the intriguing possibility that inhibitors of VEGF action may prove beneficial not only for the neovascular and permeability complications of diabetes, but also for the prevention of retinopathy progression.

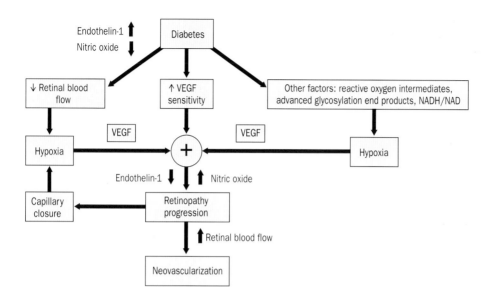

11-5-3 VEGF in Ischemia-Induced Neovascularization

Direct evidence that VEGF expression is necessary for ischemia-induced retinal neo-vascularization and NVI in animals has been obtained using three different agents that inhibit VEGF. These include VEGF-receptor chimeric proteins,[85] neutralizing antibodies,[86] and antisense phosphorothio-ate oligodeoxynucleotides.[87] These VEGF inhibitors suppressed ischemia-induced intraocular neovascularization by as much as 77% in up to 100% of animals studied. The average magnitude of inhibition was approximately 50%. Similar results were obtained for NVI in primates (Figures 11-14A,B)[86] and retinal neovascularization in mice (Figures 11-14C,D).[85] No toxicity was evident by light-microscopic evaluation in these studies of relatively short duration. As discussed earlier, VEGF overexpression in the photoreceptors of transgenic mice

Figure 11-13 *In early diabetes, molecules such as endothelin-1 and nitric oxide reduce retinal blood flow. Combined with oxidative stress, this reduced blood flow may produce initial hypoxic stimulus for VEGF expression. Diabetic state further enhances retinal VEGF sensitivity, inducing vascular abnormalities characteristic of NPDR. Positive feedback loop occurs as development of ischemic areas creates localized hypoxia and further stimulates VEGF production. Downregulation of endothelin-1 and nitric oxide by VEGF further increases retinal blood flow as retinopathy advances. Once vascular damage results in extensive retinal ischemia, VEGF concentrations become high enough to induce intraocular neovascularization.*

Redrawn from Clermont AC, Aiello LP, Mori F, et al: Vascular endothelial growth factor and severity of nonproliferative diabetic retinopathy mediate retinal hemodynamics in vivo: a potential role for vascular endothelial growth factor in the progression of nonproliferative diabetic retinopathy. Am J Ophthalmol 1997;124:433–446. Copyright 1997, with permission from Elsevier Science.

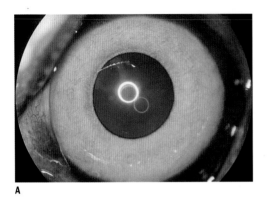

A

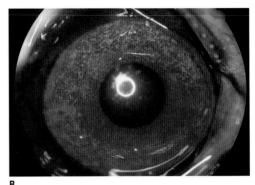

B

Figure 11-14 *Retinal ischemia in primate characteristically produces NVI, while similar ischemia in neonatal mouse produces retinal neovascularization. VEGF-neutralizing antibodies injected into vitreous of primates with retinal ischemia produced by laser retinal vein occlusion result in marked suppression of NVI (A, normal yellow iris color), which is usually observed in eyes not receiving inhibitor (B, abnormal red iris color).*

Parts A and B reproduced with permission from Tolentino MJ, Miller JW, Gragoudas, ES, et al: Vascular endothelial growth factor is sufficient to produce iris neovascularization and neovascular glaucoma in a nonhuman primate. Arch Ophthalmol *1996;114:964–970. Copyright 1996, American Medical Association.*

was sufficient to produce extensive retinal neovascularization (see Figure 11-9).[72,73]

These data demonstrate that, although the neovascular response is undoubtedly modulated by a wide variety of factors, VEGF appears necessary and sufficient to induce retinal and iris angiogenesis, particularly as a sequela of the retinal ischemia characteristic of diabetic retinopathy. In addition, these findings strongly suggest that any agent that blocks VEGF action would result in a significant, although perhaps not complete, reduction in intraocular neovascularization.

11-6

BASIC MECHANISMS AND TARGETS

The detailed biochemical mechanisms that underlie the intracellular processes permitting VEGF expression and signaling are becoming better understood. One important area, from a potential therapeutic standpoint, is the mechanism by which hypoxia increases VEGF expression. The endogenous nucleoside adenosine appears to serve an important role in this regard.[88–92] Hy-

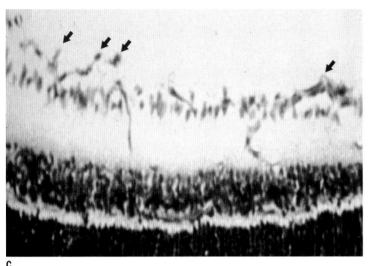

C

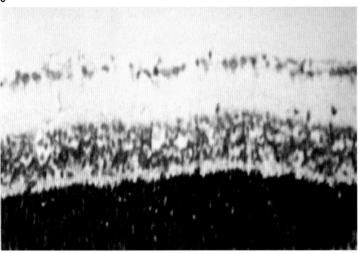

D

Figure 11-14 *(C) Similarly, VEGF-receptor chimeric protein, which binds to VEGF and inhibits its action, was injected intravitreally into neonatal mice with retinal ischemia. These animals universally develop retinal neovascularization in absence of VEGF inhibition (arrows). (D) However, intravitreal injection of VEGF-receptor chimeric protein reduced retinal neovascularization, as shown here in contralateral eye of same animal.*

Parts C and D reproduced with permission from Aiello LP, Pierce EA, Foley ED, et al: Suppression of retinal neovascularization in vivo by inhibition of vascular endothelial growth factor (VEGF) using soluble VEGF-receptor chimeric proteins. Proc Natl Acad Sci USA *1995;92: 10457–10461. Copyright 1995, National Academy of Sciences, U.S.A.*

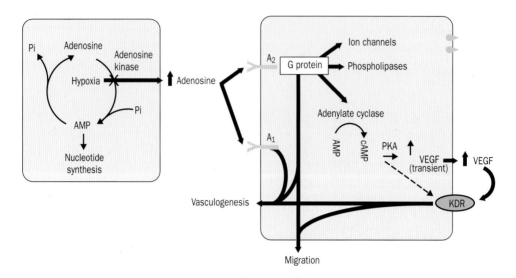

Figure 11-15 *Hypoxia reduces activity of adenosine kinase, resulting in increased release of adenosine, which primarily binds to A$_2$ receptor, activating adenylate cyclase through a G protein coupled mechanism. Resulting increase in intracellular cAMP (cyclic adenosine monophosphate) activates protein kinase A (PKA), ultimately resulting in increased expression of VEGF through as-yet-unidentified mechanisms. Adenosine A$_2$-receptor activation also induces transient decrease in VEGF receptor KDR expression (KDR = kinase domain receptor). Combined activation of both adenosine A$_2$ receptor and KDR synergistically increases cell migration, while contributions of both adenosine receptors and KDR result in synergistic increase in vasculogenesis. Pi = inorganic phosphate.*

Redrawn with permission from Aiello LP: Molecular mechanisms of growth factor action in diabetic retinopathy. Curr Opin Endocrinol Diabetes *1999;6:146–156. Also modified with permission from Aiello LP: Clinical implications of vascular growth factors in proliferative retinopathies.* Curr Opin Ophthalmol *1997;8:19–31.*

poxia increases adenosine concentrations several-fold[88,90,91] by inhibiting the enzyme adenosine kinase, which usually converts adenosine to AMP (adenosine monophosphate) (Figure 11-15).[93] In retinal endothelial cells, the specific adenosine receptors that mediate the induction of VEGF expression have been identified. In addition, several of the molecules involved in the intracellular signaling of the adenosine stimulus have been identified and include adenylate cyclase and protein kinase A (PKA).[92] The adenosine receptors also work in concert with the VEGF receptor to increase endothelial cell migration and vessel formation.[91]

Thus, inhibition of adenosine or its receptors would be expected to suppress VEGF expression under hypoxic conditions and decrease subsequent vasculogenesis. Inhibitors of adenosine receptors do have this action in cell culture, suggesting that they might prove useful in the treatment of diabetic retinopathy.[89–92] Much more study is required to determine the actual clinical applicability of these agents.

The growth factor bFGF was studied extensively as a probable mediator of angiogenesis in diabetic retinopathy, until the transgenic-mice data discussed earlier made it unlikely that the induction of neovascularization was its primary role.[30] However, the mitogenic actions of bFGF and VEGF are potently synergistic both in vivo[31] and in vitro.[32,33] The mechanism of this synergy has been partly elucidated. As shown in Figure 11-16, bFGF increases VEGF[94,95] and VEGF receptor expression (KDR = kinase domain receptor).[96] (FGFR = fibroblast growth factor receptor.) VEGF activity is closely correlated with cellular KDR expression. Even under conditions where KDR expression is low and VEGF's stimulatory activity is minimal, bFGF dramatically increases KDR expression, subsequently allowing VEGF to efficiently induce both mitogenesis and further KDR expression. Induction of VEGF receptor expression by bFGF requires activation of the enzyme protein kinase C (PKC) and mitogen-activated protein (MAP) kinase. VEGF can also increase both thrombin[97] and plasminogen activator expression,[98] which can release bioactive bFGF from the extracellular matrix and further potentiate the response.[99]

These data demonstrate that the VEGF receptor KDR is a critical regulating component of the VEGF pathway and suggest that compounds inhibiting its function or reducing its expression are likely to be effective inhibitors of the neovascularization associated with diabetes. This approach has already proven successful in animals by suppressing angiogenesis, endothelial cell proliferation, tumor growth, tumor metastasis, and cancer-associated mortality.[87,100–106]

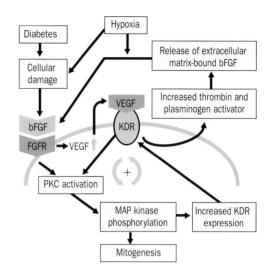

Figure 11-16 *Both diabetes and hypoxia can result in cellular damage that releases intracellular bFGF, allowing binding to its receptors on cell surface with subsequent activation of protein kinase C (PKC) and mitogen-activated protein (MAP) kinase. MAP kinase activation results in mitogenesis and also increases VEGF receptor KDR expression. Under conditions where VEGF receptor KDR is limiting, VEGF may have little mitogenic effect. However, bFGF stimulation under these conditions increases KDR expression, subsequently permitting VEGF action. VEGF also activates PKC and MAP kinase pathway, resulting in mitogenesis. In addition, VEGF increases thrombin and plasminogen activator expression, which releases extracellular matrix–bound bFGF, further potentiating response.*

Redrawn with permission from Aiello LP: Molecular mechanisms of growth factor action in diabetic retinopathy. Curr Opin Endocrinol Diabetes *1999;6:146156.*

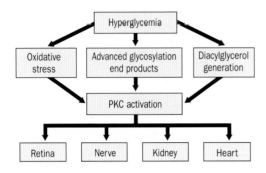

Figure 11-17 *Hyperglycemia increases oxidative stress, diacylglycerol, and advanced glycosylation end-product formation. All of these actions can ultimately result in PKC activation in tissues primarily affected by diabetes: retina, nerve, kidney, and heart.*

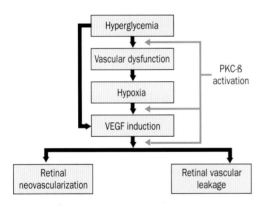

Figure 11-18 *Hyperglycemia of diabetes induces vascular dysfunction, leading to hypoxia and induction of VEGF expression. It is thought that VEGF mediates much of retinal neovascularization and retinal vascular leakage, which are characteristic of diabetic retinopathy. Activation of PKC is critical event in three of these steps, as indicated in figure. Thus, inhibition of PKC-β would be expected to reduce hyperglycemia-induced retinal complications by acting at numerous locations along this pathway.*

11-7

ROLE OF PROTEIN KINASE C

The hyperglycemia of diabetes mellitus results in numerous metabolic changes, including increases in oxidative stress, advanced glycosylation end products, and diacylglycerol. Although each of these alterations can elicit numerous biological effects, one of their shared outcomes is an activation of PKC (Figure 11-17). PKC is present in many body tissues and exists in numerous related, but structurally different, isoforms.[6] Different isoforms predominate in different body tissues, and they can respond differently to various cytokines. In diabetes, PKC activation is observed in the tissues where complications are most prevalent, including the retina, peripheral nerves, kidneys, and heart.

Within the eye, the beta isoform of PKC is of particular interest. As discussed above, the hyperglycemia of diabetes is thought to induce considerable vascular dysfunction, leading to retinal hypoxia and increased VEGF expression, which subsequently mediates both intraocular neovascularization and increased vasopermeability (Figure 11-18).

Early in the course of diabetes, PKC-β is activated in the retina by the hyperglycemia-induced de novo synthesis of diacylglycerol, the physiologic activator of PKC.[107] This PKC activation appears to account for several biochemical abnormalities associated with the diabetic state, presumably leading to progression of diabetic retinopathy. PKC activation is also a critical step in the hypoxic and hyperglycemic stimulation of VEGF expression[108,109] and in VEGF enhancement of endothelial cell survival.[110] Finally, as discussed below, PKC-β activation is required for VEGF to induce its proliferative and permeability effects.[78,111,112] Thus, inhibition of PKC-β would be expected to block the hyperglycemia-induced expression of VEGF at multiple points along the pathway, resulting in an ameliorating effect on diabetes-induced vascular complications.

11-8

PROTEIN KINASE C INHIBITORS

The development of a PKC-β-isoform-selective inhibitor (LY333531) has provided extensive data to substantiate this supposition.[113] Physiologic concentrations of VEGF induced rapid, dose-dependent increases in retinal PKC activity with translocation of PKC-α, -βII, and -δ isoforms from the cytosolic (inactive) to the membranous (active) fraction.[111] In cell culture, VEGF-induced retinal endothelial cell growth is inhibited by LY333531 (see Figure 11-7). Oral ingestion of LY333531 in pigs with laser-induced occlusion of the retinal veins suppressed the development of subsequent retinal neovascularization and was well tolerated by the animals (Figure 11-19A).[112]

Retinal vascular permeability also appears to be mediated by PKC, because both physiologic concentrations of VEGF and direct activation of PKC result in a rapid 3- to 5-fold increase in retinal vascular permeability in rats (see Figure 11-10).[78] In this model, intravitreal and orally administered PKC-β inhibitor greatly suppressed VEGF-

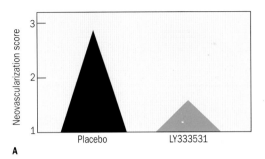

Figure 11-19 *Laser-induced occlusion of retinal veins in pig produces widespread retinal ischemia, with subsequent development of retinal neovascularization. (A) Pigs receiving control diet or diet including PKC-β-selective inhibitor LY333531 were evaluated for development of subsequent neovascularization, utilizing combined subjective and objective score incorporating clinical, angiographic, and light-microscopic evaluation. Retinal neovascularization was suppressed in animals receiving oral PKC-β inhibitor. P = 0.04.*

Part A derived from Danis RP, Bingaman DP, Jirousek M, Yang Y: Inhibition of intraocular neovascularization caused by retinal ischemia in pigs by PKCbeta inhibition with LY333531. Invest Ophthalmol Vis Sci *1998;39: 171–179.*

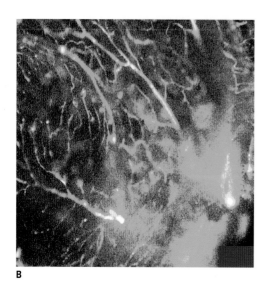

B

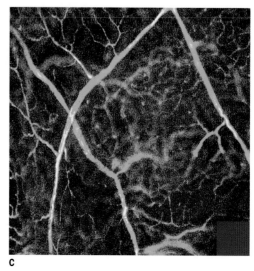

C

Figure 11-19 *Intravitreal injection of VEGF increases retinal vascular permeability in rats. (B) Fluorescein-conjugated dextran of approximately same molecular weight as albumin becomes permeable through retinal vasculature after addition of physiologic concentrations of VEGF. (C) However, when rats are fed diet containing LY333531 for 1 week prior to evaluation, ability of VEGF to induce retinal vascular permeability is markedly reduced.*

Parts B and C reproduced with permission from Aiello LP, Bursell SE, Clermont A, et al: Vascular endothelial growth factor–induced retinal permeability is mediated by protein kinase C in vivo and suppressed by an orally effective beta-isoform-selective inhibitor. Diabetes *1997;46:1473–1480.*

induced permeability (Figures 11-19B,C). The orally ingested PKC-β-isoform-selective inhibitor LY333531 was well tolerated and did not induce any overt toxicity.

Because PKC-β activation is induced by hyperglycemia and is a critical step in the development of vascular dysfunction, VEGF expression, and VEGF signal transduction, the inhibition of PKC-β by LY333531 would be expected to ameliorate diabetes-induced vascular complications by several mechanisms. Indeed, orally ingested LY333531 ameliorates diabetes-induced abnormalities of retinal blood flow, glomerular filtration rate, and albumin excretion rate in animals (Figure 11-20).[114] These findings, and a lack of clinically significant adverse events in initial human safety studies, have supported the initiation of multicenter, randomized, placebo-controlled clinical trials to determine the therapeutic potential of LY333531 as a noninvasive and nondestructive inhibitor of the progression of diabetic retinopathy and DME.

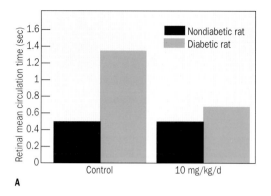

A

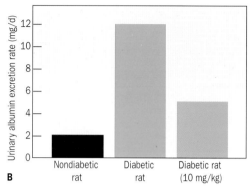

B

11-9

CURRENT STATUS
OF NOVEL THERAPEUTIC AGENTS

Advances in the development and preclinical testing of antiangiogenic agents have been rapid. Many large pharmaceutical and biotechnology companies currently have active programs devoted to the identification, development, and testing of novel antiangiogenic approaches.[115] Table 11-4 is a partial list of these agents, which are either in or presumably entering clinical trials.

The majority of therapeutic indications undergoing initial clinical evaluation are directed toward the suppression of vascular neoplasms. However, several antiangiogenic agents are now being evaluated for ophthalmic indications. Thalidomide has been in clinical trials for several years to assess its effectiveness in suppressing the choroidal neovascularization associated with age-related macular degeneration.[116,117] The PKC-β-selective inhibitor LY333531 is currently the subject in a multinational, randomized, double-masked, placebo-controlled clinical trial to assess the molecule's effect on PDR and DME. Integrin and growth-hormone

Figure 11-20 *Ingestion of PKC-β inhibitor LY333531 was evaluated in diabetic and nondiabetic rats for its effect on typical diabetes-induced abnormalities, including changes in (A) retinal blood flow (P <0.001) and (B) urinary albumin excretion rate (P <0.05). Mean retinal blood circulation time is abnormally increased in control diabetic rats. However, in diabetic rats fed 10 mg/kg per day of LY333531, diabetes-induced change in retinal circulation time is ameliorated. Similarly, diabetic rats have increased urinary albumin excretion rate. However, 1 week of oral treatment with LY333531 significantly normalizes this abnormality.*

Redrawn with permission from Ishii H, Jirousek MR, Koya D, et al: Amelioration of vascular dysfunctions in diabetic rats by an oral PKC beta inhibitor. Science 1996;272:728–731.

TABLE 11-4

Antiangiogenic Molecules Nearing or in Human Clinical Trials*

Indication	Antiangiogenic Molecule	Approximate Status
Ocular		
ARMD (wet)	Thalidomide	In clinical trials
PDR	PKC-β inhibitor (LY333531)	In clinical trials
	Growth-hormone antagonists	Nearing or in clinical trials
	Integrin antagonists	Nearing or in clinical trials
DME	PKC-β inhibitor (LY333531)	In clinical trials
Malignant pterygium	Angiostatic steroids	Nearing or in clinical trials
Nonocular		
Primarily for carcinomas	Taxol	All in clinical trials
	TNP-470 (AGM-1470)	
	Interleukin-12	
	Vitaxin	
	Pentosan polysulfate	
	Batimastat/ISV-120	
	Marimastat	
	Platelet factor 4 (PF4)	
	Tecogalan (DS4152, SP-PG)	
	Suramin	
	Carboxy-amidi triazole	
	CM101	
	Neovastat	
	SU101, SU5416	

*Because many molecules/trials are proprietary, indications and status are approximate and list is partial.

Source: *Adapted with permission from Casey R, Li WW: Factors controlling ocular angiogenesis. Am J Ophthalmol 1997; 124:521–529. Copyright 1997, with permission from Elsevier Science.*

antagonists are presumably nearing clinical trial in diabetic retinopathy as well. The first demonstration that pharmacologic intervention may be effective in diabetic retinopathy will need to await the results of these clinical investigations.

11-10

FUTURE HURDLES FOR ANTIANGIOGENIC THERAPY

Although the data supporting the use of antiangiogenic agents in humans for the treatment of PDR are compelling, several as-yet-unresolved issues are critical if these approaches are to achieve routine clinical application. The method of drug delivery is important. Local delivery would presumably have fewer side effects than would systemic administration, but achieving adequate concentrations of these agents at the retina is difficult using the local approach. Intravitreal injections allow for delivery of high intraocular concentrations of an agent, but repeated injections for the treatment of a lifelong disease such as diabetic retinopathy are suboptimal due to the sequential risks of endophthalmitis and retinal detachment. This drawback is especially notable for the treatment of diabetic retinopathy in light of the remarkable effectiveness of current laser photocoagulation, a noninvasive and relatively well-tolerated intervention.

Even if systemic therapy is attempted, it is not known whether excessive inhibition of VEGF in the adult will lead to side effects due to a physiologically required low basal expression of VEGF in the eye or other tissues. If true, careful titration of the extent of VEGF inhibition would be necessary and the therapeutic window could be small. Such strategies would almost certainly be necessary in the neonatal eye, where VEGF directs appropriate retinal vascular development.[55,60] Antiangiogenic agents would be expected to cause serious developmental defects if administered systemically during embryogenesis; thus, their use during pregnancy is likely to be severely restricted.

Even if a well-tolerated, easily administered antiangiogenic agent with limited toxicity were available, there would likely be instances where a normal neovascular response would be desired in the patient, and the angiosuppressive action of the retinopathy treatment might be detrimental. Although local drug delivery would obviate some of this problem, systemic administration could be problematic when extensive wound healing or vascular collateralization is required.

In patients with diabetes, this scenario could arise following significant trauma, with nonhealing ulcers, or following myocardial infarction. Initial clinical evaluation of direct myocardial gene transfer of VEGF in five patients with symptomatic myocardial ischemia resulted in reduced symptoms and improved myocardial perfusion.[118] Thus, antiangiogenic agents that can be rapidly reversed or that have short half-lives might permit prompt return of angiogenic capabilities when they are required. Finally, numerous clinical trials are necessary to determine the optimal manner in which these agents may be used. Various therapeutic scenarios include sole therapy, initial therapy prior to laser treatment, concurrent use with laser therapy, or perhaps application only if laser therapy is ineffective.

11-11

CONCLUSION

For more than half a century, there has been an excellent appreciation of the fundamental processes underlying the ocular complications of diabetes. However, only recently has an extraordinary series of scientific advances provided a detailed understanding of the molecular mechanisms involved in the evolution of diabetic retinopathy. These observations have suggested novel interventional approaches that hold promise for the development of effective, noninvasive, nondestructive, and potentially orally administered treatments of PDR, DME, and possibly the progression of NPDR. Several of these novel therapeutic modalities are either already being evaluated in clinical trials or will soon be reaching this stage.

Ultimately, the results of these clinical trials will resolve the remaining unanswered clinical issues and determine whether any of these approaches may yet prove effective or adaptable to clinical practice. However, at least in the case of PDR, the evidence supporting a major causal relationship between a growth factor and diabetic ocular complications is compelling. It is enlightening to remember that more than 20 years, before the discovery of insulin, Elliot P. Joslin, MD, routinely encouraged his diabetic patients to "Live, so that you may profit from some new discovery." Based on the scientific progress achieved in the past few years, it is possible that today's patients with diabetes may profit from a new ophthalmic frontier of pharmacologic therapy early in the twenty-first century.

REFERENCES

1. *Vision Problems in the U.S.: A Statistical Analysis.* New York: National Society to Prevent Blindness; 1980.

2. Ferris FL: How effective are treatments for diabetic retinopathy? *J Am Med Assoc* 1993;269: 1290–1291.

3. Greene DA, Sima AA, Stevens MJ: Aldose reductase inhibitors: an approach to the treatment of diabetic nerve damage. *Diabetes Metab Rev* 1993;9:189–217.

4. Brownlee M: The pathological implications of protein glycation. *Clin Invest Med* 1995;18: 275–281.

5. Baynes JW, Thorpe SR: Role of oxidative stress in diabetic complications: a new perspective on an old paradigm. *Diabetes* 1999;48:1–9.

6. Koya D, King GL: Protein kinase C activation and the development of diabetic complications. *Diabetes* 1998;47:859–866.

7. Horton MA: The alpha v beta 3 integrin "vitronectin receptor." *Int J Biochem Cell Biol* 1997;29:721–725.

8. King GL, Shiba T, Oliver J, et al: Cellular and molecular abnormalities in the vascular endothelium of diabetes mellitus. *Annu Rev Med* 1994;45: 179–188.

9. Gartner S, Henkind P: Neovascularization of the iris (rubeosis iridis). *Surv Ophthalmol* 1978; 22:291–312.

10. Henkind P: Ocular neovascularization: the Krill memorial lecture. *Am J Ophthalmol* 1978;85: 287–301.

11. Early Treatment Diabetic Retinopathy Study Research Group: Fluorescein angiographic risk factors for progression of diabetic retinopathy. ETDRS Report Number 13. *Ophthalmology* 1991;98:834–840.

12. Early Treatment Diabetic Retinopathy Study Research Group: Classification of diabetic retinopathy from fluorescein angiograms. ETDRS Report Number 11. *Ophthalmology* 1991;98: 807–822.

13. Branch Vein Occlusion Study Group: Argon laser scatter photocoagulation for prevention of neovascularization and vitreous hemorrhage in branch vein occlusion: a randomized clinical trial. *Arch Ophthalmol* 1986;104:34–41.

14. Aiello LM, Wand M, Liang G: Neovascular glaucoma and vitreous hemorrhage following cataract surgery in patients with diabetes mellitus. *Ophthalmology* 1983;90:814–820.

15. Michaelson IC: The mode of development of the vascular system of the retina, with some observations on its significance for certain retinal diseases. *Trans Ophthalmol Soc UK* 1948;68: 137–180.

16. Ashton N: Retinal neovascularization in health and disease. *Am J Ophthalmol* 1957;44: 7–24.

17. Friedlander M, Theesfeld CL, Sugita M, et al: Involvement of integrins alpha v beta 3 and alpha v beta 5 in ocular neovascular diseases. *Proc Natl Acad Sci USA* 1996;93:9764–9769.

18. O'Reilly MS, Holmgren L, Shing Y, et al: Angiostatin: a novel angiogenesis inhibitor that mediates the suppression of metastases by a Lewis lung carcinoma. *Cell* 1994;79:315–328.

19. O'Reilly MS, Boehm T, Shing Y, et al: Endostatin: an endogenous inhibitor of angiogenesis and tumor growth. *Cell* 1997;88:277–285.

20. Grant MB, Caballero S, Tarnuzzer RW, et al: Matrix metalloproteinase expression in human retinal microvascular cells. *Diabetes* 1998;47: 1311–1317.

21. De La Paz MA, Itoh Y, Toth CA, Nagase H: Matrix metalloproteinases and their inhibitors in human vitreous. *Invest Ophthalmol Vis Sci* 1998; 39:1256–1260.

22. Brown D, Hamdi H, Bahri S, Kenney MC: Characterization of an endogenous metalloproteinase in human vitreous. *Curr Eye Res* 1994;13: 639–647.

23. Burgess WH, Maciag T: The heparin-binding (fibroblast) growth factor family of proteins. *Annu Rev Biochem* 1989;58:575–606.

24. Vlodavsky I, Folkman J, Sullivan R, et al: Endothelial cell–derived basic fibroblast growth factor: synthesis and deposition into subendothelial extracellular matrix. *Proc Natl Acad Sci USA* 1987;84:2292–2296.

25. Abraham JA, Mergia A, Whang JL, et al: Nucleotide sequence of a bovine clone encoding the angiogenic protein, basic fibroblast growth factor. *Science* 1986;233:545–548.

26. Kandel J, Bossy-Wetzel E, Radvanyi F, et al: Neovascularization is associated with a switch to the export of bFGF in the multistep development of fibrosarcoma. *Cell* 1991;66:1095–1104.

27. McNeil PL, Muthukrishnan L, Warder E, D'Amore PA: Growth factors are released by mechanically wounded endothelial cells. *J Cell Biol* 1989;109:811–822.

28. Gao H, Hollyfield JG: Basic fibroblast growth factor (bFGF) immunolocalization in the rodent outer retina demonstrated with an anti–rodent bFGF antibody. *Brain Res* 1992;585:355–360.

29. Sivalingam A, Kenney J, Brown GC, et al: Basic fibroblast growth factor levels in the vitreous of patients with proliferative diabetic retinopathy. *Arch Ophthalmol* 1990;108:869–872.

30. Ozaki H, Okamoto N, Ortega S, et al: Basic fibroblast growth factor is neither necessary nor sufficient for the development of retinal neovascularization. *Am J Pathol* 1998;153:757–765.

31. Asahara T, Bauters C, Zheng LP, et al: Synergistic effect of vascular endothelial growth factor and basic fibroblast growth factor on angiogenesis in vivo. *Circulation* 1995;92:II365–II371.

32. Goto F, Goto K, Weindel K, Folkman J: Synergistic effects of vascular endothelial growth factor and basic fibroblast growth factor on the proliferation and cord formation of bovine capillary endothelial cells within collagen gels. *Lab Invest* 1993;69:508–517.

33. Pepper MS, Ferrara N, Orci L, Montesano R: Potent synergism between vascular endothelial growth factor and basic fibroblast growth factor in the induction of angiogenesis in vitro. *Biochem Biophys Res Commun* 1992;189:824–831.

34. LeRoith D, Roberts CT Jr: Insulin-like growth factors. *Ann NY Acad Sci* 1993;692:1–9.

35. Poulsen JE: Diabetes and anterior pituitary insufficiency: final course and postmortem study of a diabetic patient with Sheehan's syndrome. *Diabetes* 1966;15:73–77.

36. Poulsen JE: The Houssay phenomenon in man: recovery from retinopathy in a case of diabetes with Simmonds' disease. *Diabetes* 1953;2:7–12.

37. Sharp PS, Fallon TJ, Brazier OJ, et al: Long-term follow-up of patients who underwent yttrium-90 pituitary implantation for treatment of proliferative diabetic retinopathy. *Diabetologia* 1987;30:199–207.

38. Smith LE, Kopchick JJ, Chen W, et al: Essential role of growth hormone in ischemia-induced retinal neovascularization. *Science* 1997; 276:1706–1709.

39. Katsura Y, Okano T, Noritake M, et al: Hepatocyte growth factor in vitreous fluid of patients with proliferative diabetic retinopathy and other retinal disorders. *Diabetes Care* 1998; 21:1759–1763.

40. Senger DR, Galli SJ, Dvorak AM, et al: Tumor cells secrete a vascular permeability factor that promotes accumulation of ascites fluid. *Science* 1983;219:983–985.

41. Keck PJ, Hauser SD, Krivi G, et al: Vascular permeability factor, an endothelial cell mitogen related to PDGF. *Science* 1989;246:1309–1312.

42. Leung DW, Cachianes G, Kuang WJ, et al: Vascular endothelial growth factor is a secreted angiogenic mitogen. *Science* 1989;246:1306–1309.

43. Ferrara N, Houck KA, Jakeman LB, et al: The vascular endothelial growth factor family of polypeptides. *J Cell Biochem* 1991;47:211–218.

44. Williams B: Vascular permeability/vascular endothelial growth factors: a potential role in the pathogenesis and treatment of vascular diseases. *Vasc Med* 1996;1:251–258.

45. Miller JW, Adamis AP, Aiello LP: Vascular endothelial growth factor in ocular neovascularization and proliferative diabetic retinopathy. *Diabetes Metab Rev* 1997;13:37–50.

46. Aiello LP: Clinical implications of vascular growth factors in proliferative retinopathies. *Curr Opin Ophthalmol* 1997;8:19–31.

47. Aiello LP: Vascular endothelial growth factor: 20th-century mechanisms, 21st-century therapies. *Invest Ophthalmol Vis Sci* 1997;38:1647–1652.

48. Thieme H, Aiello LP, Takagi H, et al: Comparative analysis of vascular endothelial growth factor receptors on retinal and aortic vascular endothelial cells. *Diabetes* 1995;44:98–103.

49. Aiello LP, Northrup JM, Keyt BA, et al: Hypoxic regulation of vascular endothelial growth factor in retinal cells. *Arch Ophthalmol* 1995;113:1538–1544.

50. de Vries C, Escobedo JA, Ueno H, et al: The fms-like tyrosine kinase, a receptor for vascular endothelial growth factor. *Science* 1992;255:989–991.

51. Millauer B, Wizigmann-Voos S, Schnurch H, et al: High affinity VEGF binding and developmental expression suggest Flk-1 as a major regulator of vasculogenesis and angiogenesis. *Cell* 1993;72:835–846.

52. Adamis AP, Shima DT, Yeo KT, et al: Synthesis and secretion of vascular permeability factor/vascular endothelial growth factor by human retinal pigment epithelial cells. *Biochem Biophys Res Commun* 1993;193:631–638.

53. Simorre-Pinatel V, Guerrin M, Chollet P, et al: Vasculotropin-VEGF stimulates retinal capillary endothelial cells through an autocrine pathway. *Invest Ophthalmol Vis Sci* 1994;35:3393–3400.

54. Dorey CK, Aouididi S, Reynaud X, et al: Correlation of vascular permeability factor/vascular endothelial growth factor with extraretinal neovascularization in the rat. *Arch Ophthalmol* 1996;114:1210–1217.

55. Stone J, Chan-Ling T, Pe'er J, et al: Roles of vascular endothelial growth factor and astrocyte degeneration in the genesis of retinopathy of prematurity. *Invest Ophthalmol Vis Sci* 1996;37:290–299.

56. Smith LE, Wesolowski E, McLellan A, et al: Oxygen-induced retinopathy in the mouse. *Invest Ophthalmol Vis Sci* 1994;35:101–111.

57. Donahue ML, Phelps DL, Watkins RH, et al: Retinal vascular endothelial growth factor (VEGF) mRNA expression is altered in relation to neovascularization in oxygen induced retinopathy. *Curr Eye Res* 1996;15:175–184.

58. Miller JW, Adamis AP, Shima DT, et al: Vascular endothelial growth factor/vascular permeability factor is temporally and spatially correlated with ocular angiogenesis in a primate model. *Am J Pathol* 1994;145:574–584.

59. Pierce EA, Avery RL, Foley ED, et al: Vascular endothelial growth factor/vascular permeability factor expression in a mouse model of retinal neovascularization. *Proc Natl Acad Sci USA* 1995;92:905–909.

60. Pierce EA, Foley ED, Smith LE: Regulation of vascular endothelial growth factor by oxygen in a model of retinopathy of prematurity. *Arch Ophthalmol* 1996;114:1219–1228.

61. Aiello LP, Avery RL, Arrigg PG, et al: Vascular endothelial growth factor in ocular fluid of patients with diabetic retinopathy and other retinal disorders. *N Engl J Med* 1994;331:1480–1487.

62. Adamis AP, Miller JW, Bernal MT, et al: Increased vascular endothelial growth factor levels in the vitreous of eyes with proliferative diabetic retinopathy. *Am J Ophthalmol* 1994;118:445–450.

63. Burgos R, Simo R, Audi L, et al: Vitreous levels of vascular endothelial growth factor are not influenced by its serum concentrations in diabetic retinopathy. *Diabetologia* 1997;40:1107–1109.

64. Pe'er J, Folberg R, Itin A, et al: Upregulated expression of vascular endothelial growth factor in proliferative diabetic retinopathy. *Br J Ophthalmol* 1996;80:241–245.

65. Armstrong D, Augustin AJ, Spengler R, et al: Detection of vascular endothelial growth factor and tumor necrosis factor alpha in epiretinal membranes of proliferative diabetic retinopathy, proliferative vitreoretinopathy and macular pucker. *Ophthalmologica* 1998;212:410–414.

66. Chen YS, Hackett SF, Schoenfeld CL, et al: Localisation of vascular endothelial growth factor and its receptors to cells of vascular and avascular epiretinal membranes. *Br J Ophthalmol* 1997;81:919–926.

67. Frank RN, Amin RH, Eliott D, et al: Basic fibroblast growth factor and vascular endothelial growth factor are present in epiretinal and choroidal neovascular membranes. *Am J Ophthalmol* 1996;122:393–403.

68. Malecaze F, Clamens S, Simorre-Pinatel V, et al: Detection of vascular endothelial growth factor messenger RNA and vascular endothelial growth factor–like activity in proliferative diabetic retinopathy. *Arch Ophthalmol* 1994;112:1476–1482.

69. Tang S, Le-Ruppert KC, Gabel VP: Proliferation and activation of vascular endothelial cells in epiretinal membranes from patients with proliferative diabetic retinopathy: an immunohistochemistry and clinical study. *Ger J Ophthalmol* 1994;3:131–136.

70. Schneeberger SA, Hjelmeland LM, Tucker RP, Morse LS: Vascular endothelial growth factor and fibroblast growth factor 5 are colocalized in vascular and avascular epiretinal membranes. *Am J Ophthalmol* 1997;124:447–454.

71. Tolentino MJ, Miller JW, Gragoudas ES, et al: Vascular endothelial growth factor is sufficient to produce iris neovascularization and neovascular glaucoma in a nonhuman primate. *Arch Ophthalmol* 1996;114:964–970.

72. Tobe T, Okamoto N, Vinores MA, et al: Evolution of neovascularization in mice with overexpression of vascular endothelial growth factor in photoreceptors. *Invest Ophthalmol Vis Sci* 1998;39:180–188.

73. Okamoto N, Tobe T, Hackett SF, et al: Transgenic mice with increased expression of vascular endothelial growth factor in the retina: a new model of intraretinal and subretinal neovascularization. *Am J Pathol* 1997;151:281–291.

74. Senger DR, Connolly DT, Van de Water L, et al: Purification and NH2-terminal amino acid sequence of guinea pig tumor-secreted vascular permeability factor. *Cancer Res* 1990;50:1774–1778.

75. Murata T, Ishibashi T, Khalil A, et al: Vascular endothelial growth factor plays a role in hyperpermeability of diabetic retinal vessels. *Ophthalmic Res* 1995;27:48–52.

76. Murata T, Nakagawa K, Khalil A, et al: The relation between expression of vascular endothelial growth factor and breakdown of the blood–retinal barrier in diabetic rat retinas. *Lab Invest* 1996;74:819–825.

77. Tolentino MJ, Miller JW, Gragoudas ES, et al: Intravitreous injections of vascular endothelial growth factor produce retinal ischemia and microangiopathy in an adult primate. *Ophthalmology* 1996;103:1820–1828.

78. Aiello LP, Bursell SE, Clermont A, et al: Vascular endothelial growth factor–induced retinal permeability is mediated by protein kinase C in vivo and suppressed by an orally effective beta-isoform-selective inhibitor. *Diabetes* 1997;46:1473–1480.

79. Antonetti DA, Barber AJ, Khin S, et al: Vascular permeability in experimental diabetes is associated with reduced endothelial occludin content: vascular endothelial growth factor decreases occludin in retinal endothelial cells. *Diabetes* 1998;47:1953–1959.

80. Kevil CG, Payne DK, Mire E, Alexander JS: Vascular permeability factor/vascular endothelial cell growth factor–mediated permeability occurs through disorganization of endothelial junctional proteins. *J Biol Chem* 1998;273:15099–15103.

81. Boulton M, Foreman D, Williams G, McLeod D: VEGF localisation in diabetic retinopathy. *Br J Ophthalmol* 1998;82:561–568.

82. Amin RH, Frank RN, Kennedy A, et al: Vascular endothelial growth factor is present in glial cells of the retina and optic nerve of human subjects with nonproliferative diabetic retinopathy. *Invest Ophthalmol Vis Sci* 1997;38:36–47.

83. Gerhardinger C, Brown LF, Roy S, et al: Expression of vascular endothelial growth factor in the human retina and in nonproliferative diabetic retinopathy. *Am J Pathol* 1998;152:1453–1462.

84. Clermont AC, Aiello LP, Mori F, et al: Vascular endothelial growth factor and severity of nonproliferative diabetic retinopathy mediate retinal hemodynamics in vivo: a potential role for vascular endothelial growth factor in the progression of nonproliferative diabetic retinopathy. *Am J Ophthalmol* 1997;124:433–446.

85. Aiello LP, Pierce EA, Foley ED, et al: Suppression of retinal neovascularization in vivo by inhibition of vascular endothelial growth factor (VEGF) using soluble VEGF-receptor chimeric proteins. *Proc Natl Acad Sci USA* 1995;92:10457–10461.

86. Adamis AP, Shima DT, Tolentino MJ, et al: Inhibition of vascular endothelial growth factor prevents retinal ischemia–associated iris neovascularization in a nonhuman primate. *Arch Ophthalmol* 1996;114:66–71.

87. Robinson GS, Pierce EA, Rook SL, et al: Oligodeoxynucleotides inhibit retinal neovascularization in a murine model of proliferative retinopathy. *Proc Natl Acad Sci USA* 1996;93:4851–4856.

88. Fischer S, Sharma HS, Karliczek GF, Schaper W: Expression of vascular permeability factor/vascular endothelial growth factor in pig cerebral microvascular endothelial cells and its upregulation by adenosine. *Brain Res Mol Brain Res* 1995;28:141–148.

89. Fischer S, Knoll R, Renz D, et al: Role of adenosine in the hypoxic induction of vascular endothelial growth factor in porcine brain derived microvascular endothelial cells. *Endothelium* 1997;5:155–165.

90. Hashimoto E, Kage K, Ogita T, et al: Adenosine as an endogenous mediator of hypoxia for induction of vascular endothelial growth factor mRNA in U-937 cells. *Biochem Biophys Res Commun* 1994;204:318–324.

91. Lutty GA, Mathews MK, Merges C, McLeod DS: Adenosine stimulates canine retinal microvascular endothelial cell migration and tube formation. *Curr Eye Res* 1998;17:594–607.

92. Takagi H, King GL, Robinson GS, et al: Adenosine mediates hypoxic induction of vascular endothelial growth factor in retinal pericytes and endothelial cells. *Invest Ophthalmol Vis Sci* 1996;37:2165–2176.

93. Bontemps F, Vincent MF, Van den Berghe G: Mechanisms of elevation of adenosine levels in anoxic hepatocytes. *Biochem J* 1993;290:671–677.

94. Stavri GT, Zachary IC, Baskerville PA, et al: Basic fibroblast growth factor upregulates the expression of vascular endothelial growth factor in vascular smooth muscle cells: synergistic interaction with hypoxia. *Circulation* 1995;92:11–14.

95. Milanini J, Vinals F, Pouyssegur J, Pages G: p42/p44 MAP kinase module plays a key role in the transcriptional regulation of the vascular endothelial growth factor gene in fibroblasts. *J Biol Chem* 1998;273:18165–18172.

96. Pepper MS, Mandriota SJ: Regulation of vascular endothelial growth factor receptor-2 (Flk-1) expression in vascular endothelial cells. *Exp Cell Res* 1998;241:414–425.

97. Zucker S, Mirza H, Conner CE, et al: Vascular endothelial growth factor induces tissue factor and matrix metalloproteinase production in endothelial cells: conversion of prothrombin to thrombin results in progelatinase A activation and cell proliferation. *Int J Cancer* 1998;75: 780–786.

98. Mandriota SJ, Pepper MS: Vascular endothelial growth factor–induced in vitro angiogenesis and plasminogen activator expression are dependent on endogenous basic fibroblast growth factor. *J Cell Sci* 1997;110:2293–2302.

99. Benezra M, Vlodavsky I, Ishai-Michaeli R, et al: Thrombin-induced release of active basic fibroblast growth factor–heparan sulfate complexes from subendothelial extracellular matrix. *Blood* 1993;81:3324–3331.

100. Witte L, Hicklin DJ, Zhu Z, et al: Monoclonal antibodies targeting the VEGF receptor-2 (Flk1/KDR) as an anti-angiogenic therapeutic strategy. *Cancer Metastasis Rev* 1998;17:155–161.

101. Zhu Z, Rockwell P, Lu D, et al: Inhibition of vascular endothelial growth factor–induced receptor activation with anti-kinase insert domain-containing receptor single-chain antibodies from a phage display library. *Cancer Res* 1998;58: 3209–3214.

102. Ruckman J, Green LS, Beeson J, et al: 2'-Fluoropyrimidine RNA-based aptamers to the 165-amino acid form of vascular endothelial growth factor (VEGF165): inhibition of receptor binding and VEGF-induced vascular permeability through interactions requiring the exon 7-encoded domain. *J Biol Chem* 1998;273: 20556–20567.

103. Goldman CK, Kendall RL, Cabrera G, et al: Paracrine expression of a native soluble vascular endothelial growth factor receptor inhibits tumor growth, metastasis, and mortality rate. *Proc Natl Acad Sci USA* 1998;95:8795–8800.

104. Siemeister G, Schirner M, Reusch P, et al: An antagonistic vascular endothelial growth factor (VEGF) variant inhibits VEGF-stimulated receptor autophosphorylation and proliferation of human endothelial cells. *Proc Natl Acad Sci USA* 1998;95:4625–4629.

105. Kong HL, Hecht D, Song W, et al: Regional suppression of tumor growth by in vivo transfer of a cDNA encoding a secreted form of the extracellular domain of the flt-1 vascular endothelial growth factor receptor. *Hum Gene Ther* 1998; 9:823–833.

106. Strawn LM, McMahon G, App H, et al: Flk-1 as a target for tumor growth inhibition. *Cancer Res* 1996;56:3540–3545.

107. Xia P, Inoguchi T, Kern TS, et al: Characterization of the mechanism for the chronic activation of diacylglycerol–protein kinase C pathway in diabetes and hypergalactosemia. *Diabetes* 1994;43:1122–1129.

108. Mazure NM, Chen EY, Laderoute KR, Giaccia AJ: Induction of vascular endothelial growth factor by hypoxia is modulated by a phosphatidylinositol 3-kinase/Akt signaling pathway in Ha-ras-transformed cells through a hypoxia inducible factor-1 transcriptional element. *Blood* 1997;90:3322–3331.

109. Williams B, Gallacher B, Patel H, Orme C: Glucose-induced protein kinase C activation regulates vascular permeability factor mRNA expression and peptide production by human vascular smooth muscle cells in vitro. *Diabetes* 1997;46:1497–1503.

110. Gerber HP, McMurtrey A, Kowalski J, et al: Vascular endothelial growth factor regulates endothelial cell survival through the phosphatidylinositol 3′-kinase/Akt signal transduction pathway: requirement for Flk-1/KDR activation. *J Biol Chem* 1998;273:30336–30343.

111. Xia P, Aiello LP, Ishii H, et al: Characterization of vascular endothelial growth factor's effect on the activation of protein kinase C, its isoforms, and endothelial cell growth. *J Clin Invest* 1996;98:2018–2026.

112. Danis RP, Bingaman DP, Jirousek M, Yang Y: Inhibition of intraocular neovascularization caused by retinal ischemia in pigs by PKCbeta inhibition with LY333531. *Invest Ophthalmol Vis Sci* 1998;39:171–179.

113. Jirousek MR, Gillig JR, Gonzalez CM, et al: (S)-13-[(dimethylamino)methyl]-10,11,14,15-tetrahydro-4,9:16, 21-dimetheno-1H, 13H-dibenzo[e,k]pyrrolo[3,4-h][1,4,13]oxadiazacyclohexadecene-1,3(2H)-d ione (LY333531) and related analogues: isozyme selective inhibitors of protein kinase C beta. *J Med Chem* 1996;39:2664–2671.

114. Ishii H, Jirousek MR, Koya D, et al: Amelioration of vascular dysfunctions in diabetic rats by an oral PKC beta inhibitor. *Science* 1996;272:728–731.

115. Casey R, Li WW: Factors controlling ocular angiogenesis. *Am J Ophthalmol* 1997;124:521–529.

116. Kenyon BM, Browne F, D'Amato RJ: Effects of thalidomide and related metabolites in a mouse corneal model of neovascularization. *Exp Eye Res* 1997;64:971–978.

117. Kruse FE, Joussen AM, Rohrschneider K, et al: Thalidomide inhibits corneal angiogenesis induced by vascular endothelial growth factor. *Graefes Arch Klin Exp Ophthalmol* 1998;236:461–466.

118. Losordo DW, Vale PR, Symes JF, et al: Gene therapy for myocardial angiogenesis: initial clinical results with direct myocardial injection of phVEGF165 as sole therapy for myocardial ischemia. *Circulation* 1998;98:2800–2804.

Abstracts of Major Collaborative Multicenter Trials for Diabetic Retinopathy*

Compiled by

Nauman A. Chaudhry, MD
Homayoun Tabandeh, MD
Harry W. Flynn, Jr, MD

A-1

DIABETIC RETINOPATHY STUDY (DRS)

1. Diabetic Retinopathy Study Research Group: Preliminary report on effects of photocoagulation therapy. *Am J Ophthalmol* 1976;81:383–396. Copyright 1976. Reprinted with permission from Elsevier Science.

Summary Analyses of visual acuity and visual field results in the DRS provide evidence that photocoagulation treatment as carried out according to the study protocol (extensive "scatter" photocoagulation and focal treatment of new vessels) is of benefit in preventing severe visual loss, over a 2-year followup period, in eyes with proliferative retinopathy. Location of new vessels relative to the disc, severity of new vessels, and the presence of hemorrhage (vitreous or pre-retinal) all proved to be important prognostic factors. On the basis of these findings, these steps have been taken: All patients in the study have been informed of results to date and given an explanation of their implications. Photocoagulation treatment will be considered for the initially untreated eyes which now or in the future fulfill any one of the following criteria: (**1**) moderate or severe new vessels on or within 1 disc diameter of the optic disc; (**2**) mild new vessels on or within 1 disc diameter of the optic disc if fresh hemorrhage is present; and (**3**) moderate or severe new vessels elsewhere if fresh hemorrhage is present. Followup of all patients will continue to allow long-term comparison between the argon and xenon treatment techniques employed. Further analyses of accumulating data will be performed to evaluate more completely the efficacy of photocoagulation therapy.

---

*If an abstract was not published, the concluding section of the report has been reprinted (for example, Summary).

2. Diabetic Retinopathy Study Research Group: Photocoagulation treatment of proliferative diabetic retinopathy: the second report of Diabetic Retinopathy Study findings. *Ophthalmology* 1978; 85;82–106. Courtesy of *Ophthalmology*.

Abstract Data from the DRS show that photocoagulation, as used in the study, reduced the rate of development of severe visual loss and inhibited the progression of retinopathy. These beneficial effects were noted to some degree in all those stages of diabetic retinopathy which were included in the study. Some deleterious effects of treatment were also found, including losses of visual acuity and constriction of peripheral visual field. The risk of these harmful effects was considered acceptable in eyes with retinopathy in the moderate or severe proliferative stage when the risk of severe visual loss without treatment was great. In early proliferative or severe nonproliferative retinopathy, when the risk of severe visual loss without treatment was less, the risks of harmful treatment effects assumed greater importance. In these earlier stages, DRS findings have not led to a clear choice between prompt treatment and deferral of treatment unless and until progression to a more severe stage occurs. The purpose of this interim report is to present the data on which these conclusions are based. More detailed reports of study findings will appear in the future.

3. Diabetic Retinopathy Study Research Group: Four risk factors for severe visual loss in diabetic retinopathy: the third report from the Diabetic Retinopathy Study. *Arch Ophthalmol* 1979;97: 654–655. Copyright 1979, American Medical Association.

Abstract The DRS Research Group has so far identified four retinopathy factors that increase the 2-year risk of developing severe visual loss. The risk grows as the number of risk factors increases. Eyes with three or more risk factors (eyes with "high-risk characteristics") are at a much higher risk than eyes with two or fewer factors. The DRS protocol was changed in 1976 to require consideration of treatment for these "high-risk" eyes.

4. Diabetic Retinopathy Study Research Group: Photocoagulation treatment of proliferative diabetic retinopathy: a short report of long range results. DRS Report Number 4. In: *Proceedings of the 10th Congress of the International Diabetes Federation*. Amsterdam: Excerpta Medica; 1980.

Summary The 4-year followup information presented in this report confirms our previous general conclusion that photocoagulation treatment, as used in the DRS, reduces the risk of severe visual loss by more than 50% and extends this conclusion to the mildest stages of retinopathy included in the study. The reduction of the rate of severe visual loss remains somewhat greater in the xenon treatment group than in the argon group, but its magnitude is not sufficient to outweigh the more frequent occurrence of harmful side effects of the DRS xenon technique. Study findings continue to support prompt treatment when proliferative retinopathy is moderately severe. Persistent decreases in visual acuity resulted from study treatment techniques with sufficient frequency to suggest caution in applying them to eyes with mild proliferative or severe nonproliferative retinopathy. For eyes in these stages of retinopathy, DRS findings do not provide a clear choice between prompt treatment and deferral of treatment unless and until progression to a more severe stage occurs.

5. Diabetic Retinopathy Study Research Group: Photocoagulation treatment of proliferative diabetic retinopathy: relationship of adverse treatment effects to retinopathy severity. DRS Report Number 5. *Dev Ophthalmol* 1981;21:248–261.

Summary Xenon arc photocoagulation, as carried out in the DRS, is attended by an increased risk of severe macular damage secondary to vitreoretinal traction. This risk is of particular importance in eyes with severe fibrous proliferation and/or localized traction retinal detachment. Little evidence was found of such an effect following argon laser photocoagulation, although some, mostly less serious, visual acuity decreases were attributable to this treatment as well. After 4 years of followup, the beneficial effect of xenon photocoagulation in reducing the risk of severe visual loss outweighed its harmful effect, even in eyes with severe fibrous proliferation and/or traction retinal detachment. A beneficial effect of approximately equal magnitude was present in the argon group.

6. Diabetic Retinopathy Study Research Group: Design, methods, and baseline results. DRS Report Number 6. *Invest Ophthalmol Vis Sci* 1981;21: 149–209. Copyright 1981, Association for Research in Vision and Ophthalmology.

Summary The DRS is a collaborative clinical trial supported by the NEI. The main objectives of the DRS were the following three questions: (**1**) Does photocoagulation help prevent severe visual loss from proliferative diabetic retinopathy? (**2**) Is there a difference with respect to efficacy and safety between two treatment techniques: (**a**) extensive scatter treatment with the argon laser plus focal treatment of surface new vessels, elevated new vessels, and new vessels on or near the disc; or (**b**) extensive scatter treatment with the xenon arc plus focal treatment of surface new vessels? (**3**) Are there some stages of retinopathy in which treatment is helpful but others in which it is of no value or harmful? Fifteen clinical centers participated in the DRS. Patient recruitment started in April 1972, and the last patient was treated in September 1975; a total of 1758 patients were enrolled. Patients enrolled in the study had one eye randomly assigned to prompt photocoagulation with either argon or xenon and the other eye to no treatment. The primary response variable was visual acuity, but visual fields and changes in the retina and vitreous were also considered in the evaluation of treatment. All completed study forms and fundus photograph readings were sent to the Coordinating Center for editing, analysis, and storage. The DRS data were reviewed by the Data Monitoring Committee for evidence of adverse and beneficial treatment effects. The following are highlights of the characteristics of the patients enrolled in this study: (**1**) Patients were predominantly white, and there were slightly more men than women. (**2**) The age distribution of the enrolled patients was bimodal, with peaks at 20 to 29 years and 50 to 59 years of age. (**3**) Approximately 45% of the patients could be classified as juvenile-onset diabetics. (**4**) Two thirds of the patients had borderline or definite hypertension, on the basis of supine blood pressure readings at entry. (**5**) Visual acuity was equal to or better than 20/20 in approximately half of the eyes, and there was approximately the same distribution of visual acuity levels for all four groups of eyes: eyes assigned to argon treatment; eyes assigned to xenon treatment; and the fellow eyes of patients in each of these groups. (**6**) Over 90% of the eyes had intraocular pressure 20 mm Hg or less. (**7**) Fifty percent of the eyes had NVD [neovascularization of the disc], and nearly 75% had NVE [neovascularization elsewhere] as determined by the ophthalmic examination at initial visit 1. (**8**) Twenty-five percent had definite macular edema involving the center of the macula with or without cystoid changes as identified by the ophthalmic examination at baseline. On the basis of the baseline variables considered, there was no evidence of lack of comparability of the patients assigned to argon and xenon or lack of comparability of the four groups of eyes at baseline. Two previous reports contained the findings that led to the protocol changes in 1976 and 1977. Additional papers dealing with assessment of treatment effects are being prepared for publication.

7. Diabetic Retinopathy Study Research Group: A modification of the Airlie House classification of diabetic retinopathy. DRS Report Number 7. *Invest Ophthalmol Vis Sci* 1981;21:210–226. Copyright 1981, Association for Research in Vision and Ophthalmology.

Summary A modification of the Airlie House classification of diabetic retinopathy is described in detail. The classification uses a combination of standard stereoscopic photographs and written definitions to grade more than 20 lesions on a three- to six-step scale.

8. Diabetic Retinopathy Study Research Group: Photocoagulation treatment of proliferative diabetic retinopathy: clinical application of Diabetic Retinopathy Study (DRS) findings. DRS Report Number 8. *Ophthalmology* 1981;88:583–600. Courtesy of *Ophthalmology*.

Abstract Additional followup confirms previous reports from the DRS that photocoagulation, as used in the study, reduces the risk of severe visual loss by 50% or more. Decreases of visual acuity of one or more lines and constriction of peripheral visual field due to treatment were also observed in some eyes. These harmful effects were more frequent and more severe following the DRS xenon technique. The 2-year risk of severe visual loss without treatment outweighs the risk of harmful treatment effects for two groups of eyes: (**1**) eyes with new vessels and preretinal or vitreous hemorrhage; and (**2**) eyes with new vessels on or within 1 disc diameter of the optic disc (NVD) [neovascularization of the disc] equaling or exceeding ¼ to ⅓ disc area in extent . . . , even in the absence of preretinal or vitreous hemorrhage. For eyes with these characteristics, prompt treatment is usually advisable. For eyes with less severe retinopathy, DRS findings do not provide a clear choice between prompt treatment or deferral unless progression to these more severe stages occurs.

9. Diabetic Retinopathy Study Research Group: Assessing possible late treatment effects in stopping a clinical trial early: a case study. DRS Report Number 9. *Control Clin Trials* 1984;5:373–381. Copyright 1984. Reprinted with permission from Elsevier Science.

Abstract Suppose a fixed-sample trial in a disease with a long response time shows a statistically significant benefit of the experimental treatment before patients have completed the planned followup period. The question may then arise—and did arise in the DRS—whether the observed early benefit of treatment may be offset at some time in the future by the subsequent development of harmful treatment effects. If this question raises serious concerns, then the investigators are faced with a dilemma. If the trial is stopped because of the observed early treatment benefit and the treatment is administered to the untreated control group as well as to patients outside the study and if the treatment is later found to have deleterious effects, then it may ultimately do more harm than good to patients. Moreover, the fact that the treatment is harmful may never become known. If, on the other hand, the trial is not stopped and the treatment proves to have no deleterious effects, then the control group and patients outside the study would be harmed because the treatment was withheld. We show how, in the DRS, this very problem was formulated and resolved. First, a severe, delayed harmful treatment effect was postulated. Projections based on this postulation showed that the early gains were so great that they were unlikely to be offset—ever. Based in part on these projections, the following decisions were made: (**1**) the study protocol would be changed so as to allow treatment of the untreated control group, and (**2**) patients would continue to be followed in order to make possible the detection of late, harmful treatment effects, should they develop.

10. Diabetic Retinopathy Study Research Group: Factors influencing the development of visual loss in advanced diabetic retinopathy. DRS Report Number 10. *Invest Ophthalmol Vis Sci* 1985; 26:983–991. Copyright 1985, Association for Research in Vision and Ophthalmology.

Abstract Natural history data from the DRS were examined by multivariate methods to determine which baseline characteristics could predict the occurrence of severe visual loss (SVL) in eyes originally assigned to no treatment. The presence and extent of new blood vessels on the optic disc (NVD) [neovascularization of the disc] had the strongest association with SVL. Several other ocular characteristics also were strongly associated with visual outcome. In the absence of NVD at baseline, the degree of intraretinal hemorrhages and microaneurysms (HMA) had the strongest association with development of SVL. Macular edema was a factor in determining visual loss to 20/200 but not SVL (less than 5/200). Among systemic characteristics, urinary protein was the best predictor of visual outcome, but none were as good as the major ocular variables.

11. Diabetic Retinopathy Study Research Group: Intraocular pressure following panretinal photocoagulation for diabetic retinopathy. DRS Report Number 11. *Arch Ophthalmol* 1987;105: 807–809. Copyright 1987, American Medical Association.

Abstract Data collected during the first 5 years after randomization in the DRS were analyzed to determine the effect of panretinal photocoagulation on intraocular pressure (IOP). At each followup visit, median IOP was identical for the treated and untreated eyes. Mean IOP rose slightly in each group. The proportion of untreated eyes with IOP above 30 mm Hg at two consecutive visits was twice that of the treated eyes (2% versus 1%). These data show that panretinal photocoagulation reduces the risk of subsequent intraocular hypertension, apparently by preventing the development of neovascular glaucoma.

12. Diabetic Retinopathy Study Research Group: Macular edema in Diabetic Retinopathy Study patients. DRS Report Number 12. *Ophthalmology* 1987;94:754–760. Courtesy of *Ophthalmology*.
Abstract Results from the DRS demonstrate that scatter photocoagulation is associated with some loss of visual acuity soon after treatment. This visual loss is especially prominent in eyes with pre-existing macular edema. It is also associated with the intensity of treatment. Reducing macular edema by focal photocoagulation before initiating scatter treatment and dividing scatter treatment into multiple sessions with less intense burns may decrease the risk of the visual loss associated with photocoagulation.

13. Diabetic Retinopathy Study Research Group: Factors associated with visual outcome after photocoagulation for diabetic retinopathy. DRS Report Number 13. *Invest Ophthalmol Vis Sci* 1989;30:23–28. Copyright 1989, Association for Research in Vision and Ophthalmology.
Abstract Six risk factors for severe visual loss despite panretinal (scatter) photocoagulation were identified by analyzing data collected during the first 5 years after randomization in the DRS. Proportional hazards regression revealed NVD (neovascularization on/around the optic disc) to be the most important risk factor. The risk of severe visual loss rose with increasing NVD, hemorrhages/microaneurysms, retinal elevation, proteinuria, and hypoglycemia and fell with increasing "treatment density." These results are similar to previous DRS findings on untreated eyes. The importance of "treatment density" as an independent predictor of visual outcome is a new finding and lends support to the common clinical practice of repeating photocoagulation if initial treatment does not reduce or stabilize retinal neovascularization.

14. Diabetic Retinopathy Study Research Group: Indications for photocoagulation treatment of diabetic retinopathy. DRS Report Number 14. *Int Ophthalmol Clin* 1987;27:239–253. Courtesy of Lippincott-Raven Publishers.
Conclusions When photocoagulation is to be undertaken in the hope of reducing the risk of severe visual loss, the principal factor influencing the decision between prompt treatment and deferral of treatment with continued careful followup is the presence of DRS high-risk characteristics. The situation is particularly urgent when there is a threat that dispersion or recurrence of vitreous hemorrhage may soon preclude treatment or when new vessels in the anterior chamber angle pose the threat of neovascular glaucoma. Intraretinal changes should also be considered; when they are severe in both eyes, prompt initiation of treatment in one is attractive. When macular edema is present in an eye needing scatter photocoagulation, it may be desirable to treat the edema with focal or grid photocoagulation first, if scatter treatment is not urgent.

A-2

EARLY TREATMENT DIABETIC RETINOPATHY STUDY (ETDRS)

1. Early Treatment Diabetic Retinopathy Study Research Group: Photocoagulation for diabetic macular edema. ETDRS Report Number 1. *Arch Ophthalmol* 1985;103:1796–1806. Copyright 1985, American Medical Association.
Abstract Data from the ETDRS show that focal photocoagulation of "clinically significant" diabetic macular edema substantially reduces the risk of visual loss. Focal treatment also increases the chance of visual improvement, decreases the frequency of persistent macular edema, and causes only minor visual field losses. In this randomized clinical trial, which was supported by the National Eye Institute, 754 eyes that had macular edema and mild-to-moderate diabetic retinopathy were randomly assigned to focal argon laser photocoagulation, while 1490 such eyes were randomly assigned to deferral of photocoagulation. The beneficial effects of treatment demonstrated in this trial suggest that all eyes with clinically significant diabetic macular edema should be considered for focal photocoagulation. Clinically significant macular edema is defined as retinal thickening that involves or threatens the center of the macula (even if visual acuity is not yet reduced) and is assessed by stereoscopic contact lens biomicroscopy or stereoscopic photography. Followup of all ETDRS patients continues without other modifications in the study protocol.

2. Early Treatment Diabetic Retinopathy Study Research Group: Treatment techniques and clinical guidelines for photocoagulation of diabetic macular edema. ETDRS Report Number 2. *Ophthalmology* 1987;94:761–774. Courtesy of *Ophthalmology.*

Abstract The ETDRS has recently shown that argon laser photocoagulation treatment is beneficial in reducing the risk of visual loss from clinically significant diabetic macular edema. The ETDRS treatment consisted of a combination of focal treatment to individual leaking microaneurysms and grid treatment to areas of diffuse leakage and capillary nonperfusion. These techniques are described in detail, and the concepts of "clinically significant macular edema" and "treatable lesions" are defined. Guidelines for the application of ETDRS findings to clinical practice are discussed.

3. Early Treatment Diabetic Retinopathy Study Research Group: Techniques for scatter and local photocoagulation treatment of diabetic retinopathy. ETDRS Report Number 3. *Int Ophthalmol Clin* 1987;27:254–264. Courtesy of Lippincott-Raven Publishers.

Comments ETDRS techniques for scatter and local photocoagulation evolved from those of the DRS [Diabetic Retinopathy Study], which were based on those of many previous investigators. The full scatter and local protocols presented here are, we believe, suitable whenever photocoagulation is undertaken for PDR [proliferative diabetic retinopathy] or severe NPDR [nonproliferative diabetic retinopathy]. We believe that followup treatment is important and that the clinical guidelines outlined in the protocol are suitable for widespread application.

4. Early Treatment Diabetic Retinopathy Study Research Group: Photocoagulation for diabetic macular edema. ETDRS Report Number 4. *Int Ophthalmol Clin* 1987;27:265–272. Courtesy of Lippincott-Raven Publishers.

Comments The combination of focal and grid photocoagulation used in the ETDRS led to a reduction in the occurrence of visual acuity decrease (doubling of the visual angle) by approximately 50% to 70% in eyes with retinal thickening or associated hard exudate involving or threatening the center of the macula and visual acuity of 20/200 or better. ETDRS photocoagulation for macular edema emphasized focal treatment, with attempts to close larger microaneurysms directly, and followup treatment. In applying these results to clinical practice, it is important to remember that the comparisons presented are between prompt photocoagulation and indefinite deferral of photocoagulation, regardless of the course followed. In clinical practice, the decision is between prompt photocoagulation and deferral with careful followup, with reconsideration of this decision at each visit. Factors to be taken into account include the degree to which the center of the macula in involved or threatened by thickening or hard exudate, the proximity of focal leaks requiring treatment to the center, and visual acuity. . . .

4a. Early Treatment Diabetic Retinopathy Study Research Group: Case reports to accompany Early Treatment Diabetic Retinopathy Study Reports 3 and 4. *Int Ophthalmol Clin* 1987;27: 273–333. Courtesy of Lippincott-Raven Publishers.

Summary The principles exemplified by the preceding case reports are summarized below. (**1**) Although the presence of DRS [Diabetic Retinopathy Study] high-risk characteristics is the single most important indication for initiating scatter photocoagulation, intraretinal lesions suggesting ischemia (soft exudates, IRMA [intraretinal microvascular abnormalities], venous beading, arteriolar abnormalities, and moderately severe hemorrhages and/or microaneurysms) are also important. When these lesions are severe, rapid progression is likely, and initiation of scatter photocoagulation should be considered for at least one eye, even when new vessels are absent or mild (Cases 3, 5, 9, and

11). Both eyes should be followed carefully, whether treated or not, and special attention to blood pressure and renal status may be important. When these intraretinal lesions are mostly absent or mild, progression of PDR [proliferative diabetic retinopathy] may be very slow (Cases 1, 6, and 7). (**2**) NVD [neovascularization of the disc] is the single most important prognostic feature of diabetic retinopathy, and when it is well established (ie, greater than or equal to DRS Standard Photograph 10A), the indication for initiation of scatter photocoagulation is strong (Cases 7, 8, 10, and 11). (**3**) NVE [neovascularization elsewhere] in the absence of vitreous or preretinal hemorrhage or the severe intraretinal lesions listed in item 1 are a weaker indication for photocoagulation, and careful observation of such eyes is a reasonable alternative to prompt treatment. (**4**) The *initial* vitreous or preretinal hemorrhage in eyes with PDR is rarely so large that photocoagulation cannot be carried out before a subsequent larger hemorrhage occurs, *provided patients report symptoms and are examined promptly.* In such cases it is prudent to treat the lower quadrants first, if possible, before they become obscured by hemorrhage (Cases 3 to 7 and 9 to 11). (**5**) Even after full scatter photocoagulation, with burns placed no more than one-half burn diameter apart, there is ample room for additional treatment between scars, and this often seems to be effective in encouraging regression of new vessels that remain or recur after the completion of the initial treatment. Such additional scatter treatment may be concentrated in areas of NVE (Cases 2 and 5) or applied throughout the fundus (Cases 4 and 9 to 11). Extension of scatter photocoagulation into the posterior pole also appears to be effective sometimes (Case 8). (**6**) Knowledge of the tendency for new vessels to follow a cycle of proliferation and regression is important when considering additional scatter treatment when new vessels fail to regress or recur after initial scatter treatment. With this tendency in mind, the goal of photocoagulation set for such eyes can be the more realistic one of containing new vessels rather than completely eliminating them (Cases 2, 4, and 10). With such a goal it is less likely that peripheral field will be destroyed. (**7**) Familiarity with the typical course followed by posterior vitreous detachment in eyes with PDR is also important. Prior to posterior vitreous detachment, proliferation of new vessels is paralleled by increasing vitreoretinal adhe-

sions, but this is not the case when new vessels grow along the detached posterior vitreous surface or arise from the retina in areas where the vitreous is detached. Only occasionally do sheets of new vessels and fibrous tissue capable of causing retinal distortion secondary to their contraction proliferate on the retinal surface after posterior vitreous detachment. An eye in which new vessels and fibrous proliferations are limited mostly to the detached posterior vitreous surface is at little risk of traction retinal detachment and, if severe vitreous hemorrhage occurs, is a good candidate for vitrectomy (Cases 2, 10, and 11). Small patches of new vessels are sometimes avulsed completely from the retina, and the vitreous hemorrhage accompanying this event frequently is the last to occur (Cases 5 to 7). (**8**) Elevated new vessels seem less easily influenced by scatter photocoagulation than those on the surface of the retina (Cases 2, 10, and 11). (**9**) Because the size of photocoagulation burns is influenced not only by spot size setting, but also by strength of the burns (dependent on both power and duration as well as clarity of the media), the total number of scatter burns at a specified setting is not a satisfactory measure of the amount of treatment applied (Cases 4, 5, and 8). (**10**) Narrowing of retinal vessels frequently accompanies quiescence of retinopathy (Cases 4, 5, and 7 to 9). (**11**) Strong local confluent photocoagulation of NVE may cause noticeable scotomas, including nerve fiber bundle defects (Cases 3 and 7). (**12**) There is no doubt that photocoagulation improves the outlook for maintaining visual acuity in eyes with diabetic macular edema and that, for eyes with clinically significant macular edema, prompt treatment is preferable to permanent nontreatment. But progression often is slow (Case 14, left eye), and occasionally spontaneous improvement occurs (Cases 3, 11, 16 [right eye], and 18), so that deferral of treatment and careful followup may often be a useful strategy, particularly when thickening of the center of the macula is absent or equivocal or lesions to be treated are close to it (Cases 17, 18, and 20). (**13**) In view of the adverse effect that scatter photocoagulation often has, at least temporarily, on macular edema, it may be desirable in eyes needing such treatment to carry out focal or grid treatment for macular edema be-fore (or at least concurrently with) scatter treatment (Cases 3 and 11). Note that Case 12 did well with no treatment for macular edema. (**14**) Hard exudates not infrequently increase temporarily when macular edema decreases (spontaneously or after grid or focal treatment), and this may threaten the center of the macula (Cases 11 and 16). (**15**) The ETDRS protocol emphasized careful followup after initial treatment for macular edema, with re-treatment whenever clinically significant macular edema and treatable lesions were present (Case 15). (**16**) Fluorescein leakage without retinal thickening *does not constitute* macular edema (Case 19). [Emphases in original.]

5. Early Treatment Diabetic Retinopathy Study Research Group: Detection of diabetic macular edema: ophthalmoscopy versus photography. ETDRS Report Number 5. *Ophthalmology* 1989; 96:746–751. Courtesy of *Ophthalmology*.

Abstract Clinical and photographic methods were used to assess retinopathy during the examinations of diabetic patients enrolled in the ETDRS. In analyzing available data from eyes randomly selected for deferral of treatment, the authors compare the clinical detection (including contact lens biomicroscopy) with photographic detection (30° stereoscopic color fundus photographs) of diabetic macular edema. Based on clinical detection, 53% (1778 patients) had hard exudates within 1 disc diameter (DD) of the center of the macula, 56% (1868 patients) had retinal thickening within this region, and 31% (1027 patients) had thickening at the center of the macula. These analyses show agreements of 83%, 78%, and 83% between retinal specialists and photographic graders when assessing these three characteristics, respectively. Agreement was 81% in the detection of macular edema for which treatment is indicated (clinically significant macular edema). Each method has its advantages, but in general there was close agreement between these methods, particularly for clinically significant macular edema, which supports the reliability of each method.

6. Early Treatment Diabetic Retinopathy Study Research Group: C-peptide and the classification of diabetes mellitus patients in the Early Treatment Diabetic Retinopathy Study. ETDRS Report Number 6. *Ann Epidemiol* 1993;3:9–17. Copyright 1993. Reprinted with permission from Elsevier Science.

Abstract The ETDRS, conducted at 22 clinical centers during the period 1980 to 1989, collected baseline data on C-peptide levels after ingestion of Sustacal in 582 patients with diabetes mellitus, prior to enrollment in the trial. Data on several clinical factors associated with diabetes were also collected from all 3711 enrolled patients. C-peptide data were used to develop sets of clinical criteria for the classification of ETDRS patients and to compare and contrast definitions of type of diabetes used in previous studies. The distribution of C-peptide levels was strikingly bimodal, suggesting a division of study participants into two groups—those with levels at 80 pmol/L or less and those with more than 80 pmol/L of C-peptide after Sustacal ingestion. Constellations of clinical characteristics that could serve as proxies for C-peptide level were ascertained. The result was two sets of clinically developed definitions for type of diabetes in the ETDRS. According to the more restrictive set of definitions, three groups were identified, compared to two groups using the "broad" set of definitions. Discriminant analysis was also used to classify ETDRS patients, yielding similar results. A comparison of definitions of type of diabetes used in the ETDRS and in previous studies revealed that even in the absence of C-peptide data, clinically derived definitions provided good discrimination between type 1 and type 2 diabetes.

7. Early Treatment Diabetic Retinopathy Study Research Group: Early Treatment Diabetic Retinopathy Study design and baseline patient characteristics. ETDRS Report Number 7. *Ophthalmology* 1991;98:741–756. Courtesy of *Ophthalmology*.

Abstract The ETDRS, a multicenter collaborative clinical trial supported by the National Eye Institute, was designed to assess whether argon laser photocoagulation or aspirin treatment can reduce the risk of visual loss or slow the progression of diabetic retinopathy in patients with mild-to-severe nonproliferative or early proliferative diabetic retinopathy. The 3711 patients enrolled in the ETDRS were assigned randomly to either aspirin (650 mg per day) or placebo. One eye of each patient was assigned randomly to early argon laser photocoagulation, and the other to deferral of photocoagulation. Both eyes were to be examined at least every 4 months, and photocoagulation was to be initiated in eyes assigned to deferral as soon as high-risk proliferative retinopathy was detected. Examination of a large number of baseline ocular and patient characteristics indicated that there were no important differences between randomized treatment groups at baseline.

8. Early Treatment Diabetic Retinopathy Study Research Group: Effects of aspirin treatment on diabetic retinopathy. ETDRS Report Number 8. *Ophthalmology* 1991;98:757–765. Courtesy of *Ophthalmology.*

Abstract Aspirin treatment did not alter the course of diabetic retinopathy in patients enrolled in the ETDRS. In this randomized clinical trial supported by the National Eye Institute, 3711 patients with mild-to-severe nonproliferative or early proliferative diabetic retinopathy were assigned randomly to either aspirin (650 mg per day) or placebo. Aspirin did not prevent the development of high-risk proliferative retinopathy and did not reduce the risk of visual loss, nor did it increase the risk of vitreous hemorrhage. This was true both for eyes assigned randomly to deferral of photocoagulation and for eyes assigned randomly to early argon laser photocoagulation. The ETDRS results indicate that for patients with mild-to-severe nonproliferative or early proliferative diabetic retinopathy, it is likely that aspirin has no clinically important beneficial effects on the progression of retinopathy. The data also show that aspirin 650 mg per day had no clinically important harmful effects for diabetic patients with retinopathy. These findings suggest there are no ocular contraindications to aspirin when required for cardiovascular disease or other medical indications.

9. Early Treatment Diabetic Retinopathy Study Research Group: Early photocoagulation for diabetic retinopathy. ETDRS Report Number 9. *Ophthalmology* 1991;98:766–785. Courtesy of *Ophthalmology.*

Abstract The ETDRS enrolled 3711 patients with mild-to-severe nonproliferative or early proliferative diabetic retinopathy in both eyes. One eye of each patient was assigned randomly to early photocoagulation, and the other to deferral of photocoagulation. Followup examinations were scheduled at least every 4 months, and photocoagulation was initiated in eyes assigned to deferral as soon as high-risk proliferative retinopathy was detected. Eyes selected for early photocoagulation received one of four different combinations of scatter (panretinal) and focal treatment. This early treatment, compared with deferral of photocoagulation, was associated with a small reduction in the incidence of severe visual loss (visual acuity less than 5/200 at two consecutive visits), but 5-year rates were low in both the early treatment and the deferral groups (2.6% and 3.7%, respectively). Adverse effects of scatter photocoagulation on visual acuity and visual field also were observed. These adverse effects were most evident in the months immediately following treatment and were less in eyes assigned to less extensive scatter photocoagulation. Provided careful followup can be maintained, scatter photocoagulation is not recommended for eyes with mild or moderate nonproliferative diabetic retinopathy. When retinopathy is more severe, scatter photocoagulation should be considered and usually should not be delayed if the eye has reached the high-risk proliferative stage. The ETDRS results demonstrate that, for eyes with macular edema, focal photocoagulation is effective in reducing the risk of moderate visual loss, but that scatter photocoagulation is not. Focal treatment also increases the chance of visual improvement, decreases the frequency of persistent macular edema, and causes only minor visual field losses. Focal treatment should be considered for eyes with macular edema that involves or threatens the center of the macula.

10. Early Treatment Diabetic Retinopathy Study Research Group: Grading diabetic retinopathy from stereoscopic color fundus photographs: an extension of the modified Airlie House classification. ETDRS Report Number 10. *Ophthalmology* 1991;98:786–806. Courtesy of *Ophthalmology.*

Abstract The modified Airlie House classification of diabetic retinopathy has been extended for use in the ETDRS. The revised classification provides additional steps in the grading scale for some characteristics, separates other characteristics previously combined, expands the section on macular edema, and adds several characteristics not previously graded. The classification is described and illustrated, and its reproducibility between graders is assessed by calculating percentages of agreement and kappa statistics for duplicate gradings of baseline color nonsimultaneous stereoscopic fundus photographs. For retinal hemorrhages and/or microaneurysms, hard exudates, new vessels, fibrous proliferations, and macular edema, agreement was substantial (weighted kappa: 0.61 to 0.80). For soft exudates, intraretinal microvascular abnormalities, and venous beading, agreement was moderate (weighted kappa: 0.41 to 0.60). A double grading system, with adjudication of disagreements of two or more steps between duplicate gradings, led to some improvement in reproducibility for most characteristics.

11. Early Treatment Diabetic Retinopathy Study Research Group: Classification of diabetic retinopathy from fluorescein angiograms. ETDRS Report Number 11. *Ophthalmology* 1991;98: 807–822. Courtesy of *Ophthalmology*.

Abstract The ETDRS included use of nonsimultaneous stereoscopic fluorescein angiography to assess severity of characteristics such as capillary loss and fluorescein leakage and to guide treatment of macular edema. Two 30° photographic fields were taken, extending along the horizontal meridian from about 25° nasal to the disc to about 20° temporal to the macula, and a classification system was constructed to allow assessment of selected characteristics. This classification system relies on comparisons with standard and example photographs to evaluate the presence and severity of capillary loss and dilation, arteriolar abnormalities, leakage of fluorescein dye (including characterization of source), abnormalities of the retinal pigment epithelium, cystoid changes, and several other features. The classification is described and illustrated, and its reproducibility between graders assessed by calculating percentages of agreement and kappa statistics for duplicate gradings of baseline angiograms. Agreement was substantial (weighted kappa: 0.61 to 0,80) for severity of fluorescein leakage and cystoid spaces, and moderate (weighted kappa: 0.41 to 0.60) for capillary loss, capillary dilation, narrowing/pruning of arteriolar side branches, staining of arteriolar walls, and source of fluorescein leakage (microaneurysms versus diffusely leaking capillaries).

12. Early Treatment Diabetic Retinopathy Study Research Group: Fundus photographic risk factors for progression of diabetic retinopathy. ETDRS Report Number 12. *Ophthalmology* 1991;98:823–833. Courtesy of *Ophthalmology*.

Abstract In the ETDRS, a randomized clinical trial sponsored by the National Eye Institute, one eye of each patient was assigned to early photocoagulation and the other to deferral of photocoagulation (ie, careful followup and initiation of photocoagulation only if high-risk proliferative retinopathy developed). This design allowed observation of the natural course of diabetic retinopathy in the initially untreated eye. Gradings of baseline stereoscopic fundus photographs of eyes with nonproliferative retinopathy assigned to deferral of photocoagulation were used to examine the power of various abnormalities and combinations of abnormalities to predict progression to proliferative retinopathy in photographs taken at the 1-, 3-, and 5-year followup visits. Severity of intraretinal microvascular abnormalities, hemorrhages and/or microaneurysms, and venous beading were found to be the most important factors in predicting progression. On the basis of these analyses and other considerations, a retinopathy severity scale was developed. This scale, which divides diabetic retinopathy into 13 levels ranging from absence of retinopathy to severe vitreous hemorrhage, can be used to describe overall retinopathy severity and change in severity over time.

13. Early Treatment Diabetic Retinopathy Study Research Group: Fluorescein angiographic risk factors for progression of diabetic retinopathy. ETDRS Report Number 13. *Ophthalmology* 1991; 98:834–840. Courtesy of *Ophthalmology*.

Abstract In the ETDRS, a multicenter clinical trial sponsored by the National Eye Institute, one eye of each patient was assigned randomly to early photocoagulation and the other to deferral of photocoagulation (ie, careful followup and initiation of photocoagulation only if high-risk proliferative retinopathy developed). This design allowed observation of the natural course of diabetic retinopathy in the initially untreated eye. Gradings of baseline stereoscopic fluorescein angiograms of these eyes were used to examine relationships of angiographic characteristics with each other, with retinopathy severity level and macular edema status graded from color photographs, and with risk of progression from nonproliferative to proliferative retinopathy during 1 to 5 years of followup. Fluorescein leakage (particularly diffuse), capillary loss and dilation, and various arteriolar abnormalities were associated with retinopathy severity and with the likelihood of progression to proliferative retinopathy during followup. Severity of fluorescein leakage was strongly associated with macular edema.

14. Early Treatment Diabetic Retinopathy Study Research Group: Aspirin effects on mortality and morbidity in patients with diabetes mellitus. ETDRS Report Number 14. *J Am Med Assn* 1992; 268:1292–1300. Copyright 1992, American Medical Association.

Abstract *Objectives:* This report presents information on the effects of aspirin on mortality, the occurrence of cardiovascular events, and the incidence of kidney disease in the patients enrolled in the ETDRS. *Study design:* This multicenter, randomized clinical trial of aspirin versus placebo was sponsored by the National Eye Institute. *Patients:* Patients (N = 3711) were enrolled in 22 clinical centers between April 1980 and July 1985. Men and women between the ages of 18 and 70 years with a clinical diagnosis of diabetes mellitus were eligible. Approximately 30% of all patients were considered to have type 1 diabetes mellitus, 31% type 2, and in 39% type 1 or 2 could not be determined definitely. *Intervention:* Patients were randomly assigned to aspirin or placebo (two 325-mg tablets once per day). *Main outcome measures:* Mortality from all causes was specified as the primary outcome measure for assessing the systemic effects of aspirin. Other outcome variables included cause-specific mortality and cardiovascular events. *Results:* The estimate of relative risk for total mortality for aspirin-treated patients compared with placebo-treated patients for the entire study period was 0.91 (99% confidence interval: 0.75 to 1.11). Larger differences were noted for the occurrence of fatal and nonfatal myocardial infarction; the estimate of relative risk was 0.83 for the entire followup period (99% confidence interval: 0.66 to 1.04). *Conclusions:* The effects of aspirin on any of the cardiovascular events considered in the ETDRS were not substantially different from the effects observed in other studies that included mainly nondiabetic persons. Furthermore, there was no evidence of harmful effects of aspirin. Aspirin has been recommended previously for persons at risk for cardiovascular disease. The ETDRS results support application of this recommendation to those persons with diabetes at increased risk of cardiovascular disease.

15. Early Treatment Diabetic Retinopathy Study Research Group: Impaired color vision associated with diabetic retinopathy. ETDRS Report Number 15. *Am J Ophthalmol* 1999;128:612–617. Copyright 1999. Reprinted with permission from Elsevier Science.

Abstract *Purpose:* To report color vision abnormalities associated with diabetic retinopathy. *Methods:* Color vision function was measured at baseline in 2701 patients enrolled in the ETDRS, a randomized trial investigating photocoagulation and aspirin in the treatment of diabetic retinopathy. Hue discrimination was measured by the Farnsworth-Munsell 100-Hue test, and errors in color vision were reported as the square root of the total 100-Hue (SQRT 100-Hue) score. *Results:* Approximately 50% of the ETDRS population had color vision scores (SQRT 100-Hue score) worse than 95% of the normal population reported by Verriest and associates. The factors most strongly associated with impaired hue discrimination were macular edema severity, age, and presence of new vessels. A tritan-like defect was prominent and increased in magnitude with increasing severity of macular edema. However, many patients had color discrimination impairment without macular edema. *Conclusions:* Impaired color vision is a common observation among participants enrolled in the ETDRS. Compared with published data on normal subjects, approximately 50% of the patients in the ETDRS had abnormal hue discrimination. Macular edema severity, age, and presence of new vessels were the factors most strongly associated with impaired color discrimination. A titan-like defect was prominent and increased in magnitude with increasing severity of macular edema. Impaired color vision should be considered in the evaluation and counseling of patients with diabetic retinopathy.

16. Early Treatment Diabetic Retinopathy Study Research Group: Aspirin effects on the development of cataracts in patients with diabetes mellitus. ETDRS Report Number 16. *Arch Ophthalmol* 1992;110:339–342. Copyright 1992, American Medical Association.

Abstract The ETDRS, a randomized clinical trial supported by the National Eye Institute, was designed to assess the effect of photocoagulation and aspirin in 3711 patients with mild-to-severe nonproliferative or early proliferative diabetic retinopathy. Although the primary goal of the study was to evaluate the effect of photocoagulation and aspirin on diabetic retinopathy, the study also provided an opportunity to evaluate the effects of aspirin on the development of cataract. No evidence showed that aspirin use reduced the risk of development of cataract requiring extraction (4.1% versus 4.3% in patients assigned to aspirin or placebo treatment, respectively; Mantel-Cox $P = .77$; relative risk: 1.05; 99% confidence interval: 0.73 to 1.51). Aspirin use also did not reduce the risk of less extensive but visually significant lens opacities developing (29.6% versus 28.3%; Mantel-Cox $P = .76$; relative risk: 0.99; 99% confidence interval: 0.85 to 1.15). ETDRS results do not support the hypothesis that aspirin (at a dose of 650 mg per day) reduces the risk of cataract development in this diabetic population.

17. Early Treatment Diabetic Retinopathy Study Research Group: Pars plana vitrectomy in the Early Treatment Diabetic Retinopathy Study. ETDRS Report Number 17. *Ophthalmology* 1992;99:1351–1357. Courtesy of *Ophthalmology*.

Abstract *Background:* The ETDRS enrolled 3711 patients with mild-to-severe nonproliferative or early proliferative diabetic retinopathy in both eyes. Patients were randomly assigned to aspirin 650 mg per day or placebo. One eye of each patient was assigned randomly to early photocoagulation, and the other to deferral of photocoagulation. Followup examinations were scheduled at least every 4 months, and photocoagulation was initiated in eyes assigned to deferral as soon as high-risk proliferative retinopathy was detected. Aspirin was not found to have an effect on retinopathy progression or rates of vitreous hemorrhage. The risk of a combined end point, severe visual loss or vitrectomy, was low in eyes assigned to deferral (6% at 5 years) and was reduced by early photocoagulation (4% at 5 years). Vitrectomy was carried out in 208 patients during the 9 years of the study. This report presents baseline and previtrectomy characteristics and visual outcome in these patients. *Methods:* Information collected at baseline and during followup as part of the ETDRS protocol was supplemented by review of clinic charts for visual acuity and ocular status immediately before vitrectomy. *Results:* Vitrectomy was performed in 208 (5.6%) of the 3711 patients (243 eyes) enrolled in the ETDRS. The 5-year vitrectomy rates for eyes grouped by their initial photocoagulation assignment were as follows: 2.1% in the early full scatter photocoagulation group, 2.5% in the early mild scatter group, and 4.0% in the deferral group. The 5-year rates of vitrectomy (in one or both eyes) were 5.4% in patients assigned to aspirin and 5.2% in patients assigned to a placebo. The indications for vitrectomy were either vitreous hemorrhage (53.9%) or retinal detachment with or without vitreous hemorrhage (46.1%). Before vitrectomy, visual acuity was 5/200 or worse in 66.7% of eyes and better than 20/100 in 6.2%. One year after vitrectomy, the visual acuity was 20/100 or better in 47.6% of eyes, including 24.0% with visual acuity of 20/40 or better. *Conclusions:* With frequent followup examinations and timely scatter (panretinal) photocoagulation, the 5-year cumulative rate of pars plana vitrectomy in ETDRS patients was 5.3%. Aspirin use did not influence the rate of vitrectomy.

18. Early Treatment Diabetic Retinopathy Study Research Group: Risk factors for high-risk proliferative diabetic retinopathy and severe visual loss. ETDRS Report Number 18. *Invest Ophthalmol Vis Sci* 1998;39:233–252. Copyright 1998, Association for Research in Vision and Ophthalmology.

Abstract *Purpose:* To identify risk factors for the development of high-risk proliferative diabetic retinopathy (PDR) and for the development of severe visual loss or vitrectomy (SVLV) in eyes assigned to deferral of photocoagulation in the ETDRS. *Methods:* Multivariable Cox models were constructed to evaluate the strength and statistical significance of baseline risk factors for development of high-risk PDR and of SVLV. *Results:* The baseline characteristics identified as risk factors for high-risk PDR were increased severity of retinopathy, decreased visual acuity (or increased extent of macular edema), higher glycosylated hemoglobin, history of diabetic neuropathy, lower hematocrit, elevated triglycerides, lower serum albumin, and, in persons with mild-to-moderate nonproliferative retinopathy, younger age (or type 1 diabetes). The predominant risk factor for development of SVLV was the prior development of high-risk PDR. The only other clearly significant factor was decreased visual acuity at baseline. In the eyes that developed SVLV before high-risk proliferative retinopathy was observed, baseline risk factors were decreased visual acuity (or increased extent of macular edema), older age (or type 2 diabetes), and female gender. *Conclusions:* These analyses supported the view that the retinopathy-inhibiting effect of better glycemic control extends across all ages, both diabetes types, and all stages of retinopathy up to and including the severe nonproliferative and early proliferative stages and the possibility that reducing elevated blood lipids and treating anemia slow the progression of retinopathy.

19. Early Treatment Diabetic Retinopathy Study Research Group: Focal photocoagulation treatment of diabetic macular edema: relationship of treatment effect to fluorescein angiographic and other retinal characteristics at baseline. ETDRS Report Number 19. *Arch Ophthalmol* 1995;113: 1144–1155. Copyright 1995, American Medical Association.

Abstract *Objective:* To determine whether the efficacy of photocoagulation treatment of diabetic macular edema may be influenced by degree of capillary closure, severity or source of fluorescein leakage, extent of retinal edema, presence of cystoid changes, or severity of hard exudates. *Patients:* Patients with mild-to-moderate nonproliferative diabetic retinopathy and macular edema definitely or questionably involving the center of the macula. *Design:* One eye of each patient was assigned to early photocoagulation; the other was assigned to deferral of photocoagulation, with followup visits scheduled every 4 months and photocoagulation to be carried out promptly if high-risk proliferative retinopathy developed. In this report, the beneficial effect of photocoagulation was examined in subgroups defined by severity of the characteristics specified above. *Results:* We found no subgroup in which eyes that were assigned to immediate focal treatment had a less favorable visual acuity outcome than those that were assigned to deferral (ie, no qualitative interaction). *Conclusions:* Focal photocoagulation should be considered for eyes with clinically significant macular edema, particularly when the center of the macula is involved or imminently threatened. Trends for treatment effect to be less in eyes with less extensive retinal thickening and less thickening at the center of the macula support our previous recommendation that, for such eyes, an initial period of close observation may be preferable to immediate treatment, particularly when most of the leakage to be treated arises close to the center of the macula, increasing the risk of damage to it from direct treatment or subsequent migration of treatment scars.

20. Early Treatment Diabetic Retinopathy Study Research Group: Effects of aspirin on vitreous/preretinal hemorrhage in patients with diabetes mellitus. ETDRS Report Number 20. *Arch Ophthalmol* 1995;113:52–55. Copyright 1995, American Medical Association.

Abstract *Objective:* To assess whether the use of aspirin exacerbates the severity or duration of vitreous/preretinal hemorrhages in patients with diabetic retinopathy. *Design:* The ETDRS, a multicenter randomized clinical trial, was designed to assess the effect of photocoagulation and aspirin on 3711 patients with mild-to-severe nonproliferative or early proliferative diabetic retinopathy. *Intervention:* Patients were randomly assigned to either an aspirin (650 mg per day) or a placebo group. One eye of each patient was randomly assigned to early photocoagulation, and the other to deferral of photocoagulation. *Main outcome measures:* The severity and duration of the vitreous/preretinal hemorrhages were determined from gradings of the annual, seven standard stereoscopic field, fundus photographs. Clinical examinations scheduled every 4 months also provided information on the presence and duration of hemorrhages. *Results:* Annual fundus photographs of eyes assigned to deferral of photocoagulation revealed vitreous/preretinal hemorrhages at some time during followup in 564 patients (30%) assigned to the placebo group and 585 patients (32%) assigned to the aspirin group ($P = .48$). Based on gradings of fundus photographs, there were no statistical differences in the severity of vitreous/preretinal hemorrhages ($P = .11$) or their rate of resolution ($P = .86$) between the groups. Clinical examination of eyes assigned to deferral of photocoagulation revealed that 721 eyes (39%) assigned to the aspirin group and 689 (37%) assigned to the placebo group had vitreous/preretinal hemorrhages during the course of the study ($P = .30$). Again, no statistically significant difference was found between the rates of resolution, as assessed clinically, between the two treatment groups ($P = .43$). *Conclusions:* As previously reported, the use of aspirin did not increase the occurrence of vitreous/preretinal hemorrhages in patients enrolled in the ETDRS. The data presented in this report demonstrate that the severity and duration of these hemorrhages were not significantly affected by the use of aspirin and that there were no ocular contraindications to its use (650 mg per day) in persons with diabetes who require it for treatment of cardiovascular disease or for other medical indications.

21. Early Treatment Diabetic Retinopathy Study Research Group: Accommodative amplitudes in the Early Treatment Diabetic Retinopathy Study. ETDRS Report Number 21. *Retina* 1995; 15:275–281. Courtesy of Lippincott-Raven Publishers.

Abstract *Purpose:* Accommodative amplitude in persons with diabetes was investigated using data collected as part of the ETDRS. *Methods:* Accommodative amplitude was measured at the baseline visit in 1058 patients who had good visual acuity and who were less than 46 years old. Risk factors for low accommodative amplitude at baseline were evaluated using multivariable linear regression. Change in accommodative amplitude after photocoagulation was evaluated using paired *t* tests and repeated measures analysis of variance for the 578 patients who underwent followup measurements at the 4-month visit. *Results:* Accommodative amplitudes in ETDRS patients were lower than normal accommodative amplitudes. Older age ($P < 0.001$) and increased duration of diabetes ($P < 0.01$) were risk factors associated with low amplitudes of accommodation in the ETDRS. Full scatter photocoagulation was associated with an apparently transient additional reduction in accommodative amplitude; a one-third diopter loss in accommodative amplitude was demonstrated only at the 4-month visit ($P < 0.001$). *Conclusion:* This study demonstrates that diabetes and duration of diabetes, along with age, are important risk factors for reduced accommodative amplitude. These factors, along with an apparently transient decrease in accommodative amplitude following scatter photocoagulation, should be considered when assessing the accommodative needs of patients with diabetes and when discussing side effects of full scatter photocoagulation.

22. Early Treatment Diabetic Retinopathy Study Research Group: Association of elevated serum lipid levels with retinal hard exudate in diabetic retinopathy. ETDRS Report Number 22. *Arch Ophthalmol* 1996;114:1079–1084. Copyright 1996, American Medical Association.

Abstract *Objective:* To evaluate the relationship between serum lipid levels, retinal hard exudate, and visual acuity in patients with diabetic retinopathy. *Design:* Observational data from the ETDRS. *Participants:* Of the 3711 patients enrolled in the ETDRS, the first 2709 enrolled had serum lipid levels measured. *Main outcome measures:* Baseline fasting serum lipid levels, best-corrected visual acuity, and assessment of retinal thickening and hard exudate from stereoscopic macular photographs. *Results:* Patients with elevated total serum cholesterol levels or serum low-density lipoprotein cholesterol levels at baseline were twice as likely to have retinal hard exudates as patients with normal levels. These patients were also at higher risk of developing hard exudate during the course of the study. The risk of losing visual acuity was associated with the extent of hard exudate even after adjusting for the extent of macular edema. *Conclusions:* These data demonstrate that elevated serum lipid levels are associated with an increased risk of retinal hard exudate in persons with diabetic retinopathy. Although retinal hard exudate usually accompanies diabetic macular edema, increasing amounts of exudate appear to be independently associated with an increased risk of visual impairment. Lowering elevated serum lipid levels has been shown to decrease the risk of cardiovascular morbidity. The observational data from the ETDRS suggest that lipid lowering may also decrease the risk of hard exudate formation and associated vision loss in patients with diabetic retinopathy. Preservation of vision may be an additional motivating factor for lowering serum lipid levels in persons with diabetic retinopathy and elevated serum lipid levels.

23. Early Treatment Diabetic Retinopathy Study Research Group: Subretinal fibrosis in diabetic macular edema. ETDRS Report Number 23. *Arch Ophthalmol* 1997;115:873–877. Copyright 1997, American Medical Association.

Abstract *Objective:* To describe the characteristics of and risk factors for subretinal fibrosis (SRF) in patients with diabetic macular edema. *Patients and methods:* A total of 109 eyes (in 96 persons) with SRF, defined as a mound or sheet of gray-to-white tissue beneath the retina at or near the center of the macula, were identified during the ETDRS, which is a randomized clinical trial of photocoagulation and aspirin treatment in patients with mild-to-severe nonproliferative or early proliferative diabetic retinopathy. The patients and the ocular characteristics of these 109 eyes, all of which had clinically significant macular edema, were compared with those of 5653 eyes in which clinically significant macular edema, but not SRF, was observed during the trial. *Results:* In 9 of 109 eyes, the development of SRF may have been directly related to focal photocoagulation. Seventy-four percent of the eyes in which SRF developed had very severe hard exudates in the macula prior to the development of SRF, while this level of hard exudates was seen in only 2.5% of the eyes with clinically significant macular edema in which SRF did not develop ($P <.001$). Of the 264 eyes with this level of hard exudates at baseline (N = 29) or during followup (N = 235), SRF developed in 30.7% of the eyes, while this complication developed in only 0.05% of 5498 eyes with clinically significant macular edema without this level of hard exudates. *Conclusions:* Subretinal fibrosis is an infrequent complication of diabetic macular edema. Although it has been reported to be associated with photocoagulation burn intensity, in only 9 of 109 eyes in which SRF developed was it located adjacent to a photocoagulation-related scar (among 4823 eyes that received focal photocoagulation for treatment of macular edema). The strongest risk factor for the development of SRF is very severe hard exudate.

24. Early Treatment Diabetic Retinopathy Study Research Group: Causes of severe visual loss in the Early Treatment Diabetic Retinopathy Study. ETDRS Report Number 24. *Am J Ophthalmol* 1999;127:137–141. Copyright 1999. Reprinted with permission from Elsevier Science.

Abstract *Purpose:* To describe the causes of and risk factors for persistent severe visual loss occurring in the ETDRS. *Methods:* The ETDRS was a randomized clinical trial investigating photocoagulation and aspirin in 3711 persons with mild-to-severe nonproliferative or early proliferative diabetic retinopathy. Severe visual loss, defined as best-corrected visual acuity of less than 5/200 on at least two consecutive 4-month followup visits, developed in 257 eyes (219 persons). Of these 257 eyes, 149 (127 persons) did not recover to 5/200 or better at any visit (persistent severe visual loss). Ocular characteristics of these eyes were compared with those of eyes with severe visual loss that improved to 5/200 or better at any subsequent visit. Characteristics of patients with severe visual loss that did and did not improve and those without severe visual loss were also compared. *Results:* Severe visual loss that persisted developed in 149 eyes of 127 persons. In order of decreasing frequency, reasons recorded for persistent visual loss included vitreous or preretinal hemorrhage, macular edema or macular pigmentary changes related to macular edema, macular or retinal detachment, and neovascular glaucoma. Compared with all patients without persistent severe visual loss, patients with persistent severe visual loss had higher mean levels of hemoglobin A_{1c} (10.4% versus 9.7%; $P = .001$) and higher levels of cholesterol (244.1 versus 228.5 mg/dL; $P = .0081$) at baseline. Otherwise, patients with persistent severe visual loss were similar to patients with severe visual loss that improved and to those without severe visual loss. *Conclusions:* Persistent severe visual loss was an infrequent occurrence in the ETDRS. Its leading cause was vitreous or preretinal hemorrhage, followed by macular edema or macular pigmentary changes related to macular edema and retinal detachment. The low frequency of persistent severe visual loss in the ETDRS is most likely related to the nearly universal intervention with scatter photocoagulation (either before or soon after high-risk proliferative diabetic retinopathy developed) and the intervention with vitreous surgery when clinically indicated.

25. Early Treatment Diabetic Retinopathy Study Research Group: Results after lens extraction in patients with diabetic retinopathy. ETDRS Report Number 25. *Arch Ophthalmol* 1999;117: 1600–1606.

Abstract was published as the monograph was going to press. For a discussion, see page 206.

For a discussion, see page 206.

A-3

DIABETIC RETINOPATHY VITRECTOMY STUDY (DRVS)

1. Diabetic Retinopathy Vitrectomy Study Research Group: Two-year course of visual acuity in severe proliferative diabetic retinopathy with conventional management. DRVS Report Number 1. *Ophthalmology* 1985;92:492–502. Courtesy of *Ophthalmology*.

Abstract Seven hundred forty-four eyes with very severe proliferative diabetic retinopathy (PDR) were followed with conventional management over a 2-year period. Decreases in visual acuity were more frequent during the first year of followup than during the second, and were related to baseline visual acuity level and retinopathy severity. After 2 years, visual acuity was less than 5/200 in 45% of eyes with more than 4 disc areas of new vessels and visual acuity of 10/30 to 10/50 at baseline, but in only 14% of eyes with traction retinal detachment not involving the center of the macula and without active new vessels or fresh vitreous hemorrhage at baseline. Vitrectomy, which was undertaken only if retinal detachment involving the center of the macula occurred or if severe vitreous hemorrhage failed to clear after a 1-year waiting period, had been carried out in 25% of eyes after 2 years of followup.

2. Diabetic Retinopathy Vitrectomy Study Research Group: Early vitrectomy for severe vitreous hemorrhage in diabetic retinopathy: two-year results of a randomized trial. DRVS Report Number 2. *Arch Ophthalmol* 1985;103:1644–1652. Copyright 1985, American Medical Association.

Abstract Six hundred sixteen eyes with recent severe diabetic vitreous hemorrhage reducing visual acuity to 5/200 or less for at least 1 month were randomly assigned to either early vitrectomy or deferral of vitrectomy for 1 year. After 2 years of followup, 25% of the early vitrectomy group had visual acuity of 10/20 or better compared with 15% in the deferral group (*P* = .01). In patients with type 1 diabetes, who were on the average younger and had more severe proliferative retinopathy, there was a clear-cut advantage for early vitrectomy, as reflected in the percentage of eyes recovering visual acuity of 10/20 or better (36% versus 12% in the deferral group, *P* = .0001). No such advantage was found in the type 2 diabetes group (16% in the early group versus 18% in the deferral group), but evidence that this advantage differed by diabetes type was of borderline significance.

3. Diabetic Retinopathy Vitrectomy Study Research Group: Early vitrectomy for severe proliferative diabetic retinopathy in eyes with useful vision: results of a randomized trial. DRVS Report Number 3. *Ophthalmology* 1988;95:1307–1320. Courtesy of *Ophthalmology.*

Abstract Three hundred seventy eyes with advanced, active, proliferative diabetic retinopathy (PDR) and visual acuity of 10/200 or better were randomly assigned to either early vitrectomy or conventional management. After 4 years of followup, the percentage of eyes with a visual acuity of 10/20 or better was 44% in the early vitrectomy group and 28% in the conventional management group. The proportion with very poor visual outcome was similar in the two groups. The advantage of early vitrectomy tended to increase with increasing severity of new vessels. In the group with the least severe new vessels, no advantage of early vitrectomy was apparent.

4. Diabetic Retinopathy Vitrectomy Study Research Group: Early vitrectomy for severe proliferative diabetic retinopathy in eyes with useful vision: clinical application of results of a randomized trial. DRVS Report Number 4. *Ophthalmology* 1988;95:1321–1334. Courtesy of *Ophthalmology.*

Abstract Six patients are described, each of whom underwent early vitrectomy for advanced, active, proliferative diabetic retinopathy (PDR) in an eye with useful vision. These cases were selected to illustrate the spectrum of retinopathy severity for which early vitrectomy should be considered and the favorable outcome that can follow this procedure. None of the eyes that had an unfavorable result after early vitrectomy is presented. The eyes most suitable for early vitrectomy are those in which both fibrous proliferations and at least moderately severe new vessels are present, and in which extensive scatter photocoagulation has already been carried out or is precluded by vitreous hemorrhage.

5. Diabetic Retinopathy Vitrectomy Study Research Group: Early vitrectomy for severe vitreous hemorrhage in diabetic retinopathy: four-year results of a randomized trial. DRVS Report Number 5. *Arch Ophthalmol* 1990;108:958–964. Published erratum appears in *Arch Ophthalmol* 1990;108:1452. Copyright 1990, American Medical Association.

Abstract Six hundred sixteen eyes with recent severe diabetic vitreous hemorrhage reducing visual acuity to 5/200 or less for at least 1 month were randomly assigned to either early vitrectomy or deferral of vitrectomy for 1 year. The proportion of eyes with visual acuity of 10/20 or better was higher in the early vitrectomy group than in the deferral group throughout the 4-year followup period. Up to the 18-month visit, the early group had a higher proportion of eyes with visual acuity of no light perception. An increased chance of obtaining good vision with early vitrectomy was clearly present in the type 1 diabetes group, particularly in patients who developed severe vitreous hemorrhage after less than 20 years of diabetes, a patient group tending to have more severe proliferative retinopathy. This advantage was not found in the type 2 diabetes group, in which patients were older and tended to have less severe retinopathy. The findings of this and previous DRVS reports support early vitrectomy in eyes known or suspected to have very severe proliferative diabetic retinopathy as a means of increasing the chance of restoring or maintaining good vision.

A-4

DIABETES CONTROL AND COMPLICATIONS TRIAL (DCCT)

1. Diabetes Control and Complications Trial Research Group: Color photography vs fluorescein angiography in the detection of diabetic retinopathy in the Diabetes Control and Complications Trial. *Arch Ophthalmol* 1987;105: 1344–1351. Copyright 1987, American Medical Association.

Abstract During eligibility screening for the DCCT, we compared stereoscopic color fundus photography and stereoscopic fluorescein angiography in the detection of diabetic retinopathy in 320 patients (mean age: 24 years [SD: 8 years]) with insulin-dependent diabetes (mean duration: 7 years [SD: 4 years]) and no or mild diabetic retinopathy. Of 153 patients classified as having no retinopathy according to color photographs of seven standard 30° fields of both eyes, 21% of the patients had evidence of retinopathy (mostly one or two microaneurysms in one eye) on review of fluorescein angiograms, including two standard 30° fields in each eye. Of those patients with no retinopathy detected on angiograms, 19% had retinopathy on review of color photographs. When used in conjunction with color photography, angiography allows a modest increase in sensitivity to the earliest signs of retinopathy, a gain potentially useful in some research applications, although not of demonstrated value in patient management.

2. Diabetes Control and Complications Trial Research Group: The effect of intensive treatment of diabetes on the development and progression of long-term complications in insulin-dependent diabetes mellitus. *N Engl J Med* 1993;329:977–986. Copyright © 1993, Massachusetts Medical Society. All rights reserved.

Abstract *Background:* Long-term microvascular and neurologic complications cause major morbidity and mortality in patients with insulin-dependent diabetes mellitus (IDDM). We examined whether intensive treatment with the goal of maintaining blood glucose concentrations close to the normal range could decrease the frequency and severity of these complications. *Methods:* A total of 1441 patients with IDDM—726 with no retinopathy at baseline (the primary-prevention cohort) and 715 with mild retinopathy (the secondary-intervention cohort)—were randomly assigned to intensive therapy administered either with an external insulin pump or by three or more daily insulin injections and guided by frequent blood glucose monitoring or to conventional therapy with one or two daily insulin injections. The patients were followed for a mean of 6.5 years, and the appearance and progression of retinopathy and other complications were assessed regularly. *Results:* In the primary-prevention cohort, intensive therapy reduced the adjusted mean risk for the development of retinopathy by 76% (95% confidence interval: 62% to 85%), as compared with conventional therapy. In the secondary-intervention cohort, intensive therapy slowed the progression of retinopathy by 54% (95% confidence interval: 39% to 66%) and reduced the development of proliferative or severe nonproliferative retinopathy by 47% (95% confidence interval: 14% to 67%). In the two cohorts combined, intensive therapy reduced the occurrence of microalbuminuria (urinary albumin excretion of ≥ 40 mg per 24 hours) by 39% (95% confidence interval: 21% to 52%), that of albuminuria (urinary albumin excretion of ≥ 300 mg per 24 hours) by 54% (95% confidence interval: 19% to 74%), and that of clinical neuropathy by 60% (95% confidence interval: 38% to 74%). The chief adverse event associated with intensive therapy was a 2- to 3-fold increase in severe hypoglycemia. *Conclusions:* Intensive therapy effectively delays the onset and slows the progression of diabetic retinopathy, nephropathy, and neuropathy in patients with IDDM.

3. Diabetes Control and Complications Trial Research Group: Effect of intensive diabetes treatment on the development and progression of long-term complications in adolescents with insulin-dependent diabetes mellitus: Diabetes Control and Complications Trial. *J Pediatr* 1994; 125:177–188. Reproduced with permission from Mosby–Year Book, Inc.

Abstract The DCCT has demonstrated that intensive diabetes treatment delays the onset and slows the progression of diabetic complications in subjects with insulin-dependent diabetes mellitus from 13 to 39 years of age. We examined whether the effects of such treatment also occurred in the subset of young diabetic subjects (13 to 17 years of age at entry) in the DCCT. One hundred twenty-five adolescent subjects with insulin-dependent diabetes mellitus but with no retinopathy at baseline (primary-prevention cohort) and 70 adolescent subjects with mild retinopathy (secondary-intervention cohort) were randomly assigned to receive either (**1**) intensive therapy with an external insulin pump or at least three daily insulin injections, together with frequent daily blood-glucose monitoring, or (**2**) conventional therapy with one or two daily insulin injections and once-daily monitoring. Subjects were followed for a mean of 7.4 years (4 to 9 years). In the primary-prevention cohort, intensive therapy decreased the risk of having retinopathy by 53% (95% confidence interval: 1% to 78%; $P = 0.048$) in comparison with conventional therapy. In the secondary-intervention cohort, intensive therapy decreased the risk of retinopathy progression by 70% (95% confidence interval: 25% to 88%; $P = 0.010$) and the occurrence of microalbuminuria by 55% (95% confidence interval: 3% to 79%; $P = 0.042$). Motor and sensory nerve conduction velocities were faster in intensively treated subjects. The major adverse event with intensive therapy was a nearly 3-fold increase of severe hypoglycemia. We conclude that intensive therapy effectively delays the onset and slows the progression of diabetic retinopathy and nephropathy when initiated in adolescent subjects; the benefits outweigh the increased risk of hypoglycemia that accompanies such treatment.

4. Diabetes Control and Complications Trial Research Group: The effect of intensive diabetes treatment on the progression of diabetic retinopathy in insulin-dependent diabetes mellitus. *Arch Ophthalmol* 1995;113:36–51. Copyright 1995, American Medical Association.

Abstract *Objective:* To determine the magnitude of the decrease in the risk of retinopathy progression observed with intensive treatment and its relationship to baseline retinopathy severity and duration of followup. *Design:* Randomized clinical trial, with 3 to 9 years of followup. *Setting and patients:* Between 1983 and 1989, 29 centers enrolled 1441 patients with insulin-dependent diabetes mellitus aged 13 to 39 years, including 726 patients with no retinopathy and a duration of diabetes of 1 to 5 years (primary-prevention cohort) and 715 patients with very mild to moderate nonproliferative diabetic retinopathy and a duration of diabetes of 1 to 15 years (secondary-intervention cohort). Ninety-five percent of all scheduled examinations were completed. *Interventions:* Intensive treatment consisted of the administration of insulin at least three times a day by injection or pump, with doses adjusted based on self–blood glucose monitoring and with the goal of normoglycemia. Conventional treatment consisted of one or two daily insulin injections. *Outcome measures:* Change between baseline and followup visits on the Early Treatment Diabetic Retinopathy Study retinopathy severity scale, assessed with masked gradings of stereoscopic color fundus photographs obtained every 6 months. *Results:* Cumulative 8.5-year rates of retinopathy progression by three or more steps at two consecutive visits were 54.1% with conventional treatment and 11.5% with intensive treatment in the primary-prevention cohort and 49.2% and 17.1% in the secondary-intervention cohort. At the 6- and 12-month visits, a small adverse effect of intensive treatment was noted ("early worsening"), followed by a beneficial effect that increased in magnitude with time. Beyond 3.5 years of followup, the risk of progression was five or more times lower with intensive treatment than with conventional treatment. Once progression occurred, subsequent recovery was at least two times more likely with intensive treatment than with conventional treatment. Treatment effects were similar in all baseline retinopathy severity subgroups. *Conclusion:* The results of the DCCT strongly support the recommendation that most patients with insulin-dependent diabetes mellitus use intensive treatment, aiming for levels of glycemia as close to the nondiabetic range as is safely possible.

5. Diabetes Control and Complications Trial Research Group: Progression of retinopathy with intensive versus conventional treatment in the Diabetes Control and Complications Trial. *Ophthalmology* 1995;102:647–661. Courtesy of *Ophthalmology.*

Abstract *Purpose:* To answer the following questions regarding the effect of intensive diabetes management on retinopathy in insulin-dependent diabetes mellitus (IDDM): (**1**) Does intensive therapy completely prevent the development of retinopathy? (**2**) Are some states of retinopathy too advanced to benefit from intensive therapy? (**3**) Are the retinopathy end points in the DCCT clinically important? and (**4**) What other factors influence the effectiveness of therapy? *Methods:* A total of 1441 patients, ranging in age from 13 to 39 years and with IDDM of 1 to 5 years' duration and no retinopathy at baseline (primary-prevention cohort) or with 1 to 15 years' duration and minimal-to-moderate nonproliferative retinopathy (secondary-intervention cohort), were assigned randomly to either intensive or conventional diabetes therapy. Intensive therapy, aimed at achieving glycemic levels as close to the normal range as possible, included three or more daily insulin injections or a continuous subcutaneous insulin infusion, guided by four or more glucose tests daily. Conventional therapy included one or two daily injections. Seven-field stereoscopic fundus photography was performed every 6 months, for a mean followup of 6.5 years (range: 4 to 9 years). *Results:* Intensive therapy reduced the risk of any retinopathy (≥ 1 microaneurysm) developing in the primary-prevention cohort (70% of intensive versus 90% of conventional treatment group; $P = 0.002$) by 27%. It reduced the risk of retinopathy developing or progressing to clinically significant degrees by 34% to 76%. Intensive therapy was most effective when initiated early in the course of IDDM. It had a substantial beneficial effect over the entire spectrum of retinopathy studied in the DCCT and, with rare exceptions, in all patient subgroups. *Conclusion:* Although intensive therapy does not prevent retinopathy completely, it has a beneficial effect that begins after 3 years of therapy on all levels of retinopathy studied in the DCCT. The reduction in risk observed in the study is translatable directly into reduced need for laser treatment and saved sight. Intensive therapy should form the backbone of any healthcare strategy aimed at reducing the risk of visual loss from diabetic retinopathy.

6. Diabetes Control and Complications Trial Research Group: The relationship of glycemic exposure (HbA_{1c}) to the risk of development and progression of retinopathy in the Diabetes Control and Complications Trial. *Diabetes* 1995;44: 968–983. Reprinted by permission.

Abstract The DCCT demonstrated that a regimen of intensive therapy aimed at maintaining near-normal blood glucose values markedly reduces the risks of development or progression of retinopathy and other complications of insulin-dependent diabetes mellitus (IDDM) when compared with a conventional treatment regimen. This report presents an epidemiological assessment of the association between levels of glycemic exposure (HbA_{1c}) before and during the DCCT with the risk of retinopathy progression within each treatment group. The initial level of HbA_{1c} observed at eligibility screening as an index of pre-DCCT glycemia and the duration of IDDM on entry were the dominant baseline predictors of the risk of progression. The shorter the duration of IDDM on entry, the greater were the benefits of intensive therapy. In each treatment group, the mean HbA_{1c} during the trial was the dominant predictor of retinopathy progression, and the risk gradients were similar in the two groups; a 10% lower HbA_{1c} (eg, 8% versus 7.2%) is associated with a 43% lower risk in the intensive group and a 45% lower risk in the conventional group. These risk gradients applied over the observed range of HbA_{1c} values and were unaffected by adjustment for other covariates. Over the range of HbA_{1c} achieved by DCCT intensive therapy, there does not appear to be a level of glycemia below which the risks of retinopathy progression are eliminated. The change in risk over time, however, differed significantly between the treatment groups, the risk increasing with time in the study in the conventional group but remaining relatively constant in the intensive group. The risks were compounded by a multiplicative effect of the level of HbA_{1c} with the duration of exposure (time in study). Total glycemic exposure was the dominant factor associated with the risk of retinopathy progression. When examined simultaneously within each treatment group, each of the components of pre-DCCT glycemic exposure (screening HbA_{1c} value and IDDM duration) and glycemic exposure during the DCCT (mean HbA_{1c}, time in study, and their interaction) were significantly associated with risk of retinopathy progression. Similar results also apply to other retinopathic, nephropathic, and neuropathic outcomes. The recommendation of the DCCT remains that intensive therapy with the goal of achieving near-normal glycemia should be implemented as early as possible in as many IDDM patients as is safely possible.

7. Diabetes Control and Complications Trial Research Group: Early worsening of diabetic retinopathy in the Diabetes Control and Complications Trial. *Arch Ophthalmol* 1998;116:874–886. Copyright 1998, American Medical Association.

Abstract *Objectives:* To document the frequency, importance of, and risk factors for "early worsening" of diabetic retinopathy in the DCCT. *Methods:* The DCCT was a multicenter, randomized clinical trial comparing intensive versus conventional treatment in insulin-dependent diabetic patients who had no-to-moderate nonproliferative retinopathy. Retinopathy severity was assessed in 7-field stereoscopic fundus photographs taken at baseline and every 6 months. For this study, worsening was defined as progression of three steps or more on the ETDRS final scale, as the development of soft exudates and/or intraretinal microvascular abnormalities, as the development of clinically important retinopathy, or as any of the above, and was considered "early" if it occurred between baseline and 12-month followup visits. *Results:* Early worsening was observed at the 6- and/or 12-month visit in 13.1% of 711 patients assigned to intensive treatment and in 7.6% of 728 patients assigned to conventional treatment (odds ratio: 2.06; $P < .001$); recovery had occurred at the 18-month visit in 51% and 55% of these groups, respectively ($P = .39$). The risk of three-step or greater progression from the retinopathy level present 18 months after entry into the trial was greater in patients who previously had had early worsening than in those who had not. However, the large long-term risk reduction with intensive treatment was such that outcomes in intensively treated patients who had early worsening were similar to or more favorable than outcomes in conventionally treated patients who had not. The most important risk factors for early worsening were higher hemoglobin A_{1c} level at screening and reduction of this level during the first 6 months after randomization. We found no evidence to suggest that more gradual reduction of glycemia might be associated with less risk of early worsening. Early worsening led to high-risk proliferative retinopathy in 2 patients and to clinically significant macular edema in 3; all responded well to treatment. *Conclusions:* In the DCCT, the long-term benefits of intensive insulin treatment greatly outweighed the risks of early worsening. Although no case of early worsening was associated with serious visual loss, our results are consistent with previous reports of sight-threatening worsening when intensive treatment is initiated in patients with long-standing poor glycemic control, particularly if retinopathy is at or past the moderate nonproliferative stage. Ophthalmologic monitoring before initiation of intensive treatment and at 3-month intervals for 6 to 12 months thereafter seems appropriate for such patients. In patients whose retinopathy is already approaching the high-risk stage, it may be prudent to delay the initiation of intensive treatment until photocoagulation can be completed, particularly if hemoglobin A_{1c} is high.

A-5

SORBINIL RETINOPATHY TRIAL (SRT)

1. Sorbinil Retinopathy Trial Research Group: A randomized trial of sorbinil, an aldose reductase inhibitor, in diabetic retinopathy. *Arch Ophthalmol* 1990;108:1234–1244. Copyright 1990, American Medical Association.

Abstract A total of 497 patients aged 18 to 56 years with insulin-dependent diabetes mellitus for 1 to 15 years were randomly assigned to take oral sorbinil or placebo and followed up for a median of 41 months. The percentage of patients whose retinopathy severity grade at maximum followup had worsened by two or more levels was not significantly different between the two treatment groups (28% in the sorbinil group and 32% in the placebo group, P = .344). The number of microaneurysms increased at a slightly slower rate in the sorbinil group than in the placebo group, with statistically significant differences at 21 (P = .046) and 30 (P = .039) months but not at the maximum followup (P = .156). About 7% of the patients assigned to take sorbinil developed a hypersensitivity reaction in the first 3 months. On the basis of these results, it is unlikely that sorbinil administered at a dosage of 250 mg daily for 3 years has a clinically important effect on the course of retinopathy in adults with insulin-dependent diabetes of moderate duration. Our data are consistent, however, with a slightly slower progression rate in the microaneurysm count among patients assigned to take sorbinil, a finding of uncertain clinical importance.

A-6

UNITED KINGDOM PROSPECTIVE DIABETES STUDY (UKPDS)

1. United Kingdom Prospective Diabetes Study Group: Intensive blood-glucose control with sulphonylureas or insulin compared with conventional treatment and risk of complications in patients with type 2 diabetes. UKPDS 33. *Lancet* 1998;352:837–853. Reprinted with permission of The Lancet.

Summary *Background:* Improved blood-glucose control decreases the progression of diabetic microvascular disease, but the effect on macrovascular complications is unknown. There is concern that sulphonylureas may increase cardiovascular mortality in patients with type 2 diabetes and that high insulin concentrations may enhance atheroma formation. We compared the effects of intensive blood-glucose control with either sulphonylurea or insulin and conventional treatment on the risk of microvascular and macrovascular complications in patients with type 2 diabetes in a randomised controlled trial. *Methods:* 3867 newly diagnosed patients with type 2 diabetes, median age 54 years (IQR [interquartile range] 48 to 60 years), who after 3 months' diet treatment had a mean of two fasting plasma glucose (FPG) concentrations of 6.1 to 15.0 mmol/L were randomly assigned intensive policy with a sulphonylurea (chlorpropamide, glibenclamide, or glipizide) or with insulin, or conventional policy with diet. The aim in the intensive group was FPG less than 6 mmol/L. In the conventional group, the aim was the best achievable FPG with diet alone; drugs were added only if there were hyperglycaemic symptoms or FPG greater than 15 mmol/L. Three aggregate end points were used to assess differences between conventional and intensive treatment: (**1**) any diabetes-related end point (sudden death, death from hyperglycaemia or hypoglycaemia, fatal or nonfatal myocardial infarction, angina, heart failure, stroke, renal failure, amputation [of at least one digit], vitreous haemorrhage, retinopathy requiring photocoagulation, blindness in one eye, or cataract extraction); (**2**) diabetes-related death (death from myocardial infarction, stroke, peripheral vascular disease, renal disease, hyperglycaemia or hypoglycaemia, and sudden death); (**3**) all-cause mortality. Single clinical end points and surrogate subclinical end points were also assessed. All analyses were by intention to treat, and frequency of hypoglycaemia was also analyzed by actual therapy. *Findings:* Over 10 years, haemoglobin A_{1c} (HbA_{1c}) was 7.0% (6.2 to 8.2) in the intensive group compared with 7.9% (6.9 to 8.8) in the conventional group—an 11% reduction. There was no difference in HbA_{1c} among agents in the intensive group. Compared with the conventional group, the risk in the intensive group was 12% lower (95% confidence interval: 1 to 21; $P = 0.029$) for any diabetes-related end point; 10% lower (–11 to 27; $P = 0.34$) for any diabetes-related death; and 6% lower (–10 to 20; $P = 0.44$) for all-cause mortality. Most of the risk reduction in the any diabetes-related aggregate end point was due to a 25% risk reduction (7 to 40; $P = 0.0099$) in microvascular end points, including the need for retinal photocoagulation. There was no difference for any of the three aggregate end points between the three intensive agents (chlorpropamide, glibenclamide, or insulin). Patients in the intensive group had more hypoglycaemic episodes than those in the conventional group on both types of analysis (both $P < 0.0001$). The rates of major hypoglycaemic episodes per year were 0.7% with conventional treatment, 1.0% with chlorpropamide, 1.4% with glibenclamide, and 1.8% with insulin. Weight gain was significantly higher in the intensive group (mean: 2.9 kg) than in the conventional group ($P < 0.001$), and patients assigned insulin had a greater gain in weight (4.0 kg) than those assigned chlorpropamide (2.6 kg) or glibenclamide (1.7 kg). *Interpretation:* Intensive blood-glucose control by either sulphonylureas or insulin substantially decreases the risk of microvascular complications, but not macrovascular disease, in patients with type 2 diabetes. None of the individual drugs had an adverse effect on cardiovascular outcomes. All intensive treatment increased the risk of hypoglycaemia.

2. United Kingdom Prospective Diabetes Study Group: Tight blood pressure control and risk of macrovascular and microvascular complications in type 2 diabetes. UKPDS 38. *Br Med J* 1998; 317:703–713. This abstract was first published in the *British Medical Journal* and is reproduced by permission of the BMJ Publishing Group.

Abstract *Objective:* To determine whether tight control of blood pressure prevents macrovascular and microvascular complications in patients with type 2 diabetes. *Design:* Randomised controlled trial comparing tight control of blood pressure aiming at a blood pressure of <150/85 mm Hg (with the use of an angiotensin-converting enzyme inhibitor, captopril, or a beta blocker, atenolol, as main treatment), with less tight control aiming at a blood pressure of <180/105 mm Hg. *Setting:* 20 hospital-based clinics in England, Scotland, and Northern Ireland. *Subjects:* 1148 hypertensive patients with type 2 diabetes (mean age: 56, mean blood pressure at entry: 160/94 mm Hg); 758 patients were allocated to tight control of blood pressure, and 390 patients to less tight control with a median followup of 8.4 years. *Main outcome measures:* Predefined clinical end points, fatal and nonfatal, related to diabetes, deaths related to diabetes, and all-cause mortality. Surrogate measures of microvascular disease included urinary albumin excretion and retinal photography. *Results:* Mean blood pressure during followup was significantly reduced in the group assigned to tight blood pressure control (144/82 mm Hg) compared with the group assigned to less tight control (154/87 mm Hg; $P <0.0001$). Reductions in risk in the group assigned to tight control compared with that assigned to less tight control were 24% in diabetes-related end points (95% confidence interval: 8% to 38%; $P = 0.0046$), 32% in deaths related to diabetes (6% to 51%; $P = 0.019$), 44% in strokes (11% to 65%; $P = 0.013$), and 37% in microvascular end points (11% to 56%; $P = 0.0092$), predominantly owing to a reduced risk of retinal photocoagulation. There was a nonsignificant reduction in all-cause mortality. After 9 years of followup, the group assigned to tight blood pressure control also had a 34% reduction in risk in the proportion of patients with deterioration of retinopathy by two steps (99% confidence interval: 11% to 50%; $P = 0.0004$) and a 47% reduced risk (7% to 70%; $P = 0.004$) of deterioration in visual acuity by three lines of the Early Treatment of Diabetic Retinopathy Study (ETDRS) chart. After 9 years of followup, 29% of patients in the group assigned to tight control required three or more treatments to lower blood pressure to achieve target blood pressures. *Conclusion:* Tight blood pressure control in patients with hypertension and type 2 diabetes achieves a clinically important reduction in the risk of deaths related to diabetes, complications related to diabetes, progression of diabetic retinopathy, and deterioration in visual acuity.

3. United Kingdom Prospective Diabetes Study Group. Glycemic control with diet, sulfonylurea, metformin, or insulin in patients with type 2 diabetes mellitus: progressive requirement for multiple therapies. UKPDS 49. *J Am Med Assoc* 1999; 281:2005–2012. Copyright 1999, American Medical Association.

Abstract *Context:* Treatment with diet alone, insulin, sulfonylurea, or metformin is known to improve glycemia in patients with type 2 diabetes mellitus, but which treatment most frequently attains target fasting plasma glucose (FPG) concentration of less than 7.8 mmol/L (140 mg/dL) or glycosylated hemoglobin A_{1c} (HbA$_{1c}$) below 7% is unknown. *Objective:* To assess how often each therapy can achieve the glycemic control target levels set by the American Diabetes Association. *Design:* Randomized controlled trial conducted between 1977 and 1997. Patients were recruited between 1977 and 1991 and were followed up every 3 months for 3, 6, and 9 years after enrollment. *Setting:* Outpatient diabetes clinics in 15 UK hospitals. *Patients:* A total of 4075 patients newly diagnosed as having type 2 diabetes ranged in age between 25 and 65 years and had a median (interquartile range) FPG concentration of 11.5 (9.0 to 14.4) mmol/L [207 (162 to 259) mg/dL], HbA$_{1c}$ levels of 9.1% (7.5% to 10.7%), and a mean (SD) body mass index of 29 (6) kg/m^2. *Interventions:* After 3 months on a low-fat, high-carbohydrate, high-fiber diet, patients were randomized to therapy with diet alone, insulin, sulfonylurea, or metformin. *Main outcome measures:* Fasting plasma glucose and HbA$_{1c}$ levels, and the proportion of patients who achieved target levels below 7% HbA$_{1c}$ or less than 7.8 mmol/L (140 mg/dL) FPG at 3, 6, or 9 years following diagnosis. *Results:* The proportion of patients who maintained target glycemic levels declined markedly over 9 years of followup. After 9 years of monotherapy with diet, insulin, or sulfonylurea, 8%, 42%, and 24%, respectively, achieved FPG levels of less than 7.8 mmol/L (140 mg/dL) and 9%, 28%, and 24% achieved HbA$_{1c}$ levels below 7%. In obese patients randomized to metformin, 18% attained FPG levels of less than 7.8 mmol/L (140 mg/dL) and 13% attained HbA$_{1c}$ levels below 7%. Patients less likely to achieve target levels were younger, more obese, or more hyperglycemic than other patients. *Conclusions:* Each therapeutic agent, as monotherapy, increased 2- to 3-fold the proportion of patients who attained HbA$_{1c}$ below 7% compared with diet alone. However, the progressive deterioration of diabetes control was such that after 3 years approximately 50% of patients could attain this goal with monotherapy, and by 9 years this declined to approximately 25%. The majority of patients need multiple therapies to attain these glycemic target levels in the longer term.

CME Accreditation

The American Academy of Ophthalmology is accredited by the Accreditation Council for Continuing Medical Education to provide continuing medical education for physicians.

CME credit hours in category 1 of the Physician's Recognition Award of the American Medical Association may be earned for completing the study of any monograph in the Ophthalmology Monographs series. The Academy designates the number of credit hours for each monograph based on the scope and complexity of the material covered.

CME Credit Report Form

The Academy designates Ophthalmology Monograph 14, *Diabetes and Ocular Disease: Past, Present, and Future Therapies,* for up to 25 credit hours. Your request for credit must be submitted within 3 years of the date of purchase. You should claim only those hours of credit that you actually spent in this educational activity. To claim credit, complete the answer sheet for the self-study examination and sign the statement below.

I hereby certify that I have spent _____ (up to 25) hours of study on this monograph and that I have completed the self-study examination.

_____
Signature   Date

Send the completed answer sheet and signed statement to:

American Academy of Ophthalmology
P.O. Box 7424
San Francisco, CA 94120-7424
ATTN: Clinical Education Division

The Academy upon request will send you a transcript of the credit claimed on this form. Check the box below if you wish credit verification now.

☐ Please send credit verification now.

PLEASE PRINT

_____
Last Name   First Name   MI

_____
Mailing Address

_____
City

_____
State   ZIP Code

_____
Telephone   ID Number*

*Your ID Number is located following your name on most Academy mailing labels, in your membership directory, and on your monthly statement of account.

OPHTHALMOLOGY MONOGRAPH 14

Diabetes and Ocular Disease: Past, Present, and Future Therapies

Circle the letter of the response option that you regard as the "best" answer to the question.

Question	Answer				Question	Answer			
1	a	b	c	d	23	a	b	c	d
2	a	b	c	d	24	a	b	c	d
3	a	b	c	d	25	a	b	c	d
4	a	b	c	d	26	a	b	c	d
5	a	b	c	d	27	a	b	c	d
6	a	b	c	d	28	a	b	c	d
7	a	b	c	d	29	a	b	c	d
8	a	b	c	d	30	a	b	c	d
9	a	b	c	d	31	a	b	c	d
10	a	b	c	d	32	a	b	c	d
11	a	b	c	d	33	a	b	c	d
12	a	b	c	d	34	a	b	c	d
13	a	b	c	d	35	a	b	c	d
14	a	b	c	d	36	a	b	c	d
15	a	b	c	d	37	a	b	c	d
16	a	b	c	d	38	a	b	c	d
17	a	b	c	d	39	a	b	c	d
18	a	b	c	d	40	a	b	c	d
19	a	b	c	d	41	a	b	c	d
20	a	b	c	d	42	a	b	c	d
21	a	b	c	d	43	a	b	c	d
22	a	b	c	d	44	a	b	c	d

SELF-STUDY EXAMINATION

The self-study examination provided for each book in the Ophthalmology Monographs series is intended for use after completion of the monograph. The examination for *Diabetes and Ocular Disease: Past, Present, and Future Therapies* consists of 44 multiple-choice questions followed by the answers to the questions and a discussion for each answer. The Academy recommends that you not consult the answers until you have completed the entire examination.

Questions

The questions are constructed so that there is one "best" answer. Despite the attempt to avoid ambiguous selections, disagreement may occur about which selection constitutes the optimal answer. After reading a question, record your initial impression on the answer sheet (facing page).

Answers and Discussions

The "best" answer to each question is provided after the examination. The discussion that accompanies the answer is intended to help you confirm that the reasoning you used in determining the most appropriate answer was correct. If you missed a question, the discussion may help you decide whether your "error" was due to poor wording of the question or to your misinterpretation. If, instead, you missed the question because of miscalculation or failure to recall relevant information, the discussion may help fix the principle in your memory.

QUESTIONS

Chapter 1

1. Which of the following cell types exhibit abnormalities in nonproliferative diabetic retinopathy?

   a. vascular endothelial cells

   b. Müller cells

   c. ganglion cells

   d. all of the above

2. Visual loss in diabetic retinopathy ultimately results from

   a. macular edema

   b. foveal ischemia

   c. neovascularization

   d. retinal neuronal damage

3. All of the following are risk factors for diabetic macular edema *except*

   a. systemic hypertension

   b. ocular hypertension

   c. hypercholesterolemia

   d. proteinuria

4. Cotton-wool spots

   a. represent impaired axonal transport of the nerve fiber layer

   b. are caused by venous leakage

   c. never occur without other clinical signs of retinopathy

   d. occur despite normal axonal transport

Chapter 2

5. In the Wisconsin Epidemiologic Study of Diabetic Retinopathy, the prevalence of legal blindness (best-corrected visual acuity of 20/200 or worse in the better eye) in people with 30 or more years of type 1 diabetes was found to be

   a. 1%

   b. 5%

   c. 12%

   d. 25%

6. The prevalences of proliferative retinopathy in persons with type 1 and type 2 diabetes after 20 or more years of diabetes are estimated to be about

   a. 5% and 50%, respectively

   b. 50% and 50%, respectively

   c. 50% and 5%, respectively

   d. 50% and 20%, respectively

7. All of the following have been shown to be consistently associated with diabetic retinopathy *except*

   a. glycosylated hemoglobin level

   b. smoking

   c. duration of diabetes

   d. diabetic nephropathy

8. All of the following have been proven by clinical trials to reduce the incidence or progression of retinopathy in people with diabetes *except*

   a. glycemic control

   b. blood pressure control

   c. panretinal photocoagulation

   d. weight loss

Chapter 3

9. The ophthalmologist credited with inventing the photocoagulation modality is

   a. Lloyd M. Aiello, MD

   b. William P. Beetham, MD

   c. Matthew D. Davis, MD

   d. Gerd Meyer-Schwickerath, MD

10. The ophthalmologist credited with developing pars plana vitreous surgery is

    a. Lloyd M. Aiello, MD

    b. William P. Beetham, MD

    c. Matthew D. Davis, MD

    d. Robert Machemer, MD

11. Early concepts for photocoagulation included

    a. direct treatment of feeder vessels

    b. barrier treatment around vessels to prevent the spread of exudates

    c. "hitting everything that was red"

    d. all of the above

12. All of the following are the reasons that clinical trials were developed to study therapies for diabetic retinopathy *except*

    a. The value of good control of diabetes and normalization of blood glucose was questioned.

    b. Better information regarding the natural history of the disease was expected to define the indications for laser and surgical treatment.

    c. The third-party payers were unwilling to reimburse for these new treatments.

    d. Increased survival of diabetic patients through improved medical measures spawned increased numbers of patients with a long enough duration of diabetes to develop retinopathy.

Chapter 4

13. In the Diabetic Retinopathy Study, harmful effects that were worse in patients undergoing photocoagulation with the xenon arc coagulator, as compared to the argon laser, included

    a. visual field loss

    b. loss of accommodative amplitude

    c. color vision

    d. difficulties with dark adaptation and driving at night

14. All of the following questions were to be answered by the Early Treatment Diabetic Retinopathy Study *except*

    a. Is aspirin use effective for preventing the progression of diabetic retinopathy?

    b. Does tight control of blood glucose enhance the effect of photocoagulation?

    c. Is photocoagulation effective for treating diabetic macular edema?

    d. Is early photocoagulation effective for treating diabetic retinopathy?

15. All of the following findings were reported by the Early Treatment Diabetic Retinopathy Study *except*

    a. Early scatter photocoagulation results in a small reduction in risk of severe visual loss (<5/200) for at least 4 months.

    b. Early scatter photocoagulation is not indicated for eyes with mild-to-moderate diabetic retinopathy.

    c. Early scatter photocoagulation may be most effective in patients with type 2 diabetes.

    d. Panretinal photocoagulation reduces the progression of diabetic macular edema.

16. Which of the following did the Diabetic Retinopathy Vitrectomy Study demonstrate for patients with nonclearing vitreous hemorrhage after 2 years of followup?

    a. The rate of final visual acuity of 20/40 or better was increased for type 1 diabetic patients with early vitrectomy.

    b. The rate of final visual acuity of 20/200 or less was decreased for type 1 diabetic patients with early vitrectomy.

    c. The rate of no light perception was increased for patients undergoing early vitrectomy.

    d. The rate of no light perception was decreased for patients undergoing early vitrectomy.

Chapter 5

17. Intravenous fluorescein angiography is most commonly helpful in identifying

    a. neovascularization of the disc

    b. neovascularization elsewhere (that is, neovascularization of the retina)

    c. microaneurysmal abnormalities prior to focal laser treatment for clinically significant macular edema

    d. tractional retinal detachment

18. Contact B-scan ultrasonography with severe proliferative diabetic retinopathy and cloudy media least commonly shows

    a. tractional retinal detachment

    b. subhyaloidal blood

    c. intravitreal blood (vitreous hemorrhage)

    d. subretinal blood

19. Fundus photography is useful for all of the following situations *except*

    a. documenting changes in retinopathy

    b. documenting an asymptomatic, newly diagnosed diabetic patient who has not yet developed retinopathy

    c. searching for early neovascular fronds in a patient with severe nonproliferative changes, as observed on clinical examination

    d. documenting the preoperative appearance of fibrovascular components

20. The most sensitive means of detecting macular thickening is

a. visual acuity testing

b. fluorescein angiography

c. indocyanine green angiography

d. clinical examination

Chapter 6

21. A patient presents with 20/25 vision and an area of macular thickening associated with leaking microaneurysms 1.5 disc areas in size 800 µm from the center of the macula. Based on guidelines from the Early Treatment Diabetic Retinopathy Study, the recommended management of this patient would be

a. observation, because the macular thickening is not within 500 µm of the center of the macula

b. focal treatment of the microaneurysms only if panretinal photocoagulation is imminent

c. focal treatment of microaneurysms, with grid photocoagulation re-treatment of any persistent macular thickening 2 to 3 weeks later

d. focal treatment of microaneurysms followed by 3 months of observation

22. All of the following statements about the initial treatment of clinically significant macular edema are true *except*

a. Grid photocoagulation may be applied to regions of diffuse macular edema.

b. Focal treatment of microaneurysms can be performed with either argon green or dye yellow laser.

c. Treatment of microaneurysms can extend to within 300 µm of the center of the macula.

d. Usually, less power is needed to achieve a burn in retina with less edema than in retina that is more edematous.

23. A patient presents with clinically significant macular edema in the right eye and a very small tuft of neovascularization on the optic nerve head (less than 0.25 disc area in size) in the left eye. Focal laser photocoagulation is applied to the right eye. According to the guidelines from the Early Treatment Diabetic Retinopathy Study, appropriate follow-up for this patient would be

a. 1 week for application of panretinal photocoagulation in the left eye

b. 6 months for reassessment of clinically significant macular edema and neovascularization of the disc

c. 2 to 3 months for monitoring clinically significant macular edema and neovascularization of the disc

d. 4 months, with fundus fluorescein angiogram ordered for reassessment of clinically significant macular edema

24. A patient with type 2 diabetes presents with a small tuft of neovascularization of the disc (less than 0.25 disc area in size) and a small subhyaloid hemorrhage tracking along the inferotemporal arcade. Which of the following statements is true?

a. Because the neovascularization of the disc is so small, it does not meet the high-risk criteria defined by the Diabetic Retinopathy Study. The patient should be re-examined in 2 to 3 months.

b. The presence of subhyaloid hemorrhage is an indication for immediate pars plana vitrectomy to prevent the development of fibrosis and traction.

c. Because this patient meets high-risk criteria, direct laser photocoagulation to the area of neovascularization should be administered.

d. Because this patient meets high-risk criteria, panretinal photocoagulation should be administered.

Chapter 7

25. Earlier surgical intervention with vitrectomy is generally recommended for all of the following situations *except*

a. when no previous laser treatment has been performed

b. when fibrovascular proliferation complexes are known to be more extensive

c. when the patient has poorly controlled systemic hypertension

d. when the fellow eye has followed a rapidly progressive course of visual loss because of diabetic retinopathy

26. The *least* common indication for vitrectomy in diabetes is

a. progressive fibrovascular proliferation

b. tractional retinal detachment

c. combined tractional and rhegmatogenous retinal detachment

d. diabetic macular edema

27. The optimal technique of vitrectomy for tractional retinal detachment secondary to diabetic retinopathy includes

a. segmentation

b. delamination

c. en bloc

d. all of the above

28. Various investigators have found that preoperative factors indicating a more favorable postoperative result with vitrectomy in diabetes include

a. age less than 40 years

b. preoperative vision better than 20/200

c. preoperative application of photocoagulation

d. all of the above

Chapter 8

29. Multicenter clinical trials have demonstrated the benefit of which of the following treatments in reducing the progression of diabetic retinopathy?

a. aspirin

b. aldose-reductase inhibitors

c. angiotensin-converting enzyme inhibitors

d. 3-hydroxy-3-methylglutaryl (HMG)/coenzyme A (CoA) inhibitors

30. All of the following are effective strategies to minimize visual loss from diabetic retinopathy *except*

a. meticulous glycemic control (goal HbA_{1c} less than 7.0%)

b. aggressive blood pressure control (goal BP less than 130/85)

c. application of laser treatment to stages of diabetic macular edema that are not clinically significant

d. regular (annual) screening by an ophthalmologist

31. As shown by the Wisconsin Epidemiologic Study of Diabetic Retinopathy, there is a relationship between the baseline HbA_{1c} and all of the following *except*

a. macular edema in the younger-onset cohort and in the older-onset cohort overall

b. visual loss in the younger-onset cohort treated with insulin

c. visual loss in the older-onset cohort treated with insulin

d. visual loss in the older-onset cohort not treated with insulin

32. The Diabetes Control and Complications Trial demonstrated all of the following *except*

a. an increase in HbA_{1c} in the more intensively controlled groups

b. a 4-fold reduction in worsening of retinopathy in the primary-prevention cohort

c. a 3-fold reduction in worsening of retinopathy in the secondary-prevention cohort

d. an increase in the number of hypoglycemic episodes in the more intensively controlled groups

Chapter 9

33. All of the following statements regarding the outcome of cataract surgery in diabetic patients without preoperative retinopathy are true *except*

a. About 85% will achieve a postoperative visual acuity of 20/40 or better.

b. About 15% will develop nonproliferative diabetic retinopathy within 1 year of surgery.

c. The risk of angiographic cystoid macular edema is higher than in nondiabetic patients.

d. The presence of angiographic cystoid macular edema always negatively impacts final visual acuity.

34. Diabetic patients with which of the following factors are less likely to have improved visual acuity following cataract surgery?

a. posterior subcapsular opacities

b. male sex

c. preoperative diabetic macular edema

d. previous vitrectomy

35. Which of the following is *least* helpful in differentiating pseudophakic cystoid macular edema from diabetic macular edema?

a. the presence of leaking microaneurysms

b. the time to onset of macular edema following cataract surgery

c. the findings on fluorescein angiography

d. the response to topical corticosteroids or nonsteroidal anti-inflammatory agents

36. Cataract surgery in diabetic patients is associated with a higher risk of which of the following complications?

a. neovascularization of the iris

b. fibrin in the anterior chamber

c. posterior capsule opacification

d. all of the above

Chapter 10

37. Corneal abnormalities seen in diabetic patients may be due to

a. decreased corneal sensitivity

b. intrinsic abnormalities of the epithelial basement membrane

c. impaired epithelial barrier function

d. all of the above

38. All of the following statements about cranial nerve palsies in diabetic patients are true *except*

a. A cranial nerve VI palsy is a common cause of motility disturbance in diabetic patients, but it may also be a sign of increased intracranial pressure.

b. A cranial nerve III palsy due to microvascular infarction may involve the pupil.

c. Cranial nerve palsies caused by microvascular disease are usually associated with pain.

d. Workup for causes other than microvascular disease is indicated if the examination reveals involvement of more than one cranial nerve, other neurologic signs, progressive deterioration, or lack of complete recovery within 3 months.

39. All of the following statements about acute optic disc edema (diabetic papillopathy) are true *except*

 a. It generally shows no correlation with the severity of diabetic retinopathy.

 b. Fluorescein angiography usually shows diffuse leakage on the disc.

 c. It typically is associated with mild visual disturbance.

 d. It usually progresses to disc neovascularization.

40. The treatment of neovascular glaucoma includes all of the following options *except*

 a. aqueous suppressants

 b. miotics

 c. panretinal photocoagulation

 d. filtration surgery with antimetabolite

Chapter 11

41. Which of the following growth factors have been implicated as contributing to diabetic retinopathy?

 a. insulin-like growth factor (IGF) and growth hormone (GH)

 b. basic fibroblast growth factor (bFGF)

 c. vascular endothelial growth factor (VEGF)

 d. all of the above

42. Which of the following attributes are thought to be important for a mediator of neovascularization in diabetic retinopathy?

 a. induced by ischemia

 b. secreted and diffusible

 c. associated with active neovascularization

 d. all of the above

43. Which of the following classes of molecules are being considered as therapies for diabetic retinopathy?

 a. vascular endothelial growth factor antagonists and growth hormone antagonists

 b. integrin antagonists

 c. angiostatin and endostatin

 d. all of the above

44. Which of the following statements is/are true?

 a. Growth factors like vascular endothelial growth factor may be important in the development of proliferative diabetic retinopathy and macular edema.

 b. Growth factors like vascular endothelial growth factor may be important in the development of the early stages of diabetic retinopathy (that is, nonproliferative diabetic retinopathy).

 c. Growth factor antagonists are entering clinical trial for the treatment of diabetic retinopathy.

 d. all of the above

ANSWERS AND DISCUSSIONS

Chapter 1

1. **Answer—d.** All retinal cell types are involved in diabetic retinopathy.

2. **Answer—d.** Vision is mediated by neurons. Vascular lesions, macular edema, tractional detachments, and macular ischemia all result in neuronal cell dysfunction and death.

3. **Answer—b.** Ocular hypertension is not a known risk factor for diabetic macular edema, but the other choices are.

4. **Answer—a.** Because cotton-wool spots have been described in the absence of clinical or fluorescein angiographic evidence of vascular occlusion and may resolve without loss of the nerve fiber layer, the leading hypothesis is that they represent ischemically induced impaired axonal transport.

Chapter 2

5. **Answer—c.** Legal blindness is common in people with diabetes. In 1980–1982, nearly 12% of those with 30 or more years of type 1 diabetes living in an 11-county area of southern Wisconsin were found to be legally blind. Many of these individuals became blind because they had severe untreated proliferative retinopathy and/or macular edema in the 1950s and 1960s, before the efficacy of photocoagulation was demonstrated. Based on the data from the Diabetic Retinopathy Study and the Early Treatment Diabetic Retinopathy Study, it is now estimated that early detection and treatment of vision-threatening retinopathy in people with either type 1 or type 2 diabetes can prevent the development of severe visual loss by 95%. Earlier institution of tight glycemic control and blood pressure control should also reduce severe visual loss by preventing the incidence and progression of severe retinopathy.

6. **Answer—c.** These estimates, from the Wisconsin Epidemiologic Study of Diabetic Retinopathy, show the strong association of severe diabetic retinopathy with duration of disease. Duration of diabetes reflects the years of exposure to high blood glucose, the most important risk factor for the development of microvascular complications. For this reason, when a patient with diabetes is first encountered, information about the date of diagnosis is important, as it will provide a rough estimate of the probability of the presence of diabetic retinopathy, proliferative retinopathy, macular edema, nephropathy, and neuropathy.

7. **Answer—b.** One would expect smoking to be associated with diabetic retinopathy because it can alter choroidal blood flow, increase platelet adhesiveness, and depress antioxidant levels, all postulated pathogenic mechanisms associated with diabetic retinopathy. However, data from most epidemiologic studies have not supported an association of retinopathy with smoking. Still, patients should be advised that diabetic patients who smoke are 2 to 3 times as likely to die from cardiovascular disease than are those who do not smoke. In addition, smoking is associated with the development of diabetic nephropathy and an increased risk of cancer.

8. **Answer—d.** The United Kingdom Prospective Diabetes Study and the Diabetes Control and Complications Trial showed the efficacy of glycemic control, the UKPDS showed the efficacy of blood pressure control, and the Diabetic Retinopathy Study and the Early Treatment Diabetic Retinopathy Study showed the efficacy of photocoagulation in preventing the progression of diabetic retinopathy. Obesity has not been shown to be associated with the incidence of diabetic retinopathy.

Chapter 3

9. **Answer—d.** Gerd Meyer-Schwickerath, MD, first used reflected sunlight and subsequently adapted high-pressure xenon arc bulbs to produce retinal photocoagulation.

10. **Answer—d.** Robert Machemer, MD, first developed the fundamental concepts, procedures, and instruments used in performing modern vitreous surgery through the pars plana.

11. **Answer—d.** All of these were early concepts for the use of photocoagulation. The leading theories today center around relieving ischemia by reducing the demand for oxygen or by stimulating diffusible factors for incompletely defined target tissues.

12. **Answer—c.** That third-party payers were unwilling to reimburse for the new treatments was not a principal concern in the 1960s and 1970s, when new treatments were conceived and tested. The other reasons represent situations or questions that were present during those decades.

Chapter 4

13. **Answer—a.** Visual field loss was clearly higher in the xenon-treated eyes: 25% had constriction of the visual field to the Goldmann IVe4 test object of 45°, compared to only 5% of argon-treated eyes. The other choices may be present with any modality of photocoagulation, but either were not tested or were similar in the Diabetic Retinopathy Study.

14. **Answer—b.** The Diabetes Control and Complications Trial and other studies have indicated that tight control reduces the rate of retinopathy progression, but the Early Treatment Diabetic Retinopathy Study did not address this issue; it did address the other three questions.

15. **Answer—d.** Panretinal photocoagulation may increase the degree of macular edema and visual loss. Strategies for minimizing these side effects include deferring panretinal photocoagulation until high-risk characteristics are present and delivering the laser treatment in multiple sessions with fewer spots per session to effect the same treatment end point.

16. **Answer—a.** The rate of achieving 20/40 or better visual acuity was higher for all types of diabetes in the study with early vitrectomy (25%) versus conventional management (15%). This difference was even more marked for the subgroup of type 1 diabetic patients (36% versus 12%). The rates of no light perception and 20/200 or worse (or better) were similar in both study groups (early vitrectomy versus conventional management).

Chapter 5

17. **Answer—c.** Neovascularization of the disc, neovascularization elsewhere, and tractional retinal detachment can typically be seen with ophthalmoscopy. Retinal hemorrhages in diabetic retinopathy can be confused with microaneurysms, but can be differentiated with fluorescein angiography. Microaneurysms are hyperfluorescent with fluorescein angiography, whereas retinal hemorrhages are hypofluorescent. Because the protocol of the Early Treatment Diabetic Retinopathy Study includes laser treatment of microaneurysms, it is important to be able to identify them.

18. **Answer—d.** Tractional retinal detachment, subhyaloidal blood, and intravitreal blood are often seen in severe cases of proliferative diabetic retinopathy. Subretinal blood occurring in the setting of diabetic retinopathy is very unusual. When it is present, subretinal blood is usually within the scenario of vitreous hemorrhage associated with rhegmatogenous retinal detachment.

19. **Answer—b.** Photography is least useful for early or preclinical stages of diabetes, because management decisions are not exercised at this level (before retinopathy is present). Stereoscopic fundus photographs may enhance the management and document the justification for intervention in all of the other circumstances.

20. **Answer—d.** Ancillary testing does not form the basis for defining clinically significant macular edema and therefore does not determine the indication for focal laser treatment.

Chapter 6

21. **Answer—d.** Based on the definition outlined by the Early Treatment Diabetic Retinopathy Study, this patient has clinically significant macular edema because the area of retinal thickening is greater than 1 disc area in size and is within 1 disc diameter of the center of the macula. Accordingly, focal laser photocoagulation would reduce the risk of severe visual loss from 35% to 13% over the course of 3 years. Treatment of this area would involve focal laser directed at microaneurysms, followed by observation for 2 to 4 months. If there is residual edema at that time, further laser photocoagulation can be considered.

22. **Answer—c.** The initial treatment of a patient with clinically significant macular edema should stay at least 500 μm from the center of the macula. Subsequent treatments may be directed at the region between 300 and 500 μm of the center of the macula. Focal laser photocoagulation close to the foveal center carries added risk of symptomatic paracentral scotomas, visually devastating choroidal neovascularization, and worsening macular ischemia by ablating the perifoveal capillary ring.

23. **Answer—c.** This patient has two separate issues. First, the patient has proliferative diabetic retinopathy in the left eye that does not meet the strict definition of high-risk proliferative diabetic retinopathy of the Diabetic Retinopathy Study. At minimum, the patient needs to be observed carefully at 2- to 3-month intervals to monitor for progression to high-risk characteristics. Under circumstances such as suspected poor patient compliance or poor outcome in the fellow eye, prompt panretinal photocoagulation may be considered in this patient. Second, the patient has been treated for clinically significant macular edema in the right eye. Typically, patients are seen 2 to 4 months after administration of focal laser for clinically significant macular edema. If there is residual edema, the clinician may consider obtaining a fluorescein angiogram prior to re-treatment to determine whether there are still actively leaking sites.

24. **Answer—d.** Even though this patient has neovascularization of the disc that is smaller in area than that shown in standard photograph 10A, the patient meets the high-risk characteristics for proliferative diabetic retinopathy on the basis of any neovascularization of the disc with associated preretinal hemorrhage. Panretinal photocoagulation in this setting would reduce the risk of severe visual loss by 50%. Pars plana vitrectomy is not needed at this time because of the small area of neovascularization of

the disc and hemorrhage. Panretinal photocoagulation can be performed in single or multiple sessions. In this case, with subhyaloid hemorrhage threatening to obscure the clinician's view for treatment, it may be appropriate to administer the complete panretinal photocoagulation over a shorter time than usual, while the media remain clear.

Chapter 7

25. **Answer—c.** The control of systemic hypertension should be optimized before performing vitrectomy to reduce intraoperative and postoperative hemorrhaging. When there has been no previous laser treatment, the higher risk of continued progression of the proliferation justifies earlier intervention. A protracted wait for clearing of vitreous hemorrhage in the presence of active fibrovascular proliferation would lower the prognosis for achieving the surgical objectives. Finally, the rapid progression, especially with suboptimal treatment, of the fellow eye indicates that more aggressive treatment is necessary and that a more conservative approach is less likely to be effective in the second eye.

26. **Answer—d.** While the distribution of indications for vitrectomy has changed with the maturation of vitrectomy and its limitations, diabetic vitreous hemorrhage is a common indication for vitrectomy. Probably the most common indication is tractional detachment. Less common, but still frequent indications include fibrovascular proliferation and

combined tractional and rhegmatogenous retinal detachment. A rare indication is diabetic macular edema; such cases are suited for vitrectomy only when prominent, taut, posterior hyaloid traction is in evidence.

27. **Answer—d.** Each of these techniques combines similar surgical objectives, albeit in a different sequence. The technique that each surgeon is most facile and comfortable with is the basic technique that should be used. Good results have been reported with all of these techniques, and similar rates of complications have also been reported with all of the techniques.

28. **Answer—d.** All of these factors have been commonly reported to be positive prognostic factors for visual improvement. The only one of these factors that can be controlled by the clinician is preoperative application of photocoagulation. Accordingly, even if the clinician is expecting that vitrectomy is likely to be necessary, attention to maximizing preoperative panretinal photocoagulation is recommended.

Chapter 8

29. **Answer—c.** The EUCLID study (EURODIAB Controlled Trial of Lisinopril in Insulin-Dependent Diabetes Mellitus) demonstrated that lisinopril, an angiotensin-converting enzyme (ACE) inhibitor, slows the progression of retinopathy. None of the other treatments listed does. In spite of this report, ACE inhibitors are not widely used for this indication.

30. **Answer—c.** The Early Treatment Diabetic Retinopathy Study showed that laser treatment for macular edema is effective only for a degree that meets the criteria for clinically significant macular edema.

31. **Answer—d.** The older-onset cohort not undergoing insulin treatment did not show a relationship between the baseline HbA_{1c} and visual loss.

32. **Answer—a.** HbA_{1c} is decreased in the more intensively controlled groups.

Chapter 9

33. **Answer—d.** Although angiographic cystoid macular edema is more common in diabetic eyes, in the absence of retinopathy, it may not significantly affect the final visual acuity.

34. **Answer—c.** The sex of the patient, the type of cataract, and the presence of a posterior capsulotomy have not been shown to adversely affect the outcome of cataract surgery. About 90% of eyes that have undergone vitrectomy have an improvement in visual acuity following cataract surgery. Eyes with preoperative macular edema have a generally poor prognosis, and only 40% achieve a postoperative visual acuity of 20/40 or better.

35. **Answer—b.** Clinical findings and findings on fluorescein angiography usually help to differentiate pseudophakic cystoid macular edema from diabetic macular edema. Pseudophakic cystoid macular edema may respond to topical corticosteroids or nonsteroidal anti-inflammatory agents, while diabetic macular edema would not. Because both pseudophakic cystoid macular edema and diabetic macular edema occur in the postoperative period, they cannot be differentiated based on time to onset.

36. **Answer—d.** Diabetic patients have a higher risk of neovascularization of the iris, pigment dispersion with precipitates on the surface of the intraocular lens, fibrin or membrane in the anterior chamber, posterior synechiae, pseudophakic pupillary block with secondary angle-closure glaucoma, and posterior capsule opacification.

Chapter 10

37. **Answer—d.** Diabetic patients often have decreased corneal sensitivity; the severity is usually correlated with the severity of retinopathy. Ultrastructural abnormalities of the diabetic corneal epithelial basement membrane include thickening of the multilaminar basement membrane, decreased hemidesmosome frequency, and decreased penetration of anchoring fibrils.

38. Answer—c. Cranial nerve palsies caused by microvascular disease may present with orbital pain in up to 20% of cases, but are usually not associated with pain during lateral gaze.

39. Answer—d. Diabetic papillopathy typically does not progress to disc neovascularization. It is important to differentiate the prominent telangiectasia of disc vessels often present in diabetic papillopathy from neovascularization of the disc. While the disc appearance usually returns to normal, diffuse or segmental atrophy may occasionally result.

40. Answer—b. Miotics are thought to facilitate aqueous outflow and, therefore, are not expected to be of benefit in conditions in which the anterior chamber angle is closed, such as neovascular glaucoma. Miotics should be avoided in neovascular glaucoma, as they may decrease the aqueous–blood barrier and exacerbate intraocular inflammation. The other choices are commonly used in clinical practice.

Chapter 11

41. Answer—d. A wide variety of growth factors have been studied for their contribution to diabetic retinopathy, and many of them have been implicated. Insulin-like growth factor 1 and growth hormone have been implicated as necessary permissive agents for the development of neovascularization. Basic fibroblast growth factor is synergistic with several other growth factors, such as vascular endothelial growth factor, and probably act to potentiate retinal neovascularization. Vascular endothelial growth factor is implicated as a major inducer of neovascularization within the eye.

42. Answer—d. Because retinal ischemia underlies many diseases characterized by retinal neovascularization, important mediators are likely to be induced by ischemia. Major mediators are likely to be secreted and diffusible in order to account for the development of neovascularization at sites distant from the avascular zones. Strong inducers of neovascularization are likely to be associated with the active phase of the disease.

43. Answer—d. Inhibitors of molecules such as vascular endothelial growth factor and growth hormone, which induce retinal neovascularization, are candidates for therapeutic evaluation. Inhibitors of molecules such as the integrins, which are required for cellular proliferation, are also likely candidates. Angiostatin and endostatin are endogenous inhibitors of angiogenesis, which may eventually prove therapeutically useful.

44. Answer—d. As detailed in the chapter, all of the above statements are true.

INDEX

NOTE: An *f* following a page number indicates a figure, and a *t* following a page number indicates a table. Drugs are listed under their generic names; when a drug trade name is listed, the reader is referred to the generic name.

A

ACE inhibitors. *See* Angiotensin-converting enzyme (ACE) inhibitors
ACG. *See* Angle-closure glaucoma
Activity/exercise, diabetic retinopathy and, 48
ADA. *See* American Diabetes Association
Adenosine
hypoxic effects on vascular endothelial growth factor and, 256–258, 258*f*
inhibitors of receptors for, in diabetic retinopathy treatment, 258–259
Adenylate cyclase, hypoxic effects on vascular endothelial growth factor and, 258, 258*f*
African Americans, diabetic retinopathy in, 37, 37*f*
Age
as cataract risk factor, 49, 50*f*, 51, 51*t*, 52*t*
at diabetes diagnosis, as diabetic retinopathy risk factor, 40
diabetic macular edema and, 34, 36*t*
diabetic retinopathy incidence and progression and, 34–35, 34*t*, 35*t*, 36*t*
as diabetic retinopathy risk factor, 38–39, 38*f*
pre-/postpubertal, as diabetic retinopathy risk factor, 40–41
visual loss/blindness incidence and, 23, 24*t*, 25*t*, 27*t*, 28*f*, 28*t*
visual loss/blindness prevalence and, 20–22, 20*t*, 21*f*, 22*f*, 23*f*
as visual loss/blindness risk factor, 26, 27*t*, 28*f*
visual outcome after cataract surgery and, 210
AION (interior ischemic optic neuropathy), in diabetic patient, 228
Alcohol consumption, diabetic retinopathy and, 48
Aldose-reductase inhibitors, diabetic retinopathy incidence/progression affected by, 8, 92, 196

American Diabetes Association (ADA)
blood pressure control recommendations of, 192
glycemic control recommendations of, 187–188, 188*t*
American Indians, diabetic retinopathy in, 36, 189
Anesthesia
for focal/grid laser treatment, 128
for panretinal photocoagulation, 137–138
Angiogenesis. *See* Neovascularization
Angiography, fluorescein, in diabetic retinopathy evaluation, 102–108, 103*t*
in mild nonproliferative retinopathy, 104–105, 104*f*
in moderate nonproliferative retinopathy with macular edema not clinically significant, 105
in moderate nonproliferative retinopathy without macular edema, 105
in severe nonproliferative diabetic retinopathy, 108
Angioscopy, fluorescein, in diabetic retinopathy evaluation, 108
Angiostatin, as mediator of diabetic retinopathy, 245*t*
Angiotensin-converting enzyme (ACE) inhibitors
current recommendations for use of, 192
diabetic eye disease incidence/progression affected by, 45–47, 92, 189–190, 190*f*, 191*f*, 192–194, 193*f*
Angle closure, after laser photocoagulation, 145
Angle-closure glaucoma (ACG), in diabetic patient, 223. *See also* Glaucoma
after cataract surgery, 203

317

Anterior ischemic optic neuropathy (AION), in
    diabetic patient, 228
Antiangiogenic agents
    current status of, 263–264, 264*t*
    future hurdles for, 264–265
Antihistamines, diabetic retinopathy incidence/
    progression affected by, 197
Antihypertensive therapy
    current recommendations for, 192
    diabetic eye disease incidence/progression
        affected by, 45–47, 92, 189–192, 297
Argon laser photocoagulation, 71, 127
    in diabetic macular edema, 117–120
        Diabetic Retinopathy Study results for, 82–84,
            82*f*, 83*t*
        history of development of, 71
        technique for diabetic macular edema and,
            129*t*
Arterioles, retinal, 2, 3*f*
Aspirin, in patients with diabetic retinopathy, 49,
    85–86, 85*f*, 85*t*, 194–195
    with dipyridamole, 195
    Early Treatment Diabetic Retinopathy Study
        statistics on, 195, 283, 285, 286, 288
Astemizole, diabetic retinopathy incidence/pro-
    gression affected by, 197
Astemizole Retinopathy Trial, 197
Astrocytes, retinal, 1–2, 2*f*
Atenolol, diabetic eye disease incidence/progres-
    sion affected by, 46–47, 92, 189–190,
    190*f*, 191*f*
Autoregulation, retinal vascular, impairment of
    in diabetic macular edema, 9, 10*f*
    in diabetic retinopathy, 2–4

B
Bacterial corneal ulcers, contact lens–associated,
    in diabetic patient, 221
Basic fibroblast growth factor (bFGF), in dia-
    betic retinopathy, 244, 245, 245*t*, 259,
    259*f*
Beta blockers
    current recommendations for use of, 192
    diabetic eye disease incidence/progression
        affected by, 45–47, 92, 189–190, 190*f*,
        191*f*
Betaxolol, for primary open-angle glaucoma in
    diabetic patient, 223
bFGF (basic fibroblast growth factor), in dia-
    betic retinopathy, 244, 245, 245*t*, 259,
    259*f*
Biomicroscopy, slit-lamp
    in diabetic macular edema evaluation, 116
    in diabetic retinopathy evaluation, 116, 117*t*
Black Americans, diabetic retinopathy in, 37, 37*f*
Blindness, diabetes-related, 19. *See also* Diabetic
    eye disease; Visual loss in diabetes
    economic costs of, 29–30
    incidence of, 23–26, 24*t*, 25*t*, 27*t*, 28*f*, 28*t*
    as predictor of death, 30–32, 30*f*, 31*f*
    prevalence of, 19–22, 20*t*, 21*f*, 22*f*, 23*f*
    rehabilitation programs and, 29–30
    risk factors for, 26–29, 27*t*, 28*f*, 28*t*
Blood-associated glaucoma, in diabetic patient,
    225–226. *See also* Glaucoma
Blood glucose control. *See also* Glycemic control
    current recommendations for, 187–188, 188*t*
    diabetic retinopathy incidence/progression
        affected by, 42–44, 43*t*, 44*t*, 69, 90–91,
        90*t*, 91*f*, 181–188, 292–296
Blood pressure, as diabetic retinopathy risk
    factor, 45–47, 46*t*
Blood pressure control
    current recommendations for, 192
    diabetic eye disease incidence/progression
        affected by, 45–47, 92, 189–192, 297
Blood–retina barrier, alterations in
    in diabetic macular edema, 9–10
    fluorescein angiography and, 103
    in preclinical diabetic retinopathy, 5

Blood vessels, retinal, 2–4, *2f, 3f*

Blue-yellow color perception, defects in, in pre-clinical diabetic retinopathy, 4, *4t*

Body mass index, diabetic retinopathy and, 48

Bruch's membrane disruption, focal/grid laser treatment of diabetic macular edema causing, 136

C

C-peptide, as diabetic retinopathy risk factor, 44–45

Calcium dobesilate, diabetic retinopathy incidence/progression affected by, 197

Capillaries, retinal, 2, *3f*
closure of, in nonproliferative diabetic retinopathy, 6
in diabetic macular edema, photocoagulation and, 120
fragility of, agents for improvement of, diabetic retinopathy incidence/progression affected by, 197

Capsulotomy, posterior, in diabetic patient, 211

Captopril, diabetic eye disease incidence/progression affected by, 46–47, 92, 189–190, *190f, 191f*

Cataract, in diabetic patient, 49–53, *50f, 51t, 52t*, 226, *227f*
incidence of, 203
management of, 203–219. *See also* Cataract surgery
vitreous hemorrhage and, 158

Cataract surgery, in diabetic patient, 203–219
complications of, 203–204, *203f, 204f*
endophthalmitis after, 230–231, *231f*
extracapsular cataract extraction versus phacoemulsification for, 208
intraocular lens choice and, 213
laser treatment of macular edema and, 148
macular edema after, treatment of, 211–213, *212f*
method of, 208–210, *214f*
posterior capsulotomy and, 211
preoperative severity of retinopathy and, 204–208, *205f, 207f, 214f*

visual acuity outcome and, 208–210, *214f*
factors affecting, 210–211
vitrectomy before, visual outcome affected by, 210–211
vitrectomy in combination with, 158–159, 207–208, 209–210, *209f*

Cholesterol, serum levels of, diabetic retinopathy and, 47, 194

Choroidal neovascularization, focal/grid laser treatment of diabetic macular edema causing, 133, 134–135*f*, 136

Cigarette smoking, diabetic retinopathy and, 47–48

Clinically significant macular edema (CSME), 105–108, *106f, 107f, 120t*
after cataract surgery, 205–207
photocoagulation for, 120–121

Collagen cross-linking, in diabetic retinopathy, 8, 13

Color fundus photography
in diabetic macular edema evaluation, 116
in diabetic retinopathy evaluation, 101–102, *102t*

Color vision, blue-yellow, defects in, in preclinical diabetic retinopathy, 4, *4t*

Consent, informed, for photocoagulation, pretreatment discussion and, 122–124, *124t, 125t*

Contact lens–associated bacterial corneal ulcers, in diabetic patient, 221

Contact lenses, for laser photocoagulation, 124–127, *126t*

Corneal diseases, in diabetic patient, 221–222, *222t, 223f*

Corneal ulcers, in diabetic patient, 221, *222f*

Cortical opacities, in diabetic patient, 49–51

Cotton-wool spots, in nonproliferative diabetic retinopathy, 7

C-peptide, as diabetic retinopathy risk factor, 44–45

Cranial nerve abnormalities, in diabetic patient, 222*t*, 229–230, 230*f*

CSME. *See* Clinically significant macular edema

Cutting probes, vitreous, for vitrectomy, 168–169

Cystoid macular edema, pseudophakic (Irvine-Gass syndrome), after cataract surgery, 148, 211–213

D

DAMAD (Dipyridamole and Aspirin Microangiopathy of Diabetes) Study, 195

DCCT. *See* Diabetes Control and Complications Trial

Delamination technique, for vitrectomy in vitreoretinal traction, 165–166, 167*f*

Diabetes Control and Complications Trial (DCCT), 90–91, 90*t*, 91*f*, 182–184, 182*f*, 183*t*, 184*f*

  abstracts of, 292–296

  glycemic control and retinopathy incidence/progression statistics in, 42, 44*t*, 69, 90–91, 90*t*, 91*f*, 182–184, 182*f*, 183*t*, 184*f*

Diabetes mellitus

  age at diagnosis of, as diabetic retinopathy risk factor, 40

  duration of

    as cataract risk factor, 51

    as diabetic retinopathy risk factor, 39, 39*f*, 40*t*, 41*t*

    visual loss/blindness prevalence and, 22, 22*f*

    as visual loss/blindness risk factor, 26, 27*t*, 28*f*

  glycemic control in. *See also* Glycemic control

    current recommendations for, 187–188, 188*t*

    diabetic retinopathy risk/progression affected by, 42–44, 43*t*, 44*t*, 69, 90–91, 90*t*, 91*f*, 181–188, 292–296

  ophthalmic examination/care and, 55–58, 56–57*t*, 58*t*, 59*t*, 94, 94*t*

Diabetic eye disease. *See also specific type*

  cataract, 49–53, 50*f*, 51*t*, 52*t*, 226, 227*f*

  cataract surgery and, 203–219

    complications of, 203–204, 203*f*, 204*f*

    extracapsular cataract extraction versus phacoemulsification for, 208

    intraocular lens choice and, 213

    laser treatment of macular edema and, 148

    macular edema after, treatment of, 211–213, 212*f*

    method of, 208–210, 214*f*

    posterior capsulotomy and, 211

    preoperative severity of retinopathy and, 204–208, 205*f*, 207*f*, 214*f*

    visual acuity outcome and, 208–210, 214*f*

      factors affecting, 210–211

    vitrectomy in combination with, 158–159, 209–210, 209*f*

  corneal, 221–222, 222*t*, 223*f*

  cranial nerve abnormalities, 222*t*, 229–230, 230*f*

  epidemiology of, 19–69, 181–182

    incidence and progression of retinopathy and, 34–35, 34*t*, 35*t*, 36*t*

    incidence of visual impairment and, 23–26, 24*t*, 25*t*, 27*t*, 28*f*, 28*t*

    prevalence of retinopathy and, 32, 33*t*

      in Wisconsin Epidemiologic Study of Diabetic Retinopathy (WESDR), 32

    prevalence of visual impairment and, 19–22, 20t, 21*f*, 22*f*, 23*f*

    retinopathy/comorbidity/mortality and, 49, 50*f*

    risk factors for retinopathy and, 36–49

    risk factors for visual loss/blindness and, 26–29, 27*t*, 28*f*, 28*t*

  glaucoma, 53–55, 53*f*, 54*t*, 222–226, 222*t*, 224*f*

  health care delivery and, 55–58, 56–57*t*, 58*t*, 59*t*, 94, 94*t*

  infectious, 222*t*, 230–232, 231*f*, 232*f*

  lens abnormalities, 222*t*, 226, 227*f*

  nonretinal, 221–237, 222*t*

  optic nerve abnormalities, 222*t*, 227–228, 227*f*, 229*f*

rehabilitation and, 29–30

socioeconomic and psychosocial factors and, 29–30

vascular endothelial growth factor induction of basic mechanisms and targets and, 256–259, 258f, 259f

    in ischemia-induced neovascularization, 255–256, 256–257f

    in nonproliferative disease, 253–254, 253f, 255f

    in proliferative disease, 248–251, 250f, 251f, 252f

visual acuity as predictor of death and, 30–32

Diabetic macular edema

    after cataract surgery

        laser photocoagulation and, 148

        treatment of, 211–213, 212f

    cataract surgery in presence of

        nonproliferative retinopathy and, 206

        proliferative retinopathy and, 206–207

    clinical evaluation of, 116

    clinically significant, 105–108, 106f, 107f, 120t

        after cataract surgery, 205–207

        photocoagulation for, 120–121

    fluorescein angiography in evaluation of, 105, 105–108, 106f, 107f

    pathogenesis of, 6, 9–10, 10f

    patient support and, 150

    with severe retinopathy, laser photocoagulation for, 146–148

    severity of, visual loss/blindness and, 29

    symptoms/medical history in, 116

    traction and, 148, 163–164

    treatment of. *See also specific type*

        clinical trials in evaluation of, 74–76, 81–99, 117

        early versus deferred, 87, 88f, 88t, 117

        laser photocoagulation, 115–153

            cataract surgery and, 148

            checklist for, 128t

            coexisting severe retinopathy and, 146–148

            complications of, 134–135f, 136–137, 137t

            lenses and focusing for, 124–127, 126t

postoperative care/followup after, 143, 144t

pretreatment discussion and, 122–124, 124t

technique for, 128–137, 129t, 130–131f, 132f, 133f, 134–135f, 136–137f

theoretical considerations and results in, 117–121, 118–119f, 120t

vitrectomy, coexisting traction and, 148, 163–164

visual loss and, 13, 13t

Diabetic maculopathy. *See* Diabetic macular edema

Diabetic papillopathy, 227–228, 227f, 229f

Diabetic retinopathy

    age at diabetes diagnosis and, 40

    age as risk factor in, 38–39, 38f

    alcohol consumption and, 48

    angiotensin-converting enzyme inhibitors affecting, 45–47, 92, 189–190, 190f, 191f, 192–194, 193f

    antihypertensive therapy affecting, 45–47, 92, 189–192, 297

    aspirin use and, 49, 85–86, 85f, 85t, 194–195, 283, 285, 286, 288

    blindness caused by. *See* Diabetic retinopathy, visual loss/blindness caused by

    blood glucose levels and, 8, 69

    body mass index and, 48

    candidate mediators of neovascularization and, 244–246, 245t

    cataract surgery and, 203–219

        severity of retinopathy and, 204–208, 205f, 207f, 214f

    cigarette smoking and, 47–48

    clinical evaluation of, 116, 117t

    with coexisting macular edema, laser photocoagulation for, 146–148

    color fundus photography in evaluation of, 101–102, 102t

Diabetic retinopathy *(cont.)*
  comorbidity/mortality and, 49, 50*f*
  diagnosis of, 116, 117*t*
    ophthalmic care recommendations and,
      55–58, 56–57*t*, 58*t*, 94, 94*t*
    ophthalmoscopy and fundus photography
      and, 102
  duration of diabetes and, 39, 39*f*, 40*t*, 41*t*
  dyslipidemic control and, 47, 92, 194, 289
  fluorescein angiography in evaluation of,
    102–108, 103*t*
  fluorescein angioscopy in evaluation of, 108
  genetic risk factors in, 37–38
  growth-factor hypothesis of neovascularization
    and, 242–244, 243*f*, 243*t*, 244*f*
  hemorrhage and, 149–150
  hyperglycemia and, 42–44, 43*t*, 44*t*, 69. *See also*
    Glycemic control
  hypertension and, 45–47, 46*t*. *See also* Anti-
    hypertensive therapy
  incidence of, 34–35, 34*t*, 35*t*, 36*t*
  insulin therapy affecting incidence/severity of,
    34–35, 35*t*, 36*t*, 45, 181–188. *See also*
    Glycemic control
  menarche and, 40–41
  metabolic pathways associated with, 7–8
  neovascular glaucoma caused by, 224–225,
    224*f*
  nephropathy and, 47
  nonproliferative. *See* Nonproliferative diabetic
    retinopathy
  pathogenesis of, 1–17
    nonproliferative disease and, 5–8, 6*t*, 7*f*, 9*f*
    proliferative disease and, 10–13, 11*f*, 11*t*, 12*f*
  patient support and, 150
  peptide status and, 44–45
  physical activity levels and, 48
  platelet inhibitors affecting, 194–196
  preclinical, 4–5, 4*t*

  pregnancy affecting, 49
  prevalence of, 32, 33*t*
    in Wisconsin Epidemiologic Study of Dia-
      betic Retinopathy (WESDR), 32
  prevention of, clinical trials in evaluation of,
    89–92, 91*f*, 93*f*, 93*t*, 94*t*
  progression of, 34–35, 34*t*, 35*t*, 36*t*
  proliferative. *See* Proliferative diabetic
    retinopathy
  protein kinase C in induction of, 8, 9*f*, 197,
    260–261, 260*f*
    KDR expression and, 259, 259*f*, 261
  proteinuria and, 47
  puberty and, 40–41
  race and, 36–37, 37*f*
  risk factors in, 36–49
  screening for, ophthalmoscopy and fundus
    photography in, 102
  serum lipid levels and, 47, 92, 194, 289
  sex (gender) and, 36
  socioeconomic status and, 48–49
  symptoms/medical history in, 116, 117*t*
  traction and, 146*f*, 148–149, 149*f*
  treatment of. *See also specific type*
    antiangiogenic therapy
      current status of, 263–264, 264*t*
      future hurdles for, 264–265
    clinical trials in evaluation of, 74–76, 81–99.
      See also specific study
    early versus deferred, 84–86, 86*f*, 86*t*, 87*f*,
      121, 123*f*
    experimental/novel, 239–273
      current status of therapeutic agents and,
        263–264, 264*t*
      medical therapies, 196–197
    historical perspective of, 239–242, 240*t*, 241*f*
    history of, 69–79
    laser photocoagulation, 115–153
      checklist for, 138*t*
      coexisting hemorrhage and, 149–150
      coexisting macular edema and, 146–148
      coexisting traction and, 147*f*, 148–149,
        149*f*

lenses and focusing for, 124–127, 126*t*
postoperative care/followup after,
143–146, 145*t*, 147*f*
pretreatment discussion and, 122–124,
125*t*
techniques for, 137–140, 138*t*, 140*t*,
141–142*f*, 142*f*
theoretical considerations and results in,
121–122, 121*t*, 122*f*, 122*t*, 123*f*
medical, 181–201
protein kinase C inhibitors in, 261–262,
261–262*f*, 263, 263*f*
vitrectomy, 155–179
clinical trials in evaluation of, 88–89, 89*t*,
286, 290–291
early versus deferred, 88–89, 89*t*, 286,
290–291
history of development of, 72–74, 73*f*
ultrasonography in evaluation of, 108–111,
109f, 110*f*
vascular endothelial growth factor in, 244, 245,
245*t*, 246
clinical associations and, 246–248, 247*f*, 249*f*
in nonproliferative disease, 8, 9*f*, 246,
253–254, 253*f*, 255*f*
in proliferative disease, 244, 245, 245*t*, 246,
248–251, 250*f*, 251*f*, 252*f*
visual loss/blindness caused by
incidence of, 23–26
mechanisms of, 13, 13*t*
prevalence of, 20*t*, 22, 23*f*
severity and, 28*t*, 29
Diabetic Retinopathy Study (DRS), 81–84, 82*f*,
82*t*, 83*f*, 83*t*, 121–122, 122*f*
abstracts/summaries of, 275–279
treatment protocols of, 138–139, 138*t*
Diabetic Retinopathy Vitrectomy Study
(DRVS), 88–89, 89*t*, 169, 170
abstracts of, 290–291
Diabetic vitreoretinopathy, ultrasonography in
management of, 108–111, 109*f*, 110*f*
Diabetic vitreous hemorrhage
aspirin use and, 85, 85*t*, 195
in diabetic vitreoretinopathy, 108, 109, 109*f*

with fibrovascular proliferation, vitrectomy
for, 156, 159, 159–160*f*
after full scatter laser photocoagulation, 146,
147*f*
vitrectomy for, 155–159, 156*f*, 156*t*, 157*f*, 158*f*
outcomes of, 169, 170*t*
Diode green lasers, for photocoagulation, 127
Diode infrared lasers, for photocoagulation, 127
Dipyridamole and Aspirin Microangiopathy of
Diabetes (DAMAD) Study, 195
DME. *See* Diabetic macular edema
Double-ring sign, in optic nerve hypoplasia, 228
DR3/DR4, as diabetic retinopathy risk factor,
37–38
Drainage devices, glaucoma, 225
DRS. *See* Diabetic Retinopathy Study
DRVS. *See* Diabetic Retinopathy Vitrectomy
Study
Dye yellow lasers, for photocoagulation, 127
Dyslipidemic control, diabetic eye disease inci-
dence/progression affected by, 92, 194,
289

E
Early Treatment Diabetic Retinopathy Study
(ETDRS), 84–87, 84*t*, 85*f*, 86*f*, 87*f*, 88*f*,
88*t*, 117, 121, 123*f*
abstracts of, 279-290
aspirin-use statistics in, 195, 283, 285, 286, 288
cataract surgery statistics in, 206
dyslipidemic control statistics in, 194, 289
ECCE. See Extracapsular cataract extraction
Economic issues, in diabetes-related visual
loss/blindness, 29–30
Edema, retinal, power requirements for photocoagulation and, 133
Electroretinography (ERG), in preclinical diabetic retinopathy, 4, 4*t*

En bloc technique, for vitrectomy in vitreo-retinal traction, 166, 167*f*

Endophthalmitis, postoperative, in diabetic patient, 172, 230–231, 231*f*

Endostatin, as mediator of diabetic retinopathy, 245*t*

ERG. *See* Electroretinography

ETDRS. See Early Treatment Diabetic Retinopathy Study

EUCLID (EURODIAB Controlled Trial of Lisinopril in Insulin-Dependent Diabetes Mellitus), 193–194, 193*f*

EURODIAB Controlled Trial of Lisinopril in Insulin-Dependent Diabetes Mellitus (EUCLID), 193–194, 193*f*

Extracapsular cataract extraction (ECCE), in diabetic patient. *See also* Cataract surgery
endophthalmitis after, 230
visual acuity outcome and, 208

Eye examinations, in diabetic patient, 55–58, 56–57*t*, 58*t*, 59*t*, 94, 94*t*

F

Fibrinoid syndrome, after vitrectomy, 164

Fibroblast growth factor, basic (bFGF), in diabetic retinopathy, 244, 245, 245*t*, 259, 259*f*

Fibrovascular proliferation (FVP)/fibrovascular membranes
in diabetic macular edema, 148
in diabetic vitreoretinopathy, 109–110, 109*f*
after vitrectomy, 164
vitrectomy for, 159–160, 159–160*f*, 161*f*
combined media opacities and, 156, 159, 159–160*f*

Filtering surgery, for glaucoma in diabetic patient, 225

"Fluctuating myopia," 226

Fluorescein angiography, in diabetic retinopathy evaluation, 102–108, 103*t*
in mild nonproliferative retinopathy, 104–105, 104*f*
in moderate nonproliferative retinopathy with clinically significant macular edema, 105–108, 106*f*, 107*f*
in moderate nonproliferative retinopathy with macular edema not clinically significant, 105
in moderate nonproliferative retinopathy without macular edema, 105
in severe nonproliferative diabetic retinopathy, 108

Fluorescein angioscopy, in diabetic patient retinopathy evaluation, 108

Fluorouracil, filtering surgery in diabetic patient and, 225

Focal/grid laser treatment, for diabetic macular edema, 128–137, 129*t*, 130–131*f*, 132*f*, 133*f*, 134–135*f*, 136–137*f*
complications of, 134–135*f*, 136–137, 137*t*
postoperative care/followup after, 143, 144*t*

Fundus photography, color
in diabetic macular edema, 116
in diabetic retinopathy, 101–102, 102*t*, 116

FVP. *See* Fibrovascular proliferation/fibrovascular membranes

G

Gender
diabetes-related visual loss/blindness and, 26
diabetic retinopathy and, 36
visual outcome after cataract surgery and, 210

Genetics, as diabetic retinopathy risk factor, 37–38

GH. *See* Growth hormone

Ghost-cell glaucoma, in diabetic patient, 225–226

Glaucoma, in diabetic patient, 53–55, 53*f*, 54*t*, 222–226, 222*t*, 224*f*
after cataract surgery, 203
after vitrectomy, 171

Glaucoma drainage devices, 225

Glial cells, retinal, 1–2, *2f*

Glucose metabolism, in diabetic retinopathy, 8, 69

Glutamate, in diabetic retinopathy, 5

Glycation end products, vascular damage in diabetic retinopathy caused by, 8

Glycemic control, diabetic retinopathy incidence/progression affected by, 42–44, 43*t*, 44*t*, 69, 90–91, 90*t*, 91*f*, 181–188, 292–296

  current recommendations for, 187–188, 188*t*

  Diabetes Control and Complications Trial (DCCT) statistics on, 90–91, 90*t*, 91*f*, 182–184, 182*f*, 183*t*, 184*f*, 292–296

  intensive insulin therapy and, 90–91, 90*t*, 91*f*, 182–184, 182*f*, 183*t*, 184*f*, 185–186, 186*f*, 187*f*, 292–296

  Stockholm Diabetes Intervention Study (SDIS) statistics on, 184–185

  United Kingdom Prospective Diabetes Study (UKPDS) statistics on, 42–43, 185–186, 186*f*, 187*f*, 296-297, 298

  Wisconsin Epidemiologic Study of Diabetic Retinopathy (WESDR) statistics on, 45, 181–182

Glycosylated hemoglobin (glycohemoglobin/hemoglobin A_{1c}), 8

  diabetic retinopathy risk/progression and, 42, 43*t*, 44, 181–182, 182–184, 182*f*, 184*f*, 186, 186*f*

    recommendations for levels of, 187–188, 188*t*

Goldmann lenses, for photocoagulation, 124–125, 126*t*

Goniophotocoagulation, for neovascular glaucoma in diabetic patient, 224–225

Green laser wavelengths, for photocoagulation, 127

Grid/focal laser treatment, for diabetic macular edema, 128–137, 129*t*, 130–131*f*, 132*f*, 133*f*, 134–135*f*, 136–137*f*

  complications of, 134–135*f*, 136–137, 137*t*

  postoperative care/followup after, 143, 144*t*

Growth factors, in neovascularization, 242–244, 243*f*, 243*t*, 244f. *See also* Vascular endothelial growth factor

  criteria for, 242, 243*t*

  stages in, 242–244, 244*f*

Growth hormone (GH), as mediator of diabetic retinopathy, 244, 245–246, 245*t*

H

H_1-receptor antagonists, diabetic retinopathy incidence/progression affected by, 197

H_2-receptor antagonists, diabetic retinopathy incidence/progression affected by, 197

HbA_{1c}. *See* Hemoglobin A_{1c} (glycohemoglobin)

HDS (Hypertension in Diabetes Study), 189–190, 190*f*, 191*f*

Health care delivery, early identification of diabetic eye disease and, 55–58, 56–57*t*, 58*t*, 59*t*, 94, 94*t*

Heinz bodies, in ghost-cell glaucoma, 225

Hemoglobin A_{1c} (glycohemoglobin), 8

  diabetic retinopathy risk/progression and, 42, 43*t*, 44, 181–182, 182–184, 182*f*, 184*f*

  recommendations for levels of, 187–188, 188*t*

Hemolytic glaucoma, in diabetic patient, 226. *See also* Glaucoma

Hemosiderotic glaucoma, in diabetic patient, 226. *See also* Glaucoma

Hepatocyte growth factor (HGF), as mediator of diabetic retinopathy, 245*t*, 246

HGF (hepatocyte growth factor), as mediator of diabetic retinopathy, 245*t*, 246

Hispanics, diabetic retinopathy in, 36–37, 37*f*

Histamine-receptor antagonists, diabetic retinopathy incidence/progression affected by, 197

HLA (human leukocyte antigens), as diabetic retinopathy risk factor, 37–38

Human leukocyte antigens (HLA), as diabetic
retinopathy risk factor, 37–38
Hyperglycemia
diabetic retinopathy risk/progression affected
by, 42–44, 43*t*, 44*t*, 69. *See also* Glycemic control
protein kinase C activation caused by, 260,
260f
Hypertension
control of
current recommendations for, 192
diabetic retinopathy incidence/progression
affected by, 45–47, 92, 189–192, 297
as diabetic retinopathy risk factor, 45–47, 46*t*
Hypertension in Diabetes Study (HDS),
189–190, 190*f*, 191*f*
Hypoxia, vascular endothelial growth factor
expression affected by, 256–258, 258*f*,
259*f*

I,J
IGF-1 (insulin-like growth factor), as mediator
of diabetic retinopathy, 244, 245
Infectious eye disease, in diabetic patient, 222*t*,
230–232, 231*f*, 232*f*
Informed consent, for photocoagulation, pretreatment discussion and, 122–124,
124*t*, 125*t*
Infrared laser wavelengths, for photocoagulation,
127
Insulin-like growth factor (IFG-1), as mediator
of diabetic retinopathy, 244, 245
Insulin therapy
diabetic macular edema affected by, 34, 36*t*
diabetic retinopathy incidence/progression affected by, 34–35, 35*t*, 36*t*, 45, 181–188
current recommendations for, 187–188, 188*t*

Diabetes Control and Complications Trial
(DCCT) statistics on, 90–91, 90*t*, 91*f*,
182–184, 182*f*, 183*t*, 184*f*, 292–296
intensive therapy and, 90–91, 90*t*, 91*f*,
182–184, 182*f*, 183*t*, 184*f*, 185–186,
186*f*, 187*f*, 292–296
Kumamoto University Study statistics on,
185
Stockholm Diabetes Intervention Study
(SDIS) statistics on, 184–185
United Kingdom Prospective Diabetes
Study (UKPDS) statistics on, 42–43,
185–186, 186*f*, 187*f*, 296–297, 298
Wisconsin Epidemiologic Study of Diabetic
Retinopathy (WESDR) statistics on,
45, 181–182
visual loss/blindness incidence and, 23, 24*t*,
25*t*, 27*t*, 28*f*, 28*t*
visual loss/blindness prevalence and, 20, 21*f*,
22
Integrins, as mediators of diabetic retinopathy,
245*t*
Intraocular lens implantation, in diabetic patient, 213
endophthalmitis after, 230
Intraocular surgery, in diabetic patient, endophthalmitis after, 172, 230–231, 231*f*
IOL. See Intraocular lens implantation
Iris neovascularization (NVI), 241*f*, 242
in diabetic patient, 224–225, 224*f*
after cataract surgery, 203, 205, 205*f*
vascular endothelial growth factor in, 246–248,
247*f*, 249*f*, 255–256, 256–257*f*
Iris retractors, for vitrectomy, 169
Iritis, after laser photocoagulation, 145
Irvine-Gass syndrome (pseudophakic cystoid
macular edema), after cataract surgery,
148, 211–213
Ischemia-induced neovascularization, vascular
endothelial growth factor in, 255–256,
256–257*f*
Ischemic retinopathies, 240, 240*t*. *See also*
Diabetic retinopathy
Isosorbide, for angle-closure glaucoma in diabetic patient, 223

K

KDR expression
  basic fibroblast growth factor affecting, 259,
      259*f*
  protein kinase C activation and, 259, 259*f*, 261
Keratitis, in diabetic patient, 221
Krypton lasers, for photocoagulation, 127
  in diabetic macular edema, 117–120
Kumamoto University Study, 185

L

Laplace's law, diabetic macular edema and,
    9, 10*f*
Laser photocoagulation
  for diabetic macular edema and diabetic
      retinopathy, 115–153
    after cataract surgery, 148, 206
    before cataract surgery, 206, 207, 208
    clinical trials in evaluation of, 81–87, 88*f*,
        88*t*, 117, 121–122
    in combined macular edema and severe
        retinopathy, 146–148
    Diabetic Retinopathy Study in evaluation
        of, 81–84, 82*f*, 82*t*, 83*f*, 83*t*, 275–279
    diagnosis/clinical evaluation and, 116, 117*t*
    Early Treatment Diabetic Retinopathy
        Study in evaluation of, 84–87, 84*t*, 85*f*,
        86*f*, 87*f*, 88*f*, 88*t*, 279–290
    early versus deferred, 86–87, 86*f*, 86*t*, 87*f*,
        88*f*, 88*t*
    focal/grid, 128–137, 129*t*, 130–131*f*, 132*f*,
        133*f*, 134–135*f*, 136–137*f*
      complications of, 134–135*f*, 136–137, 137*t*
      postoperative care/followup after, 143,
          144*t*
    history of development of, 71–72
    laser wavelengths for, 127
    lenses and focusing for, 124–126, 126*t*
    in macular edema after cataract surgery, 148
    in macular edema with traction, 148
    mechanism of action of, 72
    panretinal/scatter, 129*t*, 137–140, 138*t*, 140*t*,
        141–142*f*, 142*f*
      postoperative care/followup after,
          143–146, 145*t*, 146*f*, 147*f*

    patient support and, 150
    postoperative care/followup after, 143–146,
        144*t*, 145*t*, 146*f*, 147*f*
    pretreatment discussion and, 122–124, 124*t*,
        125*t*
    prevalence rates of, 58, 59*t*
    in proliferative retinopathy with hemor-
        rhage, 149–150
    in proliferative retinopathy with traction,
        147*f*, 148–149, 149*f*
    results in, 117–122
    symptoms and medical history and, 115–116
    techniques for, 128–140, 141–142*f*, 142*f*
    theoretical considerations and, 117–122
    visual loss/blindness incidence affected by,
        25, 26
  for neovascular glaucoma in diabetic patient,
      224–225
Laser scars, after diabetic macular edema treat-
    ment, 137
Legal blindness, diabetes-related. *See also*
      Blindness
  incidence of, 23–26, 24*t*, 25*t*, 27*t*, 28*f*, 28*t*
  as predictor of death, 30–32, 30*f*, 31*f*
  prevalence of, 19–22, 20*t*, 21*f*, 22*f*, 23*f*
Lens abnormalities. *See also specific type*
  in diabetic patient, 222*t*, 226, 227*f*
Lenses, for laser photocoagulation, 124–127,
    126*t*
Lens opacities, in diabetic patient, 49–53, 50*f*,
    51*t*, 52*t*. *See also* Cataract
  vitreous hemorrhage and, 158
Light energy, for treatment of diabetic retinopa-
    thy, 70. *See also* Photocoagulation
Light probe, for vitrectomy, 169
Lipid-lowering therapy, diabetic eye disease
    incidence/progression affected by,
    92, 194, 289
Lipids, serum levels of. *See also* Lipid-lowering
    therapy
  diabetic retinopathy and, 47, 92, 289

Lisinopril, diabetic eye disease incidence/progression affected by, 47, 92, 193–194, 193*f*

LY333531, for diabetic retinopathy treatment, 261–262, 261–262*f*, 263, 263*f*, 264*t*

M

Macular edema
  diabetic. *See* Diabetic macular edema
  pseudophakic cystoid (Irvine-Gass syndrome), after cataract surgery, 148, 211–213

Macular traction. *See also* Vitreoretinal traction
  diabetic macular edema and, 148, 163–164
  proliferative diabetic retinopathy and, 147*f*, 148–149, 149*f*

Maculopathy, diabetic. *See* Diabetic macular edema

MAs. *See* Microaneurysms

Mainster lenses, for photocoagulation, 124, 126*t*, 127

Media opacities. *See also* Cataract
  vitrectomy for
    indications for, 155–159, 156*f*, 156*t*
    outcomes of, 169–170, 170*t*
    techniques for, 165

Menarche/menstruation, diabetes onset before/after, as diabetic retinopathy risk factor, 40–41

Mexican Americans, diabetic retinopathy in, 36–37, 37*f*

Microaneurysms
  in diabetic macular edema, 10, 106, 106*f*, 107*f*
  photocoagulation in treatment of, 117, 118–119*f*, 129–131, 130–131*f*, 132*f*, 133*f*, 134–135*f*

Mitomycin C, filtering surgery in diabetic patient and, 225

Model Reporting Area (MRA)
  visual impairment incidence statistics in, 23
  visual impairment prevalence statistics in, 19, 20*t*

Mucormycosis, orbital, in diabetic patient, 231–232, 232*f*

Müller cells, retinal, 1–2, 2*f*

Myo-inositol, reduction of, in diabetic retinopathy, 8

"Myopia, fluctuating," 226

N

Neovascular glaucoma, in diabetic patient, 224–225, 224*f*. *See also* Glaucoma

Neovascularization, in diabetic patient, 10–13, 11*f*, 11*t*, 12*f*, 224–225, 224*f*, 240–242, 241*f*
  candidate mediators of, 244–246, 245*t*
  after cataract surgery, 203, 205, 205*f*, 242
  cellular events leading to, 12, 12*f*
  clinical features of, 240–242, 241*f*
  disorders associated with, 240, 240*t*
  focal/grid laser treatment of diabetic macular edema causing, 133, 134–135*f*, 136
  growth-factor hypothesis of, 242–244, 243*f*, 243*t*, 244*f*
  ischemia-induced, vascular endothelial growth factor in, 255–256, 256–257*f*
  medical approaches to prevention of, 92
  vascular endothelial growth factor in, 244, 245, 245*t*, 246
    clinical associations and, 246–248, 247*f*, 249*f*

Neovascularization of iris (NVI). *See* Iris neovascularization

Nephropathy, diabetic, diabetic retinopathy and, 47

Neurons, retinal, 1, 2*f*
  visual loss in diabetes caused by dysfunction of, 13, 13*t*

Neuropathy, anterior ischemic optic, in diabetic patient, 228

Neurotrophic ulcers, in diabetic patient, 221, 222*f*

Nonproliferative diabetic retinopathy (NPDR). *See also* Diabetic retinopathy
  cataract surgery and
    in patients with macular edema, 206

in patients without macular edema,
205–206, 205*f*, 207*f*
early versus deferred photocoagulation affecting outcome of, 86, 87*f*
fluorescein angiography in evaluation of
in mild disease, 104–105, 104*f*
in moderate disease with clinically significant macular edema, 105–108, 106*f*, 107*f*
in moderate disease with macular edema not clinically significant, 105
in moderate disease without macular edema, 105
in severe disease, 108
pathogenesis of, 5–8, 6*t*, 7*f*, 9*f*
race as risk factor in, 37
vascular endothelial growth factor in, 8, 9*f*, 246, 253–254, 253*f*, 255*f*
NPDR. *See* Nonproliferative diabetic retinopathy
NVI. *See* Iris neovascularization

0

Ocular media, visual loss in diabetes caused by abnormalities of, 13, 13*t*
Opacities, media. *See* Media opacities
Open-angle glaucoma, primary, in diabetic patient, 222–223. *See also* Glaucoma
Ophthalmoscopy, for diabetic retinopathy screening/evaluation, 102, 116, 117*t*
Optic atrophy, in diabetic patient, 228
Optic disc edema, in diabetic patient, 227–228, 227*f*, 229*f*
Optic nerve abnormalities, in diabetic patient, 222*t*, 227–228, 227*f*, 229*f*
Optic nerve hypoplasia, in children of diabetic patients, 228
Optic neuropathy, anterior ischemic, in diabetic patient, 228
Orbital mucormycosis, in diabetic patient, 231–232, 232*f*
Oxygen consumption, retinal, in diabetic macular edema, 120

P,Q

Panfunduscope lens, for photocoagulation, 125
Panretinal (scatter) photocoagulation (PRP), 12, 129*t*, 137–140, 138*t*, 140*t*, 141–142*f*, 142*f*. *See also* Laser photocoagulation
anesthetic for, 137–138
after cataract surgery, 206
before cataract surgery, 207, 208
checklist for, 138*t*
early versus deferred, 86, 86*f*, 86*t*, 87*f*, 122
history of development of, 72
lenses and focusing for, 124–127, 126*t*
mechanism of action of, 72, 121–122
postoperative care/followup after, 143–146, 145*t*, 146*f*, 147*f*
single versus multiple sessions for, 139–140
theoretical considerations and results in, 121–122, 121*t*
treatment intensity and, 140, 140*t*, 141–142*f*, 142*f*
treatment parameters for, 138–139, 138*t*
visual loss/blindness incidence affected by, 25, 26
Papillopathy, diabetic, 227–228, 227*f*, 229*f*
Pars plana lensectomy, vitrectomy combined with, 158–159
Pars plana vitrectomy. *See also* Vitrectomy
history of development of, 73–74, 73*f*
PDR. *See* Proliferative diabetic retinopathy
Pentoxifylline, diabetic retinopathy incidence/progression affected by, 196–197
Peptide status, as diabetic retinopathy risk factor, 44–45
Peribulbar anesthesia, for panretinal photocoagulation, 137–138
Pericytes, in nonproliferative diabetic retinopathy, 7
Persistent epithelial defects, in diabetic patient, 221–222, 222*f*
Phacoemulsification, in diabetic patient. *See also* Cataract surgery
endophthalmitis after, 231*f*
visual acuity outcome and, 208

Photocoagulation, for diabetic retinopathy. *See also* Laser photocoagulation
history of development of, 70
Physical activity, diabetic retinopathy and, 48
Pigment dispersion, after cataract surgery in diabetic patient, 203
Planoconcave contact lenses, for photocoagulation, 124–127, 126*t*
Platelet inhibitors, diabetic retinopathy incidence/progression affected by, 194–196
POAG. *See* Primary open-angle glaucoma
Poiseuille's law, diabetic macular edema and, 9, 10*f*
Polyol pathway activation, in diabetic retinopathy, 8
Posterior capsulotomy, in diabetic patient, 211
Posterior hyaloid attachment, diabetic macular edema and, 148, 163–164
Posterior synechiae, after cataract surgery in diabetic patient, 203, 203*f*
Preclinical retinopathy, 4–5, 4*t*
Pregnancy, diabetic retinopathy and, 49
Primary open-angle glaucoma (POAG), in diabetic patient, 222–223. *See also* Glaucoma
Proliferative diabetic retinopathy (PDR). *See also* Diabetic retinopathy
alcohol consumption and, 48
blindness caused by, 22
cataract surgery and, 206–208, 209–210
cellular events leading to, 12, 12*f*
clinical associations of vascular endothelial growth factor and, 246–248, 247*f*, 249*f*
clinical evaluation of, 116, 117*t*
with coexisting macular edema, laser photocoagulation for, 146–148
comorbidity/mortality and, 49, 50*f*
diagnosis of, 116, 117*t*
ophthalmic care recommendations and, 55–58, 56–57*t*, 58*t*

duration of diabetes and, 39, 39*f*, 40*t*, 41*t*
features of, 11*t*
genetic risk factors in, 37–38
hemorrhage and, 149–150
hyperglycemia and, 42–44, 43*t*, 44*t*. *See also* Glycemic control
hypertension and, 45–47, 46*t*. *See also* Antihypertensive therapy
incidence of, 34–35, 34*t*, 35*t*
neovascular glaucoma caused by, 224–225, 224*f*
pathogenesis of, 10–13, 11*f*, 11*t*, 12*f*
patient support and, 150
peptide status and, 44–45
race and, 36–37
sex (gender) and, 36
socioeconomic status and, 48–49
symptoms/medical history in, 116
traction and, 147*f*, 148–149, 149*f*
treatment of. *See also specific type*
laser photocoagulation, 115–153
checklist for, 138*t*
clinical trials in evaluation of, 81–86, 121–122
coexisting hemorrhage and, 149–150
coexisting macular edema and, 146–148
coexisting traction and, 147*f*, 148–149, 149*f*
early versus deferred, 86, 87*f*
lenses and focusing for, 124–127, 126*t*
postoperative care/followup after, 143–146, 145*t*, 146*f*, 147*f*
pretreatment discussion and, 122–124, 125*t*
techniques for, 137–140, 138*t*, 140*t*, 141–142*f*, 142*f*
theoretical considerations and results in, 121–122, 121*t*, 122*f*, 122*t*, 123*f*
vitrectomy, clinical trials in evaluation of, 88–89, 89*t*, 286, 290–291
vascular endothelial growth factor in, 244, 245, 245*t*, 246, 248–251, 250*f*, 251*f*, 252*f*
Protein kinase A, in hypoxic effects on vascular endothelial growth factor, 258, 258*f*

Protein kinase C
  in diabetic retinopathy, 8, 9*f*, 197, 260–261,
      260*f*
    KDR expression and, 259, 259*f*, 261
  inhibitors of, for diabetic retinopathy treat-
      ment, 261–262, 261–262*f*, 263, 263*f*,
      264*t*
Proteinuria, in diabetic nephropathy, diabetic
      retinopathy and, 47
PRP. *See* Panretinal (scatter) photocoagulation
Pseudohypopyon, in ghost-cell glaucoma, 225
Pseudophakic cystoid macular edema (Irvine-
      Gass syndrome), after cataract surgery,
      148, 211–213
Pseudophakic pupillary block, after cataract sur-
      gery in diabetic patient, 203
Puberty, diabetes onset before/after, as diabetic
      retinopathy risk factor, 40–41

R
Race, as diabetic retinopathy risk factor, 36–37,
      37*f*
Ranitidine, diabetic retinopathy incidence/pro-
      gression affected by, 197
Red laser wavelengths, for photocoagulation,
      127
Refractive error, in diabetic patient, 226
Rehabilitation programs, in diabetes-related vi-
      sual loss/blindness, 29–30
Retina
  anatomy and physiology of, 1–4, 2*f*
  in preclinical diabetic retinopathy, 4–5, 4*t*
Retinal capillaries, 2, 3*f*
  in diabetic macular edema, photocoagulation
      and, 120
Retinal circulation, 2, 3*f*
  impaired autoregulation of
    in diabetic macular edema, 9, 10*f*
    in diabetic retinopathy, 2–4
Retinal depression sign, in nonproliferative
      diabetic retinopathy, 6, 7*f*
Retinal detachment
  in diabetic vitreoretinopathy, 109–111, 110*f*
  visual loss in diabetes caused by, 13, 13*t*

after vitrectomy, 171
    second vitrectomy for, 164
  vitrectomy for, 160–163, 162*f*, 163*f*
    outcomes of, 170, 170*t*, 171*f*
Retinal edema, power requirements for photo-
      coagulation and, 133
Retinal microcirculation, 2, 3*f*
Retinal neovascularization. *See* Neovascularization
Retinal pigment epithelium (RPE), in diabetic
      macular edema, photocoagulation and,
      117, 120
Retinal vascular permeability
  protein kinase C in regulation of, 261–262
  vascular endothelial growth factor in regula-
      tion of, 250–251, 252*f*
Retinopathies
  diabetic. *See* Diabetic retinopathy
  ischemic, 240, 240*t*. *See also* Diabetic reti-
      nopathy
Retrobulbar anesthesia, for panretinal photo-
      coagulation, 137–138
Rhegmatogenous retinal detachment
  after vitrectomy, second vitrectomy for, 164
  vitrectomy for, 163, 163*f*
    outcomes of, 170, 170*t*
Rheologic agents, diabetic retinopathy incidence/
      progression affected by, 196–197
Rodenstock Panfunduscope lens, for photoco-
      agulation, 125
RPE. *See* Retinal pigment epithelium
Rubeosis iridis, with diabetic vitreous hemor-
      rhage, vitrectomy for, 157, 157*f*
Ruby laser, for photocoagulation, 71

S
Scatter (panretinal) photocoagulation, 12, 129*t*,
      137–140, 138*t*, 140*t*, 141–142*f*, 142*f*.
      See also Laser photocoagulation
  anesthetic for, 137–138
  cataract surgery complications limited by, 206
  checklist for, 138*t*

Scatter (panretinal) photocoagulation *(cont.)*
  early versus deferred, 86, 86*f*, 86*t*, 87*f*, 122
  history of development of, 72
  lenses and focusing for, 124–127, 126*t*
  mechanism of action of, 72, 121–122
  postoperative care/followup after, 143–146,
      145*t*, 146*f*, 147*f*
  single versus multiple sessions for, 139–140
  theoretical considerations and results in,
      121–122, 121*t*
  treatment intensity and, 140, 140*t*, 141–142*f*,
      142*f*
  treatment parameters for, 138–139, 138*t*
  visual loss/blindness incidence affected by,
      25, 26
Scleral buckling, for vitreoretinal traction, 166
Sclerotomy, for vitrectomy, 169
Scotomas, focal/grid laser treatment of diabetic
      macular edema causing, 133
SDIS (Stockholm Diabetes Intervention Study),
      184–185
Segmentation technique, for vitrectomy in vitreo-
      retinal traction, 165, 165–166*f*
Sex (gender)
  diabetes-related visual loss/blindness and, 26
  diabetic retinopathy and, 36
  visual outcome after cataract surgery and, 210
Slit-lamp biomicroscopy
  in diabetic macular edema evaluation, 116
  in diabetic retinopathy evaluation, 116, 117*t*
Smoking, diabetic retinopathy and, 47–48
"Snowflake" cataract, in diabetic patient, 226,
      227*f*
Socioeconomic issues/status
  in diabetes-related visual loss/blindness,
      29–30
  as diabetic retinopathy risk factor, 48–49
Sorbinil Retinopathy Trial (SRT), 92, 93*f*, 93*t*,
      196
  abstract of, 296

Sorbitol, in diabetic retinopathy, 8, 92, 196
SRT. *See* Sorbinil Retinopathy Trial
Starling's law, diabetic macular edema and, 9, 10*f*
Stockholm Diabetes Intervention Study (SDIS),
      184–185
Subcapsular cataract, posterior, in diabetic pa-
      tient, 51
Subhyaloidal hemorrhage, in diabetic retinopa-
      thy, 149–150
  vitrectomy for, 157–158, 158*f*
  outcomes of, 169
Subretinal fibrosis, focal/grid laser treatment of
      diabetic macular edema causing, 136
Synechiae, posterior, after cataract surgery in
      diabetic patient, 203, 203*f*

T
Thalidomide, for diabetic retinopathy treatment,
      263, 264*t*
Thiazide diuretics, current recommendations for
      use of, 192
Ticlopidine Microangiopathy of Diabetes
      (TIMAD) Study Group, 195–196
TIMAD (Ticlopidine Microangiopathy of Dia-
      betes) Study Group, 195–196
Traction, vitreoretinal
  diabetic macular edema and, 148, 163–164
  diabetic retinopathy and, 147*f*, 148–149, 149*f*
  vitrectomy for
      indications for, 156*t*, 159–164, 159–160*f*,
          161*f*, 162*f*, 163*f*
      outcomes of, 170, 170*t*, 171*f*
      techniques for, 165–166, 165–166*f*, 167*f*
Tractional retinal detachment
  after vitrectomy, second vitrectomy for, 164
  vitrectomy for, 160–162, 162*f*
      outcomes of, 170, 170*t*, 171*f*

U
UGDP. *See* University Group Diabetes Program
UKPDS. *See* United Kingdom Prospective Dia-
      betes Study
Ultrasonography, in diabetic retinopathy evalua-
      tion, 108–111, 109*f*, 110*f*

United Kingdom Prospective Diabetes Study (UKPDS)
abstracts/summaries of, 296–298
glycemic control and retinopathy incidence/progression statistics in, 42–43, 185–186, 186*f*, 187*f*, 296–297, 298
hypertension–retinopathy relationship statistics in, 45–47, 92, 189–190, 190*f*, 191*f*, 297
University Group Diabetes Program (UGDP), glycemic control and retinopathy incidence/progression statistics in, 42

V

Vascular endothelial growth factor (VEGF), 2, 246
in diabetic retinopathy, 244, 245, 245*t*, 246
clinical associations of, 246–248, 247*f*, 249*f*
in nonproliferative disease, 8, 9*f*, 246
in proliferative disease, 12, 12*f*, 244, 245, 245*t*, 246, 248–251, 250*f*, 251*f*, 252*f*
expression and signaling of, 256–259, 258*f*, 259*f*
inhibitors of, diabetic retinopathy incidence/progression affected by, 197, 259
in neovascularization, 243*f*, 244*f*
Vascular endothelial growth factor receptor expression
basic fibroblast growth factor affecting, 259, 259*f*
protein kinase C activation and, 259, 259*f*, 261
Vascular endothelial growth factor/vascular permeability factor (VEGF/VPF). *See also* Vascular endothelial growth factor
in diabetic retinopathy
nonproliferative, 8, 9*f*
proliferative, 12, 12*f*
Vascular permeability
protein kinase C in regulation of, 261–262
vascular endothelial growth factor in regulation of, 250–251, 252*f*
VEGF. *See* Vascular endothelial growth factor
VEGF/VPF. *See* Vascular endothelial growth factor/vascular permeability factor

Venules, retinal, 2, 3*f*
Visual loss in diabetes. *See also* Blindness, diabetes-related; Diabetic retinopathy
economic costs of, 29–30
incidence of, 23–26, 24*t*, 25*t*, 27*t*, 28*f*, 28*t*
mechanisms of, 13, 13*t*
as predictor of death, 30–32, 30*f*, 31*f*
prevalence of, 19–22, 20*t*, 21*f*, 22*f*, 23*f*
rehabilitation and, 29–30
risk factors for, 26–29, 27*t*, 28*f*, 28*t*
Vitrectomy/pars plana vitrectomy, in diabetic patient, 155–179
before cataract surgery, visual outcome affected by, 210–211
cataract surgery combined with, 158–159, 207–208, 209–210, 209*f*
clinical trials in evaluation of, 88–89, 89*t*, 286, 290–291
complications of, 171–172
second vitrectomy for, 164
outcomes of, 171
for diabetic macular edema with traction, 148, 163–164
early versus deferred, 88–89, 89*t*, 155, 156–157, 286, 290–291
endophthalmitis after, 172, 231
for hemorrhage control, 168
history of development of, 72–74, 73*f*
indications for, 155–164, 156*t*
instrumentation for, 168–169
for laser endophotocoagulation, 168
for management of severe conditions, 168
for media opacities
indications for, 155–159, 156*f*, 156*t*
outcomes of, 169–170, 170*t*
techniques for, 165
objectives of, 164–169, 165*t*
outcomes of, 169–171, 170*t*, 171*f*
public health considerations and, 172
for reproliferation, 168
for retinal breaks, 168
techniques for, 164–169, 165–166*f*, 167*f*

Vitrectomy/pars plana vitrectomy, in diabetic
patient *(cont.)*
for vitreoretinal traction
indications for, 156*t*, 159–164, 159–160*f*,
161*f*, 162*f*, 163*f*
techniques for, 165–166, 165–166*f*, 167*f*
Vitreoretinal traction, vitrectomy for
indications for, 156*t*, 159–164, 159–160*f*, 161*f*,
162*f*, 163*f*
outcomes of, 170, 170*t*, 171*f*
techniques for, 165–166, 165–166*f*, 167*f*
Vitreoretinopathy, diabetic, ultrasonography in
management of, 108–111, 109*f*, 110*f*
Vitreous-cutting probes, for vitrectomy, 168–169
Vitreous detachment
in diabetic vitreoretinopathy, 109–110, 110*f*
partial, diabetic macular edema and, 148
Vitreous hemorrhage
aspirin use and, 85, 85*t*, 195, 288
in diabetic vitreoretinopathy, 108, 109, 109*f*
with fibrovascular proliferation, vitrectomy
for, 156, 159, 159–160*f*
after full scatter laser photocoagulation, 146,
147*f*
after vitrectomy, 171
second vitrectomy for, 164
vitrectomy for, 155–159, 156*f*, 156*t*, 157*f*, 158*f*,
164
outcomes of, 169, 170*t*
Volk lenses, for photocoagulation, 124, 126*t*, 127

W
WESDR. *See* Wisconsin Epidemiologic Study of
Diabetic Retinopathy
Wide-angle viewing systems, for vitrectomy, 169
Wisconsin Epidemiologic Study of Diabetic
Retinopathy (WESDR), 181–182
cataract risk factor statistics in, 51, 51*t*, 52*t*
economic costs of blindness statistics in, 29
glaucoma risk factor statistics in, 53, 53*f*
ophthalmic care statistics in, 55, 58*t*
photocoagulation prevalence rate statistics in,
58, 59*t*

rehabilitation statistics in, 29
retinopathy comorbidity and mortality statistics in, 49, 50*f*
retinopathy incidence/progression statistics in,
34–35, 34*t*, 35*t*, 36*t*
retinopathy prevalence statistics in, 32
retinopathy risk factor statistics in
age and, 38–39, 38*f*
age at diagnosis and, 40
alcohol consumption and, 48
blood pressure and, 45, 46*t*, 47, 189
body mass index and, 48
cigarette smoking and, 47–48
duration of diabetes and, 39, 39*f*, 40*t*, 41*t*
genetics and, 38
hyperglycemia and, 42, 43*t*
insulin therapy and, 45, 181–182
peptide status and, 44–45
physical activity levels and, 48
proteinuria and nephropathy and, 47
puberty and, 40–41
race and, 26–27
serum lipid levels and, 47, 194
sex (gender) and, 36
socioeconomic status and, 48–49
visual acuity/survival statistics in, 30–32, 31*f*
visual impairment incidence statistics in,
23–26, 24*t*, 25*t*, 27*t*, 28*f*, 28*t*
visual impairment prevalence statistics in,
20–22, 22*f*, 23*f*
visual impairment risk factor statistics in,
26–29, 27*t*, 28*f*, 28*t*
Wolfram syndrome, 228

X
Xenon laser, for photocoagulation, Diabetic
Retinopathy Study results for, 82–84,
82*f*, 83*t*

Y,Z
YAG capsulotomy, diabetic macular edema affecting timing of, 148
Yellow laser wavelengths, for photocoagulation,
127

Harry W. Flynn, Jr, MD, is Professor of Ophthalmology at the Bascom Palmer Eye Institute, University of Miami School of Medicine. Dr Flynn has participated in the Diabetes 2000® project for the past decade as a member of the National Operations Committee and as an instructor for the Diabetes 2000 Course at the Annual Meeting of the American Academy of Ophthalmology. During the Early Treatment Diabetic Retinopathy Study, he served as Principal Investigator in Miami and was a member of an ETDRS executive committee. Dr Flynn's other activities for the Academy include chairing Section 12, *Retina and Vitreous*, of the Basic Clinical and Science Course (BCSC) and cochairing the Vitreoretinal Update Course before the Annual Meeting in 1997 and 1998. He has authored numerous publications on diabetic retinopathy and vitreoretinal surgery.

William E. Smiddy, MD, is Professor of Ophthalmology at the Bascom Palmer Eye Institute, University of Miami School of Medicine. Dr Smiddy received his medical degree from the Johns Hopkins University School of Medicine and finished his training at that institution. His residency in ophthalmology, as well as his fellowship in vitreoretinal surgery, was completed at the Wilmer Eye Institute. Dr Smiddy's clinical research interests include diabetic retinopathy, complications of cataract surgery, and macular disorders. He has authored or coauthored in excess of one hundred fifty original articles, twenty-five chapters, and three books.

Item No. 0210240

ISBN 1-56055-173-9